DR. SEBI HERBAL BIBLE [30 BOOKS IN 1]

The Most Complete Guide to Dr. Sebi Alkaline Diet, Natural Healing, and Non-Toxic Lifestyle. Deeply Cleanse Your Body and Boost Your Long-Term Vitality

LUNA MARIA SOLEDAD

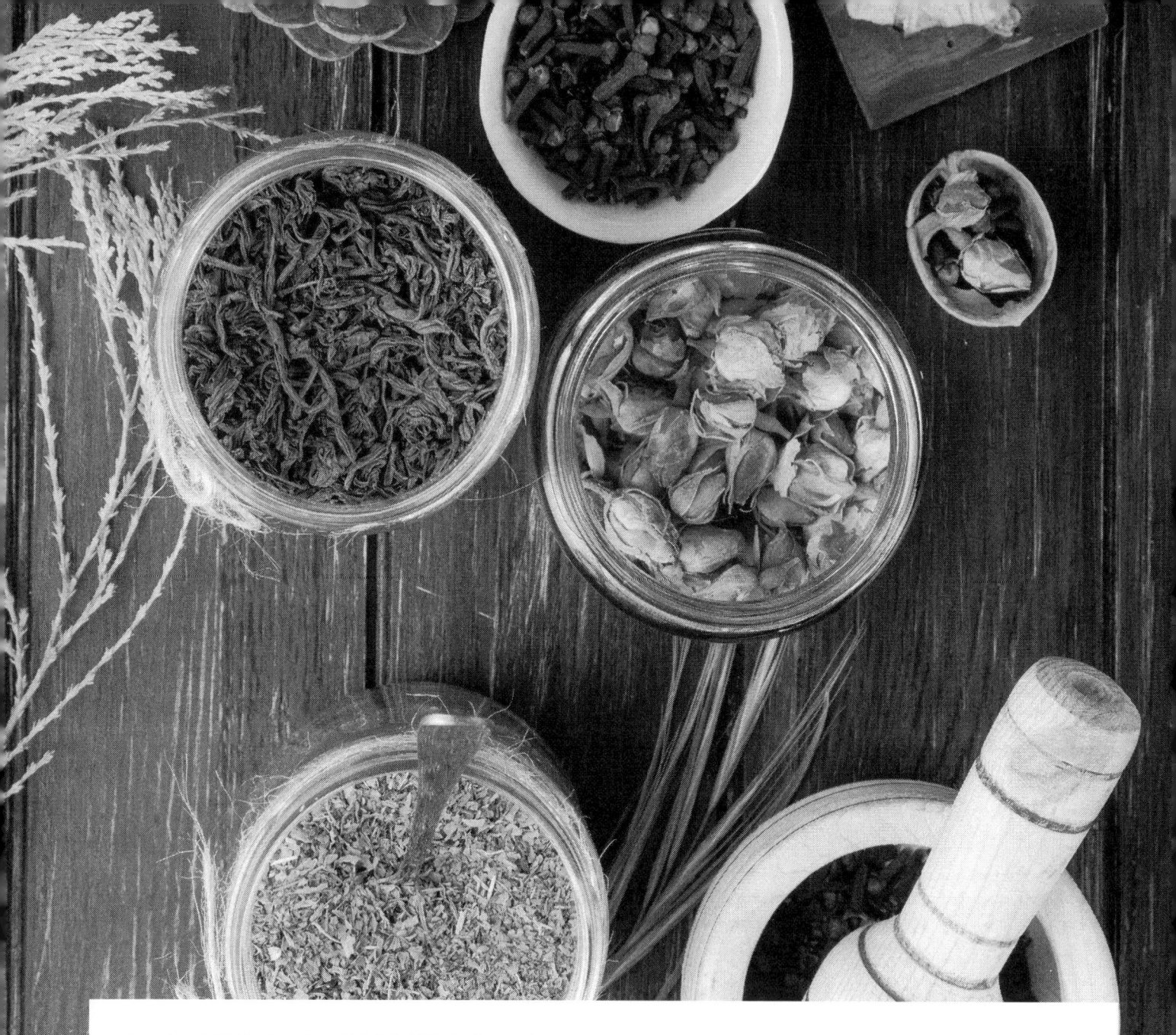

Copyright © 2024 by Luna Maria Soledad. All Rights Reserved.

This book, Dr. Sebi Herbal Bible: [30 Books in 1]: The Most Complete Guide to Dr. Sebi Alkaline Diet, Natural Healing, and Non-Toxic Lifestyle, is intended solely for informational and educational purposes. No part of this publication may be reproduced, distributed, or transmitted in any form or by any means, including photocopying, recording, or other electronic or mechanical methods, without prior written permission from the publisher.

This publication is sold with the understanding that the author and publisher are not engaged in rendering medical, legal, or other professional services. If medical or other expert assistance is required, the services of a competent professional should be sought.

Disclaimer

The information contained within this book is not authored by Dr. Sebi himself but is inspired by his teachings and philosophy. This guide is a tribute to Dr. Sebi's legacy and is not an official publication from Dr. Sebi or his estate. It is intended to provide a practical resource for understanding and applying the principles associated with Dr. Sebi's approach, including the alkaline diet, herbal remedies, and detox protocols.

The author and publisher are not medical professionals. This book is not a substitute for professional medical advice, diagnosis, or treatment. Readers should consult their healthcare provider before undertaking any new health or diet program, especially if they have pre-existing health conditions, are pregnant or nursing, or are taking medication.

While the author and publisher have made every effort to ensure the accuracy of the information provided, individual results may vary. Neither the author nor the publisher shall be held liable or responsible for any errors, omissions, or outcomes related to the use of the information in this book. The reader assumes full responsibility for their own health and wellness decisions and releases the author and publisher from any liability resulting from the use or misuse of the information herein.

All trademarks and brands mentioned within this book are the property of their respective owners and are used for clarification and reference only. The author and publisher do not claim any affiliation with or endorsement by these trademark owners.

TABLE OF CONTENTS

INTRODUCTION 10

BOOK 1
FOUNDATIONS OF DR. SEBI'S PHILOSOPHY

CHAPTER 1
DR. SEBI'S HOLISTIC VISION 13

CHAPTER 2
WHO WAS DR. SEBI? 15

CHAPTER 3
PRINCIPLES OF THE ALKALINE DIET 17

BOOK 2
UNDERSTANDING THE ALKALINE DIET

CHAPTER 1
THE ALKALINE DIET EXPLAINED 20

CHAPTER 2
ELECTRIC FOODS AND HEALTH 23

CHAPTER 3
KEY BENEFITS OF THE ALKALINE LIFESTYLE 26

BOOK 3
ALKALINE FOODS LIST

CHAPTER 1
APPROVED ALKALINE FOODS 29

CHAPTER 2
FOODS TO AVOID 31

CHAPTER 3
SOURCING AND PREPARING ALKALINE INGREDIENTS 33

BOOK 4
INTEGRATING ELECTRIC FOODS DAILY

CHAPTER 1
BUILDING AN ALKALINE PLATE 36

CHAPTER 2
ALKALINE FOODS FOR ENERGY 39

CHAPTER 3
ADAPTING RECIPES FOR FAMILY 41

BOOK 5
BASICS OF DETOXIFICATION

CHAPTER 1
WHY DETOX IS ESSENTIAL 44

CHAPTER 2
IDENTIFYING TOXINS AND THEIR EFFECTS 47

CHAPTER 3
PREPARING FOR A DETOX 50

BOOK 6
DR. SEBI'S DETOX PROTOCOLS

CHAPTER 1
DAILY DETOX HABITS 54

CHAPTER 2
STEP-BY-STEP DETOX PROGRAMS 57

CHAPTER 3
BENEFITS OF REGULAR DETOXIFICATION 59

BOOK 7
DR. SEBI'S HEALING HERBS

CHAPTER 1
INTRODUCTION TO ALKALINE HERBS 63

CHAPTER 2
PROPERTIES AND BENEFITS OF KEY HERBS 65

CHAPTER 3
ESSENTIAL HERBAL BLENDS 67

BOOK 8
DR. SEBI'S HERBAL APOTHECARY

CHAPTER 1
HERBAL REMEDIES FOR EVERYDAY HEALTH 71

CHAPTER 2
STORAGE AND PREPARATION TECHNIQUES 74

CHAPTER 3
SAFETY AND DOSAGE TIPS 76

BOOK 9
REMEDIES FOR DETOXIFICATION

CHAPTER 1
DETOX TEAS AND DECOCTIONS 78

CHAPTER 2
PREPARATION TECHNIQUES 81

CHAPTER 3
USING REMEDIES FOR REGULAR DETOX 83

BOOK 10
HERBAL REMEDIES FOR COMMON CONDITIONS

CHAPTER 1
CREATING HEALING BLENDS 86

CHAPTER 2
HERBAL SOLUTIONS FOR EVERYDAY ILLNESSES 89

CHAPTER 3
DR. SEBI'S FAVORITE REMEDIES 92

BOOK 11
CULTIVATING YOUR OWN HEALING HERBS

CHAPTER 1
GROWING ALKALINE HERBS 95

CHAPTER 2
SOIL, ENVIRONMENT, AND CARE 98

CHAPTER 3
HARVESTING AND STORAGE TIPS 101

BOOK 12
HEART HEALTH AND DR. SEBI'S PRINCIPLES

CHAPTER 1
HERBS FOR HEART HEALTH 104

CHAPTER 2
LOWERING BLOOD PRESSURE NATURALLY 107

CHAPTER 3
DIETARY TIPS FOR CARDIOVASCULAR HEALTH 109

BOOK 13
MANAGING DIABETES NATURALLY

CHAPTER 1
ALKALINE DIET'S IMPACT ON BLOOD SUGAR 112

CHAPTER 2
KEY HERBS FOR DIABETES SUPPORT 115

CHAPTER 3
DETOX AND PANCREATIC HEALTH 118

BOOK 14
SUPPORTING AUTOIMMUNE HEALTH

CHAPTER 1
FOODS AND HERBS FOR IMMUNE BALANCE 122

CHAPTER 2
DETOX PROTOCOLS FOR AUTOIMMUNE WELLNESS 125

CHAPTER 3
GUT HEALTH AND INFLAMMATION REDUCTION 128

BOOK 15
HERBAL SUPPORT FOR VIRAL INFECTIONS

CHAPTER 1
ALKALINE DIET FOR VIRAL MANAGEMENT 132

CHAPTER 2
HERBS FOR IMMUNE BOOSTING 135

CHAPTER 3
PROTOCOLS FOR VIRAL CLEANSING 138

BOOK 16
HERBS FOR STRESS AND MENTAL CLARITY

CHAPTER 1
DR. SEBI'S HERBS FOR ANXIETY 141

CHAPTER 2
ALKALINE FOODS FOR EMOTIONAL BALANCE 144

CHAPTER 3
DETOX FOR MENTAL CLARITY 147

BOOK 17
DIGESTIVE HEALTH AND DR. SEBI'S METHODS

CHAPTER 1
ALKALINE FOODS FOR GUT HEALTH 151

CHAPTER 2
REMEDIES FOR DIGESTIVE ISSUES 154

CHAPTER 3
DETOX PROTOCOLS FOR DIGESTIVE SUPPORT 157

BOOK 18
KIDNEY HEALTH SUPPORT

CHAPTER 1
HERBAL PROTOCOLS FOR KIDNEY HEALTH 161

CHAPTER 2
PREVENTING KIDNEY STONES 164

CHAPTER 3
NATURAL DETOX FOR KIDNEY SUPPORT 167

BOOK 19
CANCER PREVENTION AND MANAGEMENT

CHAPTER 1
ROLE OF ALKALINE FOODS IN CANCER PREVENTION 171

CHAPTER 2
HERBS FOR CANCER RECOVERY 174

CHAPTER 3
DETOXIFICATION PROTOCOLS FOR CANCER 177

BOOK 20
RESPIRATORY HEALTH WITH ALKALINE REMEDIES

CHAPTER 1
HERBAL TREATMENTS FOR LUNG HEALTH 181

CHAPTER 2
DETOX PROTOCOLS FOR RESPIRATORY SUPPORT 184

CHAPTER 3
PREVENTING RESPIRATORY ILLNESS 187

EXCLUSIVE INSIGHTS AND BONUS CONTENT 190

YOUR EXCLUSIVE BONUS 191

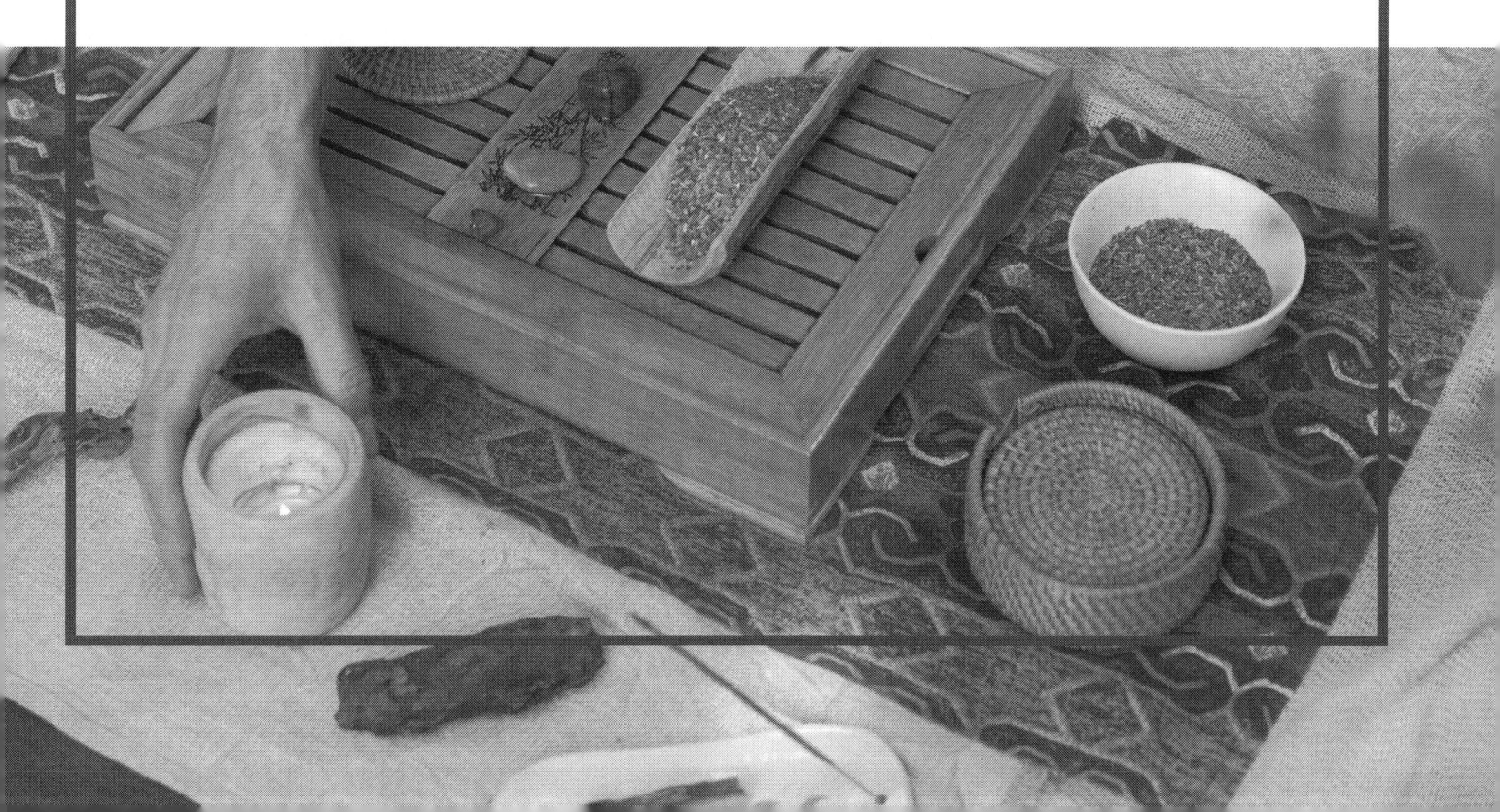

INTRODUCTION

OVERVIEW OF DR. SEBI'S PHILOSOPHY AND VISION

Dr. Sebi, born Alfredo Darrington Bowman, was a renowned herbalist and holistic health advocate who dedicated his life to helping individuals understand the healing power of nature. His approach to health and wellness was deeply rooted in the belief that the human body, when treated correctly, possesses an incredible ability to heal itself. Rather than relying on synthetic medicines and complex procedures, Dr. Sebi advocated a return to natural remedies, particularly through the use of specific herbs and a diet centered on alkaline, plant-based foods.

Dr. Sebi's journey into holistic health began as a personal quest. Suffering from conditions like asthma, diabetes, and obesity, he sought help from both Western medicine and various natural healers. Yet it was only when he encountered herbal remedies and the principles of an alkaline diet that he found the transformative health he had been seeking. This personal success inspired him to share his approach with the world, eventually developing a comprehensive system based on "electric foods" — foods that work harmoniously with the body's natural energy and structure.

The foundation of Dr. Sebi's philosophy is that illness stems from mucus buildup in the body, which can obstruct vital systems and organs. He believed that an acidic internal environment exacerbates mucus formation and leads to disease, while an alkaline environment promotes natural healing and wellness. According to Dr. Sebi, the key to maintaining health is twofold: removing toxins from the body and providing it with nutrient-dense, alkalizing foods that restore balance and vitality.

Central to Dr. Sebi's teachings is his unique understanding of bio-mineral balance. He maintained that every plant, food, and herb has a unique composition, offering specific minerals and elements that can support the body's functions. By consuming "electric" or natural foods, individuals can feed their bodies the minerals they need, thereby promoting cellular health and preventing diseases.

WHY AN ALKALINE LIFESTYLE?

The alkaline lifestyle is more than just a diet; it's a commitment to a holistic approach that prioritizes nourishing the body, mind, and spirit. But why specifically an alkaline approach? At the heart of Dr. Sebi's system is the idea that pH balance in the body is essential for optimal health. The pH scale measures the acidity or alkalinity of a substance, and the human body functions best in a slightly alkaline state, around a pH of 7.4.

1. **Reduced Mucus Formation and Inflammation**: Dr. Sebi emphasized that disease in the body often starts with mucus. Inflammation is a common precursor to many chronic diseases, including arthritis, diabetes, and heart disease. By reducing the consumption of acidic foods (such as processed meats, dairy, and refined sugars) and incorporating more alkaline options, one can help reduce mucus buildup and support a healthy inflammatory response.

2. **Enhanced Detoxification**: Living an alkaline lifestyle supports the body's natural detoxification processes. Alkaline foods, particularly raw fruits and vegetables, are rich in fiber and essential nutrients that help the liver, kidneys, and colon process toxins more effectively. With a steady intake of alkaline foods, the body can eliminate waste and toxins more efficiently, which in turn supports overall health.

3. **Improved Energy Levels**: One of the primary benefits of an alkaline diet is increased energy. By reducing heavy, hard-to-digest foods and instead focusing on nutrient-dense, alkaline options, the body can redirect its energy from processing foods to healing and maintaining optimal function. As a result, those who follow an alkaline lifestyle often report higher energy levels, improved focus, and greater vitality.

4. **Balanced Hormones and Better Mental Health**: An alkaline diet, particularly when combined with the herbs recommended by Dr. Sebi, can help regulate hormones. Hormones play a critical role in various bodily functions, from metabolism to mood. Certain alkaline foods, such as leafy greens and sea vegetables, are rich in minerals like magnesium and potassium, which are essential for hormonal balance and stress reduction. Additionally, an alkaline environment in the body supports brain health, often leading to clearer thinking, reduced anxiety, and a more stable mood.

5. **Long-Term Disease Prevention**: Dr. Sebi believed that maintaining an alkaline internal environment can protect against disease. Chronic conditions such as diabetes, high blood pressure, and even cancer thrive in an acidic environment. By neutralizing the body's pH, the alkaline lifestyle may reduce the likelihood of these diseases developing in the first place.

6. **Whole-Body Wellness**: Beyond physical health, an alkaline lifestyle encourages a harmonious connection between body, mind, and spirit. Dr. Sebi promoted mindfulness, breathing exercises, and relaxation techniques

alongside diet to help individuals fully embrace their journey to wellness.

An alkaline lifestyle is not a temporary fix but a sustainable path to a healthier life. For those who are new to the alkaline diet, it may seem challenging at first, particularly when shifting from acidic foods that have become dietary staples. However, the benefits that follow this transition often speak for themselves, bringing about a profound change in both health and mindset.

HOW TO USE THIS BOOK FOR HEALTH TRANSFORMATION

This book is designed as a comprehensive guide to understanding and implementing Dr. Sebi's alkaline lifestyle. Within these pages, you will find a blend of foundational knowledge, practical advice, and easy-to-follow protocols that can help you achieve vibrant health naturally. To make the most of this book, here's a suggested approach:

1. **Start with Understanding**: Begin by familiarizing yourself with the fundamental principles of Dr. Sebi's teachings. This includes understanding why an alkaline environment is beneficial for the body and learning which foods are considered "electric" and compatible with the body's natural chemistry. The first few sections of this book provide a solid foundation in these concepts, helping you to understand not just what to do but why it's essential.
2. **Identify Your Health Goals**: Take some time to reflect on your personal health objectives. Are you looking to improve your energy levels? Manage a specific health condition? Detoxify your body? Knowing what you hope to achieve will make it easier to tailor the protocols in this book to your needs. For example, if you are dealing with digestive issues, you can focus more closely on the chapters dedicated to gut health and detoxification.
3. **Follow the Detox Protocols**: Detoxification is central to Dr. Sebi's approach. The book provides various detox protocols, ranging from gentle daily practices to more intensive programs. If you are new to detoxing, start with a milder approach and gradually work your way up. The detox chapters offer step-by-step guidance, so even beginners can follow along comfortably.
4. **Integrate Alkaline Foods**: Transitioning to an alkaline diet doesn't have to happen overnight. You may find it easier to start by gradually incorporating more alkaline foods into your meals while reducing acidic ones. This book includes meal plans and recipes to simplify this process, allowing you to explore a variety of flavors while ensuring nutritional balance.
5. **Explore Herbal Remedies**: Dr. Sebi placed great emphasis on the use of specific herbs to support bodily functions and address common ailments. This book provides an extensive guide to herbs that Dr. Sebi endorsed, complete with preparation instructions and specific protocols. For those looking to manage conditions such as diabetes, high blood pressure, or stress, these herbal remedies can be an invaluable resource.
6. **Practice Consistency**: Health transformation doesn't happen overnight. Dr. Sebi's approach requires patience, consistency, and dedication. Consider making a gradual transition, and don't be discouraged by setbacks. This book is structured to provide support at each stage, and as you progress, you'll likely notice gradual improvements in your energy, mood, and overall health.
7. **Tailor the Information to Your Needs**: While this book is comprehensive, health is a personal journey, and everyone's needs are different. Take the information provided and adapt it to fit your unique situation. If you find certain foods or herbs resonate more with you, feel free to focus on those. The journey to wellness is flexible, and this book is a guide to help you find what works best for you.
8. **Embrace a Holistic Approach**: True health goes beyond diet alone. Dr. Sebi's philosophy was not only about food but about cultivating a balanced, holistic lifestyle. Consider incorporating practices such as meditation, mindful movement, and breathwork alongside dietary changes. Each chapter in this book offers suggestions for supporting mind, body, and spirit, helping you build a complete wellness routine.
9. **Track Your Progress**: Keeping a journal of your journey can be incredibly beneficial. Record how you feel, any changes in your symptoms, and reflections on the process. Not only does this help you stay motivated, but it also allows you to notice subtle improvements that you might otherwise overlook.
10. **Share with Your Family**: Dr. Sebi believed that a healthy lifestyle should extend beyond the individual to the family. This book includes family-friendly recipes and protocols that can benefit children, elders, and everyone in between. Encouraging your loved ones to join you on this journey can help foster a healthier, more vibrant environment for all.

This book aims to serve as a lifelong companion on your journey to wellness. While it provides a comprehensive overview, health is a continuous learning process, and there is always room to explore new insights. Whether you are here to address a specific health condition or simply to lead a more vibrant life, this guide offers the tools, inspiration, and support needed to achieve lasting wellness through the wisdom of Dr. Sebi's alkaline lifestyle.

BOOK 1
Foundations of Dr. Sebi's Philosophy

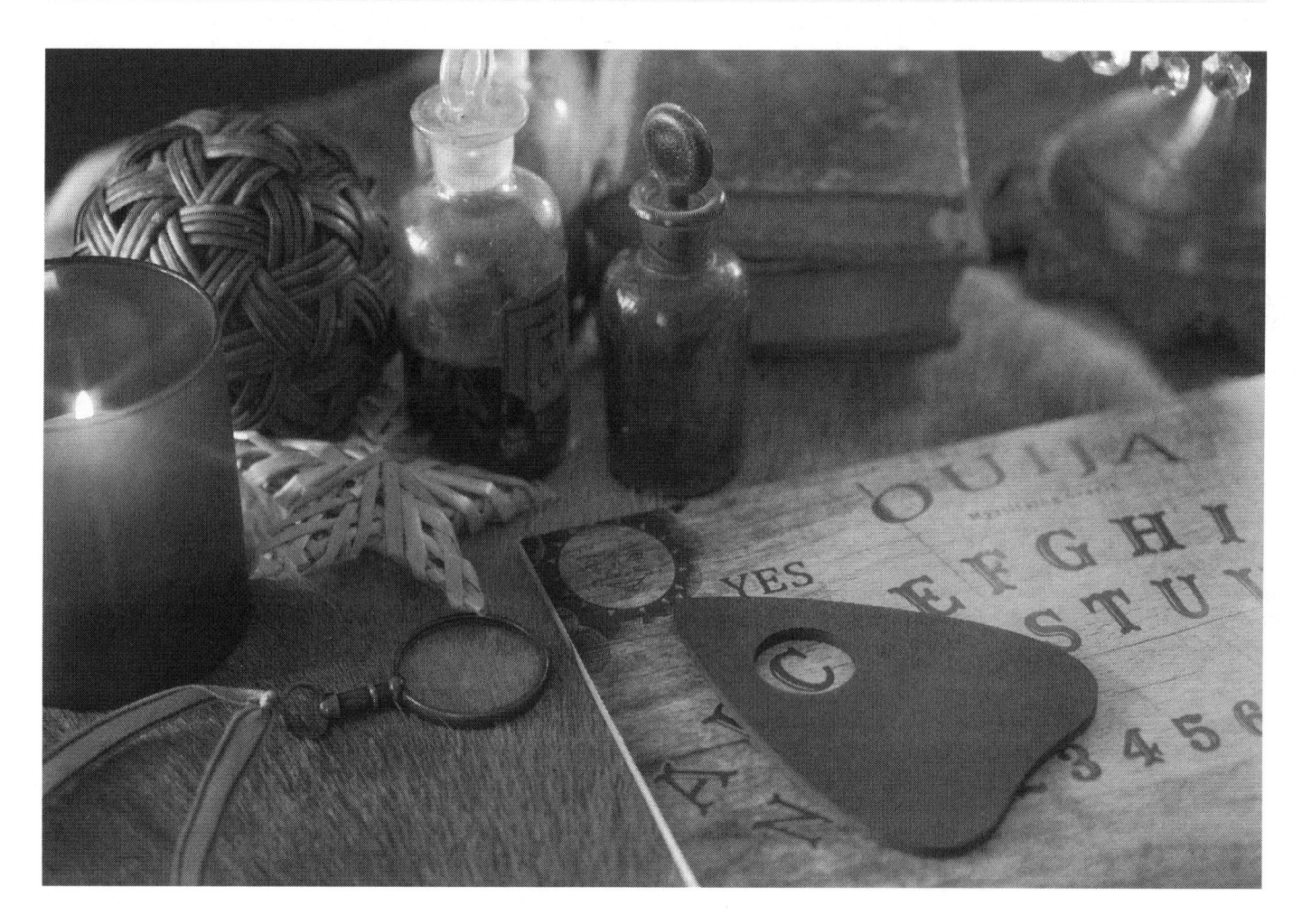

Dr. Sebi's approach to health and wellness offers a refreshingly simple yet profound perspective on the body's ability to heal. Rooted in nature and shaped by his personal journey, his philosophy empowers individuals to take control of their health by supporting the body's innate healing capacity. Unlike conventional medicine, which often focuses on treating symptoms, Dr. Sebi's methods emphasize prevention, detoxification, and nourishing the body with alkaline, plant-based foods.

In this foundational section, we'll explore the core principles of Dr. Sebi's teachings, beginning with his holistic vision for health and wellness. We'll look at who Dr. Sebi was, his journey, and how his philosophy emerged as a guide for those seeking natural healing. Through understanding his vision, you'll gain insight into how an alkaline lifestyle and a commitment to natural remedies can serve as powerful tools for achieving balance, vitality, and resilience.

CHAPTER 1
DR. SEBI'S HOLISTIC VISION

Dr. Sebi's vision for health was a profound departure from conventional practices, advocating a return to natural, whole-body wellness rooted in simplicity and nature. His philosophy wasn't merely about treating symptoms but about embracing a lifestyle that suwpports the body's ability to heal itself. According to Dr. Sebi, optimal health and longevity are achievable through a commitment to natural remedies, an alkaline diet, and detoxification practices. His approach challenged the mainstream health industry, promoting a system that empowers individuals to take control of their health by nurturing the body, mind, and spirit in harmony.

1. **Nature as the Ultimate Healer**

Dr. Sebi's philosophy starts with the belief that nature provides everything we need for optimal health. He argued that the Earth offers plants, herbs, and foods that work in synergy with the body's natural processes. By choosing foods that are whole, unprocessed, and aligned with the body's cellular structure, Dr. Sebi believed we can restore and maintain health. In his view, synthetic medications and highly processed foods disrupt the body's equilibrium, leading to a host of health issues. His philosophy was grounded in the idea that natural remedies — rather than pharmaceuticals — encourage the body to find balance and strength. For Dr. Sebi, it wasn't enough to merely alleviate symptoms. Instead, he focused on identifying and addressing the root causes of illness. He argued that by aligning ourselves with nature's wisdom, we could achieve sustainable wellness without dependency on synthetic treatments. His vision promoted natural remedies as a way to empower individuals to participate actively in their health journeys, embracing a proactive rather than reactive approach to healing.

2. **The Body as a Self-Healing System**

A cornerstone of Dr. Sebi's philosophy is the understanding that the body has an incredible, inherent ability to heal itself. He believed that the body, when supported correctly, will naturally work to repair damage, fight disease, and restore balance. In Dr. Sebi's view, the real task of any health regimen should be to remove obstacles to this natural healing process, allowing the body to operate at its best. According to Dr. Sebi, factors like poor diet, toxin exposure, and emotional stress create obstacles that interfere with the body's natural healing. His holistic approach was designed to support this self-healing mechanism by encouraging habits and practices that align with the body's needs. Detoxification, an alkaline diet, and herbal supplementation were central to his approach. By providing the body with the necessary nutrients and eliminating harmful substances, he argued that individuals could maintain resilience, resist disease, and foster long-term health.

3. **The Role of Alkalinity and Electric Foods**

Dr. Sebi introduced the concept of "electric foods" — foods that align with the body's natural electrical energy. He believed that every cell in the body has its own electrical charge and that foods with high natural energy, or bio-electricity, are crucial for cellular health. Electric foods are raw, whole, and plant-based, rich in essential minerals, enzymes, and nutrients that "charge" the body, supporting it at a cellular level. These foods, according to Dr. Sebi, help the body maintain an alkaline environment, which he believed to be the foundation of health. Alkalinity plays a pivotal role in Dr. Sebi's philosophy. He argued that an alkaline environment discourages disease and promotes healing, while an acidic environment fosters illness, inflammation, and disease progression. He observed that the typical modern diet — filled with processed foods, animal products, and refined sugars — creates an acidic environment within the body, weakening the immune system and making it more susceptible to illness. By adopting an alkaline, electric diet, Dr. Sebi believed we could restore the body's natural pH balance, reduce inflammation, and support overall vitality.

4. **Detoxification as a Pathway to Health**

Dr. Sebi's emphasis on detoxification is central to his holistic approach. He believed that toxins accumulated from food, environmental pollution, and stress burden the body, interrupting its natural functions and impairing health. Dr. Sebi's detox protocols involve both dietary changes and the use of specific herbs to cleanse the organs, tissues, and blood, ultimately supporting the body's ability to detoxify itself effectively. According to Dr. Sebi, detoxification is the first step toward restoring health because it creates a clean foundation for the body to work from. He promoted a regular regimen of cleansing to clear out obstructions, whether it's from dietary toxins, waste buildup, or environmental pollutants. His detox strategies, including fasting and herbal supplements, were developed to target key organs like the liver, kidneys, colon, and lymphatic system. By focusing on these systems, Dr. Sebi's protocols aim to remove toxins that may be inhibiting cellular health, allowing the body to function more effectively and regenerate naturally.

5. **Healing Beyond the Physical**

Dr. Sebi's holistic vision extends beyond just physical health; he saw wellness as an integration of mind, body, and spirit. He understood that mental and emotional well-being are equally crucial for overall health and that the body cannot reach its full potential if the mind is burdened with stress or negativity. To Dr. Sebi, an alkaline lifestyle includes not just diet and detox but also the cultivation of a peaceful, balanced mind. He often advocated for practices like mindfulness, breathing exercises, and spending time in nature as ways to maintain emotional health.

Dr. Sebi believed that a calm, centered mind positively influences the body's healing process, reinforcing resilience and adaptability. Emotional stress, in his view, creates an acidic state that affects cellular health, making the body more vulnerable to disease. Therefore, Dr. Sebi encouraged his followers to actively nurture their mental well-being through self-care practices, meditation, and mindful living. By fostering a positive mental state and reducing stress, Dr. Sebi believed individuals could strengthen their immunity and experience a deeper sense of wellness.

6. **Prevention as the Ultimate Form of Health Care**

Dr. Sebi's vision was not solely about treating disease; it was fundamentally about preventing it. He often emphasized that by maintaining an alkaline diet, using detoxification practices, and nourishing the body with electric foods, people could avoid many common ailments. Prevention, in Dr. Sebi's philosophy, is far more empowering than treatment because it gives individuals the knowledge and tools to sustain their health independently. Dr. Sebi taught that disease arises from imbalance, usually due to an acidic environment and toxin accumulation. His approach to prevention included lifestyle adjustments that promote balance and fortify the body against illness. Rather than reacting to health issues, Dr. Sebi encouraged adopting a lifestyle that naturally supports resilience, so the body remains prepared to resist disease. His preventive philosophy is an invitation to embrace daily practices that contribute to long-term vitality, making wellness a way of life rather than a remedy for specific conditions.

7. **Empowering People Through Knowledge and Natural Choices**

Dr. Sebi's ultimate goal was to empower people with knowledge about natural health. His vision was to put the tools of wellness into the hands of each individual, allowing them to take control of their health journeys. He believed that everyone should have access to the benefits of natural remedies and an alkaline lifestyle, and that knowledge about these practices should be freely shared. By providing simple, practical guidance and encouraging people to explore natural healing, he sought to inspire self-reliance and independence from the traditional healthcare system. At the heart of Dr. Sebi's vision is the belief that health is not a privilege but a right. He advocated for accessibility in wellness, with simple and affordable solutions that are available to everyone. His teachings emphasize the use of everyday plants, herbs, and dietary practices that people can adopt regardless of their financial or medical background. This philosophy of accessibility and empowerment has resonated with countless individuals worldwide, helping them reclaim their health and find renewed vitality through natural means.

SUMMARY OF DR. SEBI'S HOLISTIC VISION

Dr. Sebi's holistic vision is about reconnecting with nature's wisdom, supporting the body's innate healing power, and embracing a lifestyle that promotes balance and vitality. His philosophy encourages each person to be active participants in their own wellness journey, recognizing that true health extends beyond the physical to include mental and emotional harmony. By prioritizing detoxification, alkalinity, and natural remedies, Dr. Sebi believed that individuals could prevent disease, regain strength, and achieve sustainable wellness.

Dr. Sebi's approach is an invitation to simplify, to rely on nature's bounty, and to trust in the body's natural intelligence. This foundation serves as a guiding principle for all who seek a path to health that respects the body, honors the spirit, and aligns with the cycles of nature.

CHAPTER 2

WHO WAS DR. SEBI?

Dr. Sebi, born Alfredo Darrington Bowman on November 26, 1933, in the small village of Ilanga in Honduras, emerged as one of the most influential figures in natural healing and holistic health. Known for his unorthodox methods and groundbreaking views on wellness, Dr. Sebi dedicated his life to the belief that true health is attainable by aligning with nature. His work left a profound impact on countless people, challenging conventional approaches to medicine and offering an alternative rooted in the power of plants, herbs, and an alkaline lifestyle.

EARLY LIFE AND CULTURAL INFLUENCES

Growing up in Honduras, Dr. Sebi was deeply influenced by the natural world around him. His early exposure to traditional healing practices and the use of plants as medicine shaped his foundational understanding of health. In Ilanga, his grandmother, a healer herself, introduced him to the medicinal value of local plants, setting the stage for a lifelong interest in natural remedies. It was here that he first experienced the connection between health and the earth, a bond he would later advocate as essential to his philosophy of wellness.

Despite his interest in nature, Dr. Sebi did not initially pursue a path in health or wellness. He moved to the United States as a young man, where he worked various jobs, including as a steam engineer. Like many immigrants, he sought the opportunities that America promised. Yet, despite the promising life he was building, he struggled with numerous health problems that Western medicine failed to address adequately. Asthma, diabetes, impotence, and obesity plagued him, and the medications prescribed offered little relief. Frustrated and seeking alternatives, Dr. Sebi's personal health challenges became the catalyst for a life-changing journey.

THE TURNING POINT: DISCOVERY OF NATURAL HEALING

The turning point in Dr. Sebi's life came when he traveled to Mexico and met a herbalist from whom he learned about natural healing. This encounter exposed him to the idea that plants could not only relieve symptoms but also heal the root causes of disease. Inspired, Dr. Sebi returned to the wisdom of natural medicine, experimenting with herbal remedies and dietary changes. It was through these practices that he finally experienced relief from his health conditions, and for the first time, his body felt balanced and energized.

This transformation gave Dr. Sebi a new sense of purpose. He realized that natural healing had the potential to restore health in ways that conventional medicine often could not, and he was determined to share these insights with others. His healing journey would become the foundation of the wellness practices and dietary guidelines he developed, leading him to create a unique approach that integrated herbal medicine, diet, and detoxification.

DEVELOPING A UNIQUE HEALING SYSTEM: CELLULAR REVITALIZATION

Dr. Sebi's approach to health, which he later called "cellular revitalization," focused on restoring the body at a cellular level. He believed that disease arises when the body is deprived of essential minerals and nutrients, leading to imbalances and weakened immunity. To combat this, Dr. Sebi advocated a strict plant-based, alkaline diet that nourishes the body with "electric foods." He coined this term to refer to foods that align with the body's bio-electricity, which he believed was essential for optimal health.

Cellular revitalization also emphasizes the importance of detoxification. Dr. Sebi believed that toxins, particularly from processed foods, preservatives, and environmental pollutants, disrupt the body's natural balance. By using specific herbs that promote cleansing and alkalinity, his protocols aimed to help the body eliminate accumulated toxins, enabling it to reset and regain resilience. These herbs — including sea moss, burdock root, and bladderwrack — became staples in his healing system and are still widely used today by followers of his practices.

Dr. Sebi's dietary recommendations also extended to specific foods he advised against, such as dairy, meat, and processed items that he believed create an acidic environment in the body. This philosophy formed the foundation of what is now widely known as the Dr. Sebi Alkaline Diet, a lifestyle that emphasizes whole, plant-based foods that support alkalinity and detoxification.

FOUNDING THE USHA RESEARCH INSTITUTE

In the early 1980s, Dr. Sebi returned to his native Honduras and established the Usha Research Institute in La Ceiba. The institute served as a wellness retreat where people from around the world came to experience his natural healing methods firsthand. At the institute, he tested and refined his protocols, offering visitors personalized treatment plans centered on his alkaline diet, herbal supplements, and detox practices.

The Usha Research Institute soon became known as a sanctuary for those who had exhausted conventional medical treatments and were seeking an alternative path. Over the years, Dr. Sebi's work with thousands of patients helped him to expand his knowledge of herbal remedies and refine his approach further. His institute continues to operate to this day, now managed by his family, and remains a destination for individuals seeking natural healing through the methods he pioneered.

A CONTROVERSIAL FIGURE AND LEGAL CHALLENGES

Dr. Sebi's unconventional methods, particularly his claims of curing chronic diseases like diabetes, cancer, and AIDS, attracted attention — and scrutiny — from both supporters and critics. His challenges to the medical industry's conventional wisdom were met with controversy, and he was often labeled a fringe healer or pseudoscientist. However, Dr. Sebi was unapologetic in his stance, insisting that his methods were based on natural science and that the body, when treated properly, could indeed heal from severe ailments.

In 1988, Dr. Sebi was arrested and taken to court in New York on charges of practicing medicine without a license after he placed ads in newspapers claiming that he could cure AIDS. During the trial, he presented numerous witnesses and testimonies from people who attested to the efficacy of his treatments. Remarkably, the judge ruled in his favor, marking a historic legal victory that bolstered his credibility and further cemented his place in the alternative health movement. This court case elevated Dr. Sebi's profile and drew more people to his work, both in the U.S. and internationally.

LEGACY AND GLOBAL INFLUENCE

Dr. Sebi's work has had a lasting impact, particularly in communities that have been historically underserved by mainstream healthcare. His teachings have inspired countless people to adopt a plant-based diet, use herbal remedies, and explore natural approaches to health. Today, his legacy continues through his family and a community of followers who share his commitment to natural wellness. His teachings on an alkaline diet, herbal remedies, and detox protocols have gained a global following, with many people crediting his approach to their own health improvements and recovery.

Beyond his specific protocols, Dr. Sebi's influence extends to the broader conversation about health equity, accessibility, and self-empowerment. His message of self-reliance and natural healing resonates with people who feel disillusioned by conventional medicine, and his teachings serve as a reminder that health can be accessible through simple, natural practices. Dr. Sebi's methods, which emphasize the importance of lifestyle, diet, and natural resources, continue to inspire individuals to seek a balanced and proactive approach to wellness.

THE VISION FOR A HEALTHIER FUTURE

Dr. Sebi's vision was never just about treating illness; it was about fostering a culture of wellness and self-empowerment. He believed that health is a human right and that everyone deserves access to natural remedies and education about their bodies. Through his work, he sought to shift the focus from treatment to prevention, encouraging people to understand their own health and take proactive steps toward well-being.

Dr. Sebi's life and work represent a vision of health that is accessible, sustainable, and rooted in nature. His teachings continue to empower individuals to reclaim control over their health through the principles of alkalinity, detoxification, and natural nourishment. His legacy serves as an invitation to explore wellness beyond conventional means and to embrace a holistic approach to health that respects the body's innate intelligence.

Dr. Sebi's life was a testament to the power of determination, self-discovery, and a commitment to natural wellness. His journey from a young boy in Honduras to an internationally recognized healer serves as an inspiring story of resilience and purpose. Through his teachings, he opened the door to a new way of thinking about health — one that emphasizes simplicity, prevention, and self-empowerment.

Today, Dr. Sebi's work continues to impact lives worldwide, offering an alternative path to wellness that prioritizes harmony with nature, nourishment at the cellular level, and a profound respect for the body's ability to heal itself. His legacy endures as a beacon of hope and empowerment for all who seek a holistic, nature-based approach to health.

CHAPTER 3
PRINCIPLES OF THE ALKALINE DIET

The alkaline diet lies at the heart of Dr. Sebi's approach to wellness, emphasizing the importance of maintaining a balanced internal environment to promote health, vitality, and disease prevention. According to Dr. Sebi, the body operates optimally in an alkaline state, which supports cellular function, enhances energy, and reduces the buildup of mucus and toxins that contribute to illness. This chapter provides an in-depth exploration of the alkaline diet's core principles, how it fosters health, and practical ways to incorporate it into everyday life.

UNDERSTANDING PH BALANCE AND ITS IMPORTANCE

To grasp the alkaline diet's foundation, it's essential to understand the concept of pH balance. The pH scale measures the acidity or alkalinity of a substance on a scale from 0 to 14, with 7 being neutral. Anything below 7 is considered acidic, and anything above 7 is alkaline. The human body, particularly the blood, functions best when it maintains a slightly alkaline pH of approximately 7.4. Dr. Sebi believed that this slight alkalinity is essential for proper cellular function, immune resilience, and overall wellness.

Dr. Sebi argued that an acidic environment within the body promotes inflammation, mucus buildup, and disease. In contrast, an alkaline environment discourages these imbalances and supports the body's natural processes. The body's pH can be influenced by diet, stress levels, environmental factors, and lifestyle habits. By adopting a diet rich in alkaline foods, individuals can promote a balanced internal environment that discourages disease and enhances energy, clarity, and longevity.

1. **The Role of Alkaline Foods in Cellular Health**

Dr. Sebi believed that foods have an energy or "electrical charge" that directly impacts the body's cells. He referred to foods compatible with this energy as "electric foods." These foods, typically plant-based, raw, and unprocessed, are rich in natural minerals, vitamins, and enzymes that provide fuel for the body's cellular functions. According to Dr. Sebi, alkaline foods are those that support cellular health by aligning with the body's natural electrical currents. Electric foods contribute to cellular regeneration and vitality, supporting the body's natural healing and energy production. Leafy greens, fresh fruits, and certain herbs provide essential minerals like potassium, magnesium, and calcium, which are crucial for cellular activity. By consuming electric foods, individuals can enhance their cellular health, protect against cellular damage, and foster an environment conducive to healing and restoration.

2. **Eliminating Acidic Foods for Optimal Health**

In Dr. Sebi's philosophy, avoiding acidic foods is as critical as consuming alkaline ones. Acidic foods, which include processed foods, dairy, refined sugars, caffeine, and animal products, disrupt the body's natural balance and increase acidity. This acidity creates an environment that Dr. Sebi believed was ideal for mucus formation, inflammation, and the growth of disease. Processed and refined foods, in particular, are stripped of nutrients and are often high in preservatives, artificial colors, and additives that burden the body's detoxification systems. By reducing or eliminating acidic foods, the body has an opportunity to reset and focus on restoration rather than neutralizing harmful substances. Dr. Sebi argued that many modern health problems stem from excessive consumption of acidic foods, which disrupt the body's pH balance and lead to issues like digestive discomfort, fatigue, and immune dysfunction. Instead, he encouraged a focus on whole, plant-based foods that nourish and sustain the body.

3. **Mineral-Rich Foods and Their Role in the Alkaline Diet**

Dr. Sebi's approach to the alkaline diet emphasizes foods that are rich in minerals, as he believed minerals to be the "building blocks of life." Minerals such as iron, calcium, magnesium, and phosphorus are essential for numerous bodily functions, including bone health, muscle function, enzyme activation, and energy production. Foods that are naturally abundant in these minerals help the body maintain its pH balance and support the proper functioning of organs and systems. For example, iron is a critical component of red blood cells, which transport oxygen throughout the body. Alkaline foods high in iron, such as kale, watercress, and certain herbs, support blood health, energy levels, and cognitive function. Magnesium, another essential mineral, is found in foods like leafy greens and sea vegetables, which Dr. Sebi encouraged as part of a balanced diet. Magnesium aids in muscle relaxation, nervous system health, and cellular repair. By incorporating mineral-rich foods into the diet, individuals can support the body's foundational needs and promote vitality.

4. **Herbal Supplements and Natural Remedies**

In addition to alkaline foods, Dr. Sebi recommended herbal supplements to support the body's detoxification processes and boost nutrient intake. His chosen herbs, such as sea moss, burdock root, and bladderwrack, are rich in essential minerals and have detoxifying properties. Dr. Sebi's herbal protocols focus on cleansing the blood, lymphatic system, and organs to help the body eliminate waste and restore balance. Sea moss, for instance, is often referred to as a "superfood" due to its high mineral content, containing over 90 of the 102 minerals the body requires. Burdock root is known for its blood-purifying qualities, helping to remove toxins and impurities. Bladderwrack, another sea vegetable, is rich in iodine, supporting thyroid health, which is crucial for maintaining a healthy metabolism. These herbal supplements complement the alkaline diet by ensuring the body receives the nutrients necessary for optimal health and natural detoxification.

5. Mucus as the Root of Disease

A distinctive aspect of Dr. Sebi's philosophy is his view that mucus buildup is the underlying cause of disease. He believed that when the body becomes overly acidic, it produces excess mucus to protect itself, leading to congestion in vital systems and organs. This buildup, according to Dr. Sebi, obstructs natural functions and becomes a breeding ground for disease. By maintaining an alkaline diet and avoiding foods that cause mucus production, individuals can prevent the conditions in which illness thrives. Foods like dairy, processed meats, and refined sugars, Dr. Sebi argued, are some of the largest contributors to mucus formation. These foods trigger an immune response that leads to inflammation and an increase in mucus production, creating an environment that supports conditions such as respiratory infections, digestive issues, and chronic inflammation. The alkaline diet, on the other hand, emphasizes foods that discourage mucus production, allowing the body to function without obstruction and enabling a clearer path to healing and resilience.

6. Detoxification and Its Role in the Alkaline Diet

Detoxification is a vital component of the alkaline diet, as Dr. Sebi believed that regular cleansing allows the body to operate efficiently and effectively. The typical diet and lifestyle in modern society expose the body to various toxins, from processed foods to environmental pollutants. Over time, these toxins accumulate in the body, placing a strain on the liver, kidneys, and digestive system. Dr. Sebi's detox protocols often include periods of fasting, herbal teas, and cleansing diets to help the body eliminate these accumulated toxins. Fasting, in particular, allows the digestive system to rest and promotes deeper detoxification, enabling the body to focus on repairing and regenerating cells. By incorporating detoxification practices into the alkaline lifestyle, individuals can clear out toxins that disrupt cellular health and immune function, laying the foundation for improved wellness.

7. Practical Guidelines for an Alkaline Lifestyle

Transitioning to an alkaline diet may seem daunting at first, especially for those accustomed to a diet high in acidic foods. However, Dr. Sebi's principles offer practical, gradual steps to ease into the lifestyle. Rather than making abrupt changes, he recommended starting with small adjustments, such as incorporating more fresh fruits and vegetables into daily meals, drinking alkaline water, and reducing processed food intake. One approach is to focus on making one meal per day completely alkaline, then gradually increasing to two and, eventually, all meals. Substituting common acidic ingredients with alkaline alternatives can also make the transition easier. For instance, swapping refined sugars with dates or agave, replacing dairy with almond or coconut milk, and choosing leafy greens over starchy vegetables are practical changes that align with Dr. Sebi's alkaline philosophy. Meal planning is another helpful strategy for those new to the alkaline diet. Preparing meals in advance and ensuring the pantry is stocked with alkaline-friendly foods can make it easier to maintain consistency. Additionally, trying new recipes that incorporate a variety of alkaline ingredients can add flavor and excitement to meals, making the diet more enjoyable and sustainable in the long run.

8. The Holistic Benefits of an Alkaline Diet

The benefits of the alkaline diet extend beyond physical health, supporting mental clarity, emotional stability, and spiritual well-being. Dr. Sebi taught that a healthy body creates a foundation for a healthy mind, and many who follow the alkaline diet report improvements in mental focus, reduced anxiety, and a greater sense of calm. The clarity that comes with a clean diet and detoxified body can promote emotional resilience, enabling individuals to handle stress more effectively. Spiritually, Dr. Sebi believed that an alkaline lifestyle allows individuals to connect more deeply with themselves and the world around them. By living in harmony with nature and consuming foods that align with the body's needs, individuals can foster a sense of balance and peace that transcends the physical realm. This holistic approach makes the alkaline diet more than just a regimen; it becomes a way of life that fosters personal growth, self-awareness, and spiritual alignment.

CONCLUSION OF CHAPTER 3

The principles of the alkaline diet reflect Dr. Sebi's holistic approach to health, focusing on harmony, balance, and nourishment at a cellular level. By understanding and applying these principles, individuals can transform their relationship with food, their bodies, and their well-being. Through electric foods, detoxification, and a focus on alkaline nourishment, the alkaline diet offers a practical path to health that encourages the body to perform at its best, free from obstruction and excess acidity.

Dr. Sebi's alkaline diet is more than a dietary choice; it's a commitment to embracing natural wellness, respecting the body's intelligence, and empowering oneself to maintain long-term health. The following chapters will explore specific aspects of this lifestyle in greater detail, providing practical guidance and inspiration for those ready to embark on their journey toward vitality and resilience.

BOOK 2
Understanding the Alkaline Diet

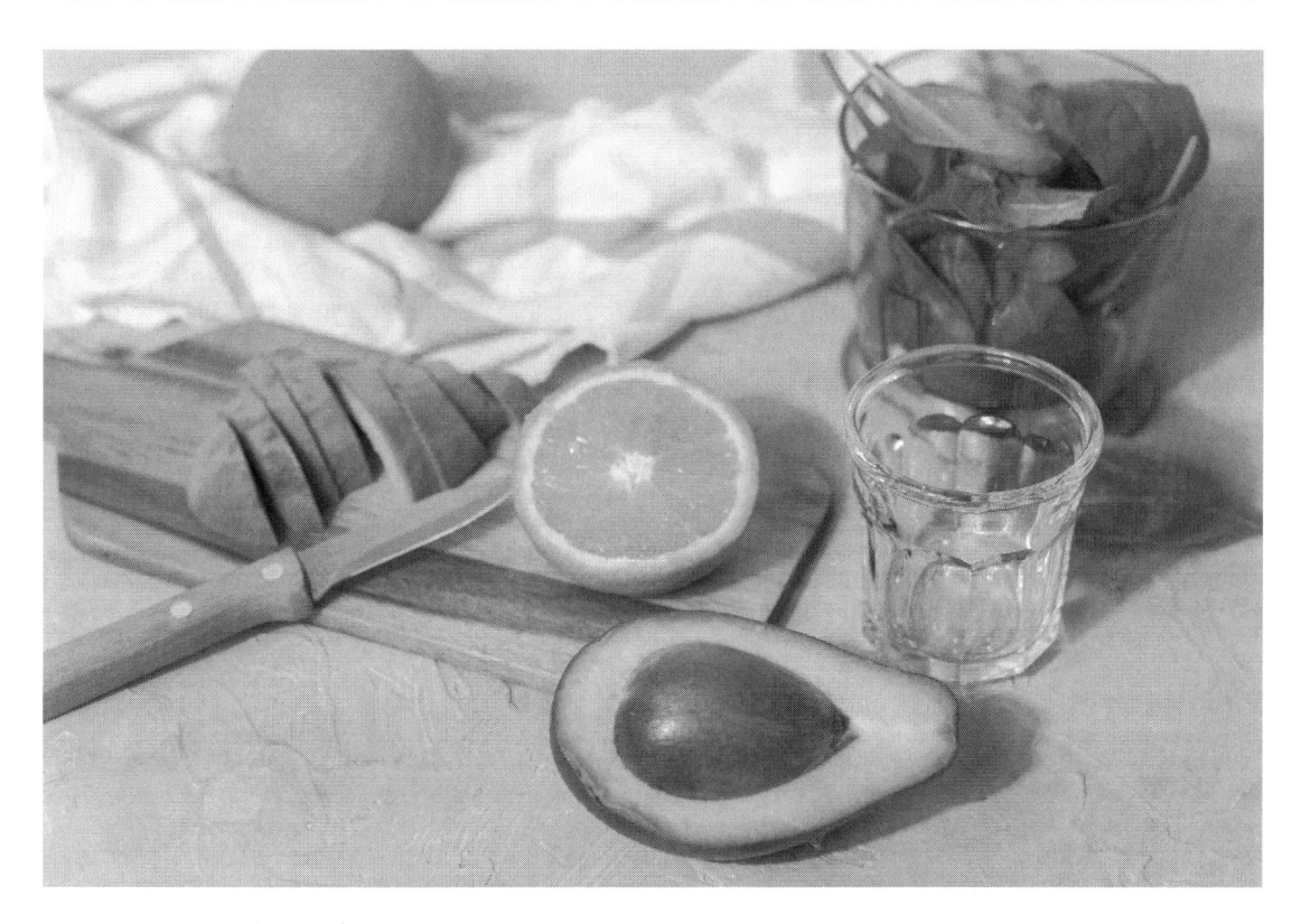

The alkaline diet forms the foundation of Dr. Sebi's approach to natural health and wellness. Rooted in the principle of pH balance, this diet emphasizes foods that support an alkaline environment within the body, fostering resilience, vitality, and healing. Dr. Sebi believed that an alkaline internal state creates conditions that discourage disease and promote cellular health, allowing the body to function at its best.

This book explores the key elements of the alkaline diet, starting with an overview of its purpose and practical applications, followed by a deep dive into the foods that support an alkaline state. Understanding how the alkaline diet works, its benefits, and its principles will empower you to make dietary choices that align with Dr. Sebi's philosophy, setting the stage for holistic wellness.

CHAPTER 1

THE ALKALINE DIET EXPLAINED

The alkaline diet, as advocated by Dr. Sebi, is based on a straightforward yet profound principle: the body thrives in an alkaline state, a state that supports energy, immunity, and natural healing processes. Dr. Sebi believed that by aligning the body with this alkaline balance, individuals could prevent illness, increase vitality, and maintain an environment that fosters long-term wellness. This chapter offers a thorough explanation of the alkaline diet, detailing how it works, why it's beneficial, and how it can be applied practically for a balanced, health-focused lifestyle.

WHAT IS THE ALKALINE DIET?

At its core, the alkaline diet emphasizes consuming plant-based, nutrient-rich foods that help the body maintain a slightly alkaline pH. The pH scale measures acidity and alkalinity on a scale from 0 to 14, with 7 being neutral. A pH below 7 is considered acidic, while above 7 is alkaline. The human body operates best at a slightly alkaline pH of around 7.4, particularly in the blood. When the body's pH is balanced, it's better equipped to resist disease, manage inflammation, and promote efficient cell function.

Dr. Sebi argued that an acidic internal environment creates conditions that encourage mucus buildup, inflammation, and disease. Foods like meat, dairy, refined sugars, caffeine, and processed items, when consumed regularly, contribute to this acidic state. In contrast, alkaline foods — fruits, vegetables, nuts, seeds, and certain grains — help neutralize acidity, creating an environment where the body can thrive. By focusing on a diet that supports alkalinity, Dr. Sebi believed that individuals could protect their health, reduce their risk of chronic conditions, and sustain greater energy and vitality.

HOW DOES THE ALKALINE DIET IMPACT THE BODY?

1. **Promoting pH Balance for Optimal Health**

One of the most significant benefits of the alkaline diet is its ability to maintain the body's pH balance. When we consume acidic foods, they release metabolic byproducts that lower the body's pH. This requires the body to work harder to restore balance, diverting energy that could otherwise be used for natural healing and restoration. When the body remains too acidic for too long, it can lead to a range of health issues, including inflammation, digestive issues, and reduced immune function. Alkaline foods, particularly those rich in minerals like magnesium, potassium, and calcium, help stabilize pH levels and buffer acidity in the body. These minerals are essential for various bodily functions, such as muscle function, nerve communication, and blood pressure regulation. By prioritizing foods that supply these minerals, individuals support cellular health, promote a balanced pH, and reduce the body's reliance on its own mineral reserves, preserving bone health and reducing the risk of conditions related to mineral depletion.

2. **Reducing Mucus Production and Inflammation**

Dr. Sebi placed a great deal of emphasis on the connection between acidity, mucus production, and disease. He argued that an acidic environment promotes mucus formation as the body's response to counteract harmful, irritating substances. While mucus serves a protective function, excessive mucus production can obstruct the airways, digestive tract, and other vital systems, creating a breeding ground for pathogens. The alkaline diet discourages foods that cause mucus buildup, like dairy products, red meat, and processed sugars. Instead, it emphasizes foods that help thin mucus and reduce inflammation, such as leafy greens, fresh fruits, and specific herbs. By limiting mucus-inducing foods, individuals may experience improved respiratory health, clearer digestion, and enhanced nutrient absorption. In this way, the alkaline diet promotes a cleaner internal environment, reducing stress on the body and enabling more efficient function across all systems.

3. **Supporting Cellular Energy and Health**

Dr. Sebi introduced the concept of "electric foods," foods that align with the body's natural electrical energy, essential for maintaining cellular health. According to Dr. Sebi, electric foods contain bioavailable minerals and nutrients that "charge" the body at a cellular level. Leafy greens, fresh fruits, nuts, seeds, and certain herbs are examples of electric foods that can replenish the body's energy stores, support enzymatic reactions, and promote cellular repair. Consuming foods rich in natural enzymes and essential nutrients ensures that cells are adequately fueled and equipped to carry out their functions. This is critical for maintaining overall vitality, as cells play an integral role in energy production, detoxification, and the repair of tissues. By prioritizing cellular health through the alkaline diet, individuals can experience improvements in energy levels, cognitive function, and physical endurance.

4. **Enhancing Detoxification and Waste Removal**

Detoxification is central to Dr. Sebi's approach to health. He believed that an accumulation of toxins and waste products, especially from acidic foods, burdens the liver, kidneys, and colon, ultimately impairing their ability to function optimally. The alkaline diet supports detoxification by reducing the intake of substances that strain the body's detox pathways, while introducing foods that facilitate waste elimination. Fiber-rich foods, particularly fruits and vegetables, promote regular bowel movements, which are essential for removing toxins and preventing waste buildup in the colon. Leafy greens and water-rich fruits help to hydrate the body and support kidney function, which is crucial for filtering waste from the bloodstream. Herbs like burdock root, sarsaparilla, and sea moss, commonly included in Dr. Sebi's herbal protocols, also play a role in cleansing the blood and supporting the liver's detoxification processes. By following an alkaline diet, individuals can enhance their body's natural ability to detoxify, reducing toxic load and promoting a healthier internal environment.

5. Improving Immune Function

A strong immune system is essential for protecting the body from infections and chronic illnesses. Dr. Sebi argued that an acidic environment weakens the immune response, making the body more susceptible to pathogens and inflammation. The alkaline diet, with its abundance of vitamins, minerals, and antioxidants, strengthens the immune system, helping the body ward off infections and recover more quickly from illness. Alkaline foods like berries, citrus fruits, and leafy greens are high in antioxidants, which protect cells from oxidative stress and reduce inflammation. These foods also provide essential nutrients like vitamin C, zinc, and iron, all of which support immune cell function and help the body mount an effective defense against disease. By maintaining an alkaline environment, individuals can fortify their immunity and reduce their vulnerability to seasonal illnesses, chronic inflammation, and other immune-related conditions.

6. Facilitating Weight Management and Metabolic Health

The alkaline diet can be a powerful tool for those seeking to achieve or maintain a healthy weight. Unlike processed foods that are high in refined sugars and unhealthy fats, alkaline foods are naturally nutrient-dense and lower in calories, helping to satisfy hunger while supporting weight management. The high fiber content in vegetables, fruits, nuts, and seeds also promotes satiety, reducing the likelihood of overeating and supporting a balanced metabolism. Moreover, many alkaline foods contain compounds that support metabolic health, such as potassium and magnesium, which are necessary for blood sugar regulation and energy production. By reducing reliance on sugary, processed foods, individuals can better regulate blood glucose levels, prevent insulin resistance, and avoid energy crashes. The result is a balanced metabolic rate, stable energy levels, and a healthier approach to weight management that is sustainable over the long term.

PRACTICAL GUIDELINES FOR FOLLOWING THE ALKALINE DIET

1. Focus on Whole, Plant-Based Foods

The foundation of the alkaline diet is rooted in consuming whole, plant-based foods that are minimally processed. These foods offer an abundance of vitamins, minerals, and antioxidants that naturally promote alkalinity. Key categories include leafy greens, cruciferous vegetables, fresh fruits, nuts, seeds, and legumes. By centering meals around these foods, individuals can ensure they're receiving the nutrients necessary to maintain an alkaline state.

2. Avoid Processed and Acidic Foods

Foods that disrupt the body's pH balance and contribute to acidity should be minimized or eliminated. These include refined sugars, processed snacks, sodas, red meat, dairy, and fried foods. Such items are often high in artificial ingredients, preservatives, and unhealthy fats, which Dr. Sebi argued interfere with the body's natural equilibrium. By avoiding these foods, individuals can reduce the body's acidic load and support a healthier, balanced state.

3. Incorporate Herbal Supplements

Dr. Sebi's approach to the alkaline diet includes the use of specific herbs that complement an alkaline lifestyle. Herbs like sea moss, bladderwrack, and burdock root are rich in minerals that promote detoxification, support cellular health, and maintain electrolyte balance. These herbs can be taken in tea, tincture, or capsule form, and are often used in Dr. Sebi's protocols to support the body's ability to cleanse and replenish itself.

4. Stay Hydrated with Alkaline Water

5.
Hydration is a critical component of the alkaline diet. Drinking alkaline water, which has a pH above 7, helps to neutralize acidity in the body and supports digestion, circulation, and detoxification. Staying hydrated assists the kidneys in filtering waste, aids in nutrient transport, and ensures that the body's cells are functioning efficiently. Many followers of the alkaline diet choose to drink alkaline water throughout the day to support these processes.

6. Transition Gradually

For those new to the alkaline diet, a gradual transition may be easier to maintain. Start by making small changes, like incorporating more fresh fruits and vegetables into meals and gradually reducing the intake of acidic foods. Over time, as the body adjusts, the shift to a fully alkaline diet can become more intuitive and manageable. Many people find that as they incorporate more alkaline foods, they naturally begin to crave healthier options, making the diet easier to sustain.

THE BROADER IMPACT OF THE ALKALINE DIET

Beyond individual health, the alkaline diet reflects a philosophy of harmony with nature and sustainable living. By prioritizing natural, plant-based foods, individuals can reduce their ecological footprint and contribute to environmental wellness. Many alkaline foods, such as organic fruits and vegetables, are less resource-intensive than animal products, making them a more sustainable dietary choice. This alignment with nature resonates with Dr. Sebi's teachings on the interconnectedness of health, environment, and community well-being.

The alkaline diet, as advocated by Dr. Sebi, is more than just a set of dietary rules; it's a lifestyle that emphasizes balance, prevention, and a deep respect for the body's natural intelligence. By understanding how the alkaline diet influences cellular health, immunity, detoxification, and energy, individuals can make informed choices that support long-term wellness.

In adopting the alkaline diet, you are embracing a holistic approach that fosters resilience, clarity, and vitality. It's a proactive step toward health that relies on nature's abundance, providing a foundation for wellness that extends beyond the physical to include mental and spiritual well-being. As we continue to explore Dr. Sebi's approach, the following chapters will offer deeper insights and practical advice to help integrate the alkaline diet seamlessly into daily life, guiding you on a journey to sustained health and harmony.

CHAPTER 2
ELECTRIC FOODS AND HEALTH

Dr. Sebi's concept of "electric foods" is one of the most distinctive elements of his dietary philosophy, central to his vision of health and vitality. According to Dr. Sebi, electric foods are natural, plant-based foods that harmonize with the body's natural "electrical" energy, supplying it with the minerals and nutrients necessary for cellular health, energy production, and disease prevention. Unlike processed and animal-based foods, which can disrupt the body's natural balance, electric foods support the body's functions at a cellular level, making them ideal for promoting overall wellness.

WHAT ARE ELECTRIC FOODS?

Electric foods, as Dr. Sebi defined them, are foods that retain their natural energy, structure, and nutrient content, which he believed aligns with the bio-electrical composition of human cells. These foods are minimally processed, typically raw or lightly cooked, and rich in minerals that are essential for the body's cellular processes. They are also usually alkaline, which supports Dr. Sebi's belief in maintaining a slightly alkaline pH in the body.

Examples of electric foods include leafy greens, certain fruits, vegetables, nuts, seeds, and some herbs. These foods are "alive" in the sense that they contain natural enzymes, nutrients, and minerals in their unaltered forms, preserving their bioavailability — meaning they are easier for the body to absorb and utilize. The concept of electric foods is tied to the idea that these natural, unprocessed foods can "charge" the body, helping it maintain energy, cellular health, and balance.

In contrast, non-electric foods — such as processed items, dairy, refined sugars, and animal products — are believed to disrupt the body's electrical balance and pH, making it more acidic. Dr. Sebi argued that these foods lack the energy and structure needed to sustain life at a cellular level, as they have often been altered or stripped of their nutrients. Electric foods, on the other hand, work in harmony with the body, supporting it with vital minerals and contributing to a state of vibrancy and health.

THE ROLE OF MINERALS IN ELECTRIC FOODS

Dr. Sebi often highlighted minerals as the "building blocks of life," and he believed they are essential for every cellular process in the body. Minerals like iron, calcium, magnesium, potassium, and phosphorus play crucial roles in supporting cellular health, muscle function, nerve signaling, and enzyme activation. Electric foods are rich in these minerals, making them ideal for nourishing the body at a foundational level.

For example, iron is crucial for the production of hemoglobin, which carries oxygen to cells throughout the body. Foods high in iron, such as watercress, kale, and certain herbs, help maintain healthy blood and energy levels. Magnesium, often found in dark leafy greens and sea vegetables, supports muscle relaxation, nerve function, and hundreds of enzymatic reactions. By consuming electric foods rich in these minerals, individuals can maintain strong cellular function, sustain energy levels, and support overall health.

Dr. Sebi placed special emphasis on the importance of maintaining a balance of alkaline minerals, as he believed they helped buffer the acidic byproducts of metabolism and the acidic nature of many foods. By eating electric foods rich in these minerals, individuals help to restore and maintain the body's pH balance, creating a favorable environment for health and disease prevention.

HOW ELECTRIC FOODS AFFECT CELLULAR HEALTH

At the core of Dr. Sebi's philosophy is the belief that health begins at the cellular level. He argued that if each cell in the body is functioning optimally, then organs, tissues, and systems will naturally follow suit. Electric foods are considered "cell food" because they nourish cells with bioavailable nutrients that the body can use immediately and efficiently. This cellular support promotes better energy production, aids in cellular repair, and protects against cellular damage.

Electric foods also contain antioxidants, which help protect cells from oxidative stress. Oxidative stress, caused by free radicals, is a primary contributor to aging and chronic disease. Fruits and vegetables high in antioxidants — such as berries, citrus fruits, and leafy greens — neutralize free radicals, helping cells maintain their integrity and reducing the risk of disease. Additionally, the natural fiber in electric foods supports detoxification, ensuring that waste products do not accumulate and interfere with cellular function.

By consistently consuming electric foods, individuals support their cells' ability to detoxify, regenerate, and produce energy. This focus on cellular health extends to overall wellness, as well-nourished cells translate into improved energy, mental clarity, and physical resilience.

THE CONNECTION BETWEEN ELECTRIC FOODS AND ENERGY PRODUCTION

Energy is an essential component of life, and Dr. Sebi believed that consuming electric foods helped the body maintain its natural "charge." Electric foods are nutrient-dense and easily digestible, which means that the body expends less energy on digestion and can direct more toward producing energy for other functions. Additionally, these foods contain the essential nutrients needed for mitochondrial health — the mitochondria being the "powerhouses" of cells where energy production occurs.

For example, potassium and magnesium, commonly found in leafy greens and certain fruits, are essential for cellular energy production and nervous system function. Potassium helps maintain fluid balance within cells and supports heart health, while magnesium is a cofactor in many energy-producing reactions in the mitochondria. By providing these vital nutrients, electric foods directly contribute to sustained energy levels, mental clarity, and physical endurance.

In contrast, processed foods and those high in refined sugars can lead to blood sugar spikes and crashes, depleting the body's energy stores and creating a cycle of fatigue and cravings. Electric foods, with their natural fiber and complex carbohydrates, promote stable blood sugar levels, providing a slow and steady release of energy that supports sustained physical and mental performance.

ELECTRIC FOODS AS NATURAL DETOXIFIERS

One of the unique advantages of electric foods is their natural ability to aid the body's detoxification processes. Many electric foods are rich in fiber, antioxidants, and water content, all of which are essential for supporting the liver, kidneys, colon, and lymphatic system in waste removal. Detoxification is a fundamental aspect of Dr. Sebi's philosophy, as he believed that accumulated toxins from food, environmental pollutants, and stress hinder the body's natural functions.

Leafy greens, fruits, and water-rich vegetables are especially beneficial for cleansing the digestive tract, preventing the buildup of waste in the colon, and reducing inflammation. Citrus fruits like lemons, for example, are alkalizing and help stimulate the liver's detoxification processes. Herbs like burdock root and dandelion, often included in Dr. Sebi's protocols, are known for their blood-purifying properties, aiding in the removal of toxins and improving circulation.

By regularly consuming electric foods, individuals can support their body's detoxification processes, maintain clearer skin, and experience improved digestion. This internal "cleanliness" not only promotes better physical health but also enhances energy and mental clarity, allowing the body to function at its best.

EXAMPLES OF ELECTRIC FOODS

Dr. Sebi recommended a wide range of electric foods that support cellular health, detoxification, and overall vitality. Some key examples include:

- **Leafy Greens**: Kale, watercress, arugula, dandelion greens, and other dark leafy greens are rich in minerals, fiber, and chlorophyll, which support blood health and cellular function.
- **Fruits**: Berries, oranges, lemons, limes, apples, and melons are high in antioxidants and provide a natural source of hydration, vitamins, and minerals.
- **Vegetables**: Zucchini, cucumbers, bell peppers, and squashes are hydrating and nutrient-rich, supporting digestive health and reducing inflammation.
- **Nuts and Seeds**: Almonds, hemp seeds, chia seeds, and walnuts provide healthy fats, protein, and minerals, supporting energy production and brain health.
- **Herbs and Spices**: Basil, thyme, oregano, and cilantro not only add flavor but also contain antioxidants and anti-inflammatory compounds that support immune function and cellular health.
- **Sea Vegetables**: Sea moss, bladderwrack, and nori are particularly valued in Dr. Sebi's protocols for their high mineral content, including iodine, which supports thyroid health.

Each of these foods plays a role in supporting the body's natural processes, from energy production to detoxification, helping to sustain a state of balance and vitality.

INCORPORATING ELECTRIC FOODS INTO DAILY LIFE

For those new to electric foods, transitioning to an electric food-focused diet may require some adjustments. Dr. Sebi suggested starting small, gradually incorporating more of these foods into daily meals. Here are some practical tips for incorporating electric foods into everyday routines:

1. **Start the Day with a Nutrient-Dense Smoothie**

Smoothies are a convenient way to introduce a variety of electric foods at once. Blending fruits like berries or apples with leafy greens such as kale or dandelion greens provides a burst of vitamins, minerals, and fiber. Adding ingredients like chia seeds or sea moss can further enhance the smoothie's nutrient profile, making it an energizing way to start the day.

2. **Replace Processed Snacks with Fresh Fruits and Nuts**

Instead of reaching for processed snacks, keep a selection of fresh fruits, nuts, and seeds on hand. These snacks are not only nutritious but also satisfying, providing a steady source of energy without the blood sugar spikes associated with sugary snacks.

3. Use Herbs and Spices to Flavor Meals

Herbs like basil, oregano, and cilantro add depth of flavor to meals while contributing beneficial compounds that support health. Using herbs regularly is an easy way to incorporate electric foods into daily life while enhancing the taste and appeal of meals.

4. Drink Alkaline Water and Herbal Teas

Staying hydrated is essential for maintaining an alkaline environment in the body. Dr. Sebi recommended drinking alkaline water and herbal teas that support detoxification, such as burdock root or dandelion tea. These beverages not only hydrate but also provide minerals and antioxidants that enhance cellular function.

5. Experiment with New Recipes

Trying new recipes that feature electric foods can make the transition enjoyable and sustainable. From salads packed with leafy greens and fresh vegetables to soups made with nutrient-rich herbs and spices, experimenting in the kitchen is a fun way to integrate electric foods while discovering flavors that you enjoy.

Incorporating electric foods into daily meals supports the body's natural energy, enhances detoxification, and strengthens immunity, promoting long-term vitality and resilience. By choosing these foods, individuals can experience benefits that extend beyond physical health, positively impacting mental clarity, mood, and overall well-being.

CHAPTER 3
KEY BENEFITS OF THE ALKALINE LIFESTYLE

Dr. Sebi's alkaline lifestyle goes beyond diet; it's a holistic approach to health that encourages balance, vitality, and disease prevention. Centered around an alkaline diet, detoxification practices, and natural living, this lifestyle aims to create an environment within the body that promotes wellness on every level. By reducing the body's acidity and embracing natural, plant-based foods, the alkaline lifestyle offers numerous physical, mental, and emotional benefits. This chapter explores these key benefits, providing a closer look at how the alkaline lifestyle supports comprehensive health and enhances overall quality of life.

1. ENHANCED ENERGY AND VITALITY

One of the primary benefits of an alkaline lifestyle is improved energy. Many people report feeling more energized after switching to an alkaline diet, and this boost in vitality stems from several factors. First, alkaline foods — especially leafy greens, fruits, and certain herbs — are rich in essential nutrients like magnesium, potassium, and iron that play a critical role in cellular energy production. These minerals help to fuel the mitochondria, the "powerhouses" of cells, which produce energy for the body.

Furthermore, an alkaline diet emphasizes whole, unprocessed foods that are easy for the body to digest. Unlike processed foods, which can strain the digestive system and create metabolic waste, electric foods are easily broken down, requiring less energy and allowing the body to focus on maintaining energy for physical and mental tasks. By minimizing the burden on digestion and maximizing nutrient intake, the alkaline lifestyle can provide a sustainable source of energy that supports day-to-day activities, workouts, and mental focus.

2. IMPROVED DIGESTION AND NUTRIENT ABSORPTION

The alkaline lifestyle promotes digestive health by reducing the intake of acidic foods that are often challenging to digest, such as meat, dairy, and processed grains. Acidic foods can lead to digestive discomfort, bloating, and inflammation in the gastrointestinal tract, disrupting the balance of gut bacteria and impairing nutrient absorption.

Alkaline foods, on the other hand, are typically high in fiber, which supports healthy digestion and keeps the digestive tract functioning smoothly. Fiber from fruits, vegetables, and whole grains encourages regular bowel movements, helping to prevent constipation and reduce the buildup of toxins in the colon. Additionally, by consuming more natural foods, the body can better absorb essential nutrients, ensuring that the vitamins and minerals it needs for cellular health are readily available. This improved digestion and nutrient absorption also contribute to higher energy levels, enhanced immunity, and a greater sense of well-being.

3. REDUCED INFLAMMATION AND PAIN RELIEF

Inflammation is a natural immune response, but when it becomes chronic, it can lead to a range of health issues, including arthritis, heart disease, and autoimmune disorders. Dr. Sebi's alkaline lifestyle helps to reduce inflammation by minimizing the consumption of acidic, inflammatory foods and emphasizing foods that naturally support an anti-inflammatory response in the body.

Many alkaline foods, such as leafy greens, berries, and herbs like turmeric and ginger, contain antioxidants and phytonutrients that fight inflammation. These compounds help to neutralize free radicals, which are harmful molecules that can damage cells and contribute to inflammation. By consuming a diet rich in anti-inflammatory, alkaline foods, individuals can experience relief from joint pain, muscle soreness, and chronic inflammatory conditions. This reduction in inflammation also supports long-term health, as it minimizes the wear and tear on the body's tissues, reducing the risk of degenerative diseases.

4. STRENGTHENED IMMUNE SYSTEM

A strong immune system is essential for fighting off infections and maintaining overall health. The alkaline lifestyle provides the body with the nutrients it needs to strengthen the immune system and enhance its response to pathogens. Many alkaline foods are rich in immune-boosting vitamins and minerals, such as vitamin C, zinc, and selenium, which support the body's defenses against viruses and bacteria.

Additionally, an alkaline environment discourages the growth of harmful pathogens, as many bacteria, viruses, and fungi thrive in acidic conditions. By maintaining an alkaline internal environment, the body is better equipped to resist infections and recover more quickly if illness does occur. Regular detoxification practices, which are often part of the alkaline lifestyle, also help to remove toxins and impurities from the body, preventing them from weakening immune function and leading to a more resilient immune response overall.

5. ENHANCED MENTAL CLARITY AND EMOTIONAL STABILITY

The alkaline lifestyle extends beyond physical health to support mental and emotional well-being. Many people who adopt an alkaline diet report feeling clearer and more focused, and this may be due to the diet's impact on brain health. The brain, like other organs, benefits from a steady supply of nutrients, including omega-3 fatty acids, antioxidants, and minerals that support cognitive function. The alkaline lifestyle provides these essential nutrients, reducing the likelihood of "brain fog" and promoting sharper mental clarity.

Furthermore, avoiding acidic foods that are high in refined sugars and unhealthy fats helps to stabilize blood sugar levels, which can have a significant impact on mood and emotional stability. Blood sugar spikes and crashes are often associated with irritability, anxiety, and fatigue. By focusing on nutrient-dense, whole foods, the alkaline lifestyle promotes balanced blood sugar levels, supporting a stable mood and helping individuals feel more emotionally balanced and in control.

6. PREVENTION OF CHRONIC DISEASES

Dr. Sebi's alkaline lifestyle emphasizes the prevention of disease by creating conditions in the body that discourage illness. Chronic conditions like diabetes, cardiovascular disease, and hypertension are often linked to lifestyle factors, including diet. Many of these conditions are exacerbated by high levels of inflammation, poor diet, and an acidic internal environment. The alkaline diet, by prioritizing foods that reduce inflammation, support vascular health, and prevent the buildup of acidic waste, offers a proactive approach to preventing these common health issues.

Alkaline foods support cardiovascular health by reducing cholesterol, regulating blood pressure, and promoting better blood flow. Fruits, vegetables, and plant-based fats provide antioxidants that protect blood vessels, reducing the risk of atherosclerosis and other cardiovascular issues. By maintaining an alkaline diet, individuals take preventative steps toward long-term health, reducing their reliance on medications and the risk of developing lifestyle-related diseases.

7. BETTER SKIN HEALTH AND REDUCED SIGNS OF AGING

The benefits of the alkaline lifestyle extend to skin health, as well. Alkaline foods are high in antioxidants, vitamins, and minerals that protect skin cells from oxidative stress, reduce inflammation, and encourage collagen production. Collagen is a protein that maintains the skin's elasticity and structure, preventing wrinkles and sagging. By consuming foods that support collagen synthesis and protect against free radical damage, individuals can promote healthier, more youthful-looking skin.

Additionally, the detoxifying effect of the alkaline diet helps to clear toxins from the bloodstream, which can improve skin clarity and reduce issues like acne, eczema, and psoriasis. The high water content of many alkaline foods, such as cucumbers, melons, and leafy greens, also keeps the skin hydrated, promoting a radiant complexion and slowing the visible effects of aging.

8. HORMONAL BALANCE AND IMPROVED REPRODUCTIVE HEALTH

Hormones play a significant role in regulating metabolism, mood, reproductive health, and various bodily functions. The alkaline lifestyle supports hormonal balance by providing the nutrients necessary for hormone production and regulation. For instance, magnesium and vitamin B6, found in leafy greens and nuts, are essential for the production and balance of hormones. By supplying the body with the right nutrients, the alkaline lifestyle can help regulate hormones naturally, reducing symptoms related to hormonal imbalances such as fatigue, mood swings, and irregular menstrual cycles.

For those interested in reproductive health, the alkaline diet provides a foundation of nutrients that support fertility and hormonal health. The reduction of processed, acidic foods helps to balance estrogen levels, which can improve fertility and reduce symptoms associated with hormonal imbalances, such as PMS and menopausal discomfort.

By adopting an alkaline lifestyle, individuals can experience a wide array of benefits that extend from physical resilience to mental clarity and emotional balance. Dr. Sebi's approach emphasizes preventive care, promoting habits and food choices that support the body's natural intelligence and capacity for health. Through the alkaline lifestyle, individuals have a pathway to not only enhanced wellness but also a life filled with vitality and peace.

BOOK 3
Alkaline Foods List

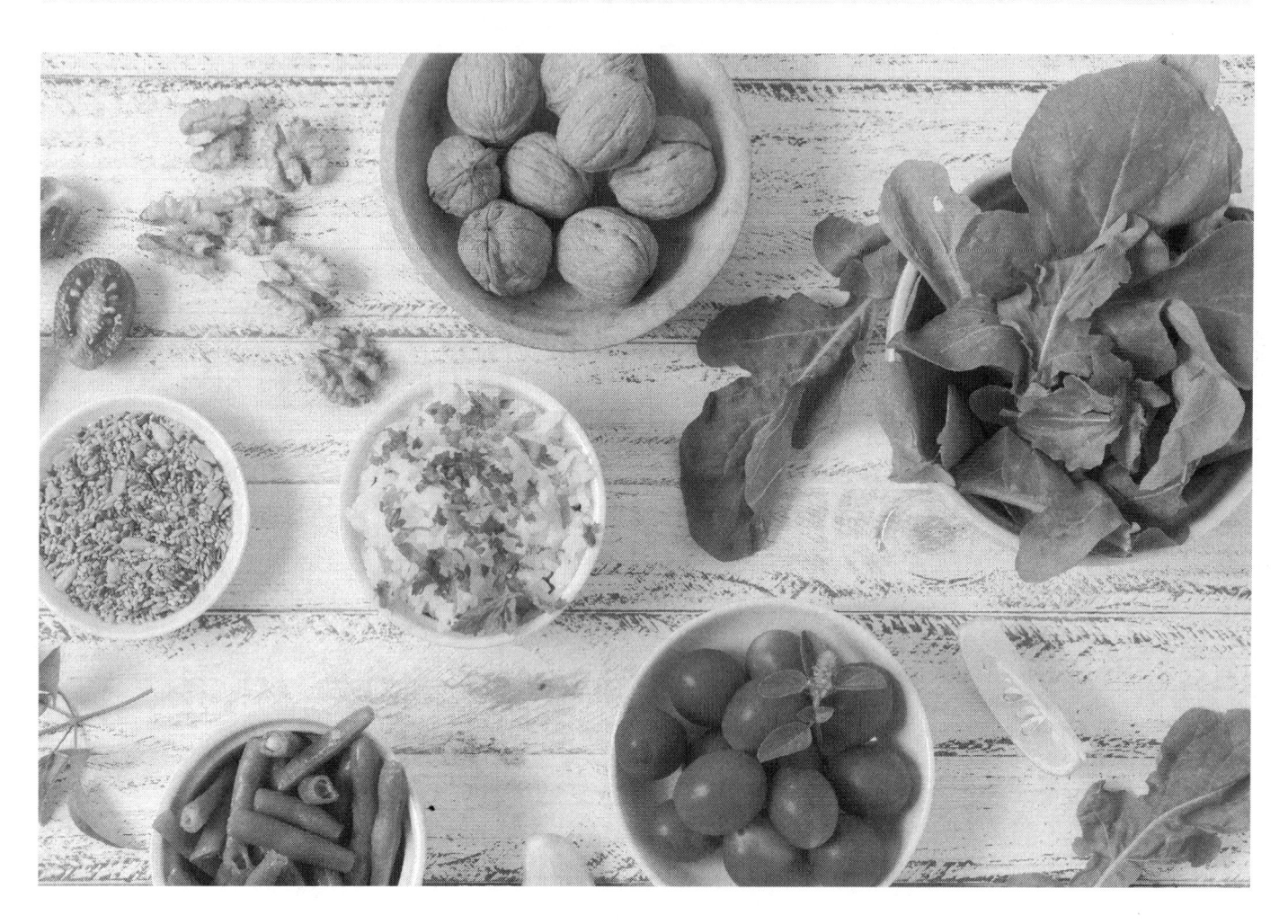

In the journey to adopt Dr. Sebi's alkaline lifestyle, understanding which foods align with an alkaline diet is essential. Dr. Sebi's list of approved alkaline foods is designed to support cellular health, reduce acidity, and maintain a balanced pH. Each food on this list is chosen for its nutrient density, natural composition, and ability to support the body's energy and detoxification processes.

This book provides a comprehensive look at the foods Dr. Sebi recommended, focusing on plant-based, nutrient-rich choices that offer a foundation for a balanced, health-promoting lifestyle. From leafy greens to fruits, vegetables, and herbs, the following chapters will explore each food group in depth, offering practical guidance on how to incorporate these foods into daily meals for optimal wellness.

CHAPTER 1
APPROVED ALKALINE FOODS

Dr. Sebi's philosophy places significant importance on consuming foods that support the body's natural balance. These "electric" or alkaline foods work with the body's cellular makeup, providing essential nutrients, minerals, and hydration to sustain health and prevent disease. Here is a guide to Dr. Sebi's approved alkaline foods, along with insights on their unique benefits and how to incorporate them into everyday meals.

1. LEAFY GREENS

Leafy greens are some of the most powerful foods for maintaining an alkaline state. These nutrient-dense plants are high in vitamins, minerals, and antioxidants that support cellular health, detoxification, and energy production. They're also rich in chlorophyll, which aids in cleansing the blood and promoting oxygenation. Dr. Sebi recommended a variety of specific greens for their alkaline properties:

- **Kale**: Kale is a nutrient powerhouse, loaded with vitamins A, C, and K, along with minerals like calcium and iron that are essential for bone health, immunity, and energy. Kale can be used in smoothies, salads, or lightly sautéed as a side dish.
- **Watercress**: Known for its slightly peppery taste, watercress is rich in vitamin C, iron, and calcium, which support blood health and cellular repair. Watercress can be added to salads, smoothies, or juices to boost nutrient intake.
- **Dandelion Greens**: High in potassium and iron, dandelion greens support liver function and help detoxify the body. They can be added to salads, stir-fried, or used as a tea for their cleansing properties.
- **Arugula**: This leafy green has a unique flavor and is high in calcium and magnesium, which aid in muscle and bone health. Arugula works well in salads or as a topping for cooked dishes.

These leafy greens can be enjoyed raw or lightly cooked, allowing for maximum nutrient retention. Adding them to meals provides a simple yet powerful way to boost alkalinity and overall health.

2. FRUITS

Fresh fruits are naturally alkaline and hydrating, making them ideal for an alkaline diet. Dr. Sebi recommended fruits with low sugar content that provide antioxidants, fiber, and essential vitamins to nourish the body and promote detoxification. Key alkaline fruits include:

- **Berries (Blueberries, Blackberries, and Strawberries)**: These berries are rich in antioxidants, vitamin C, and fiber, supporting immune health, skin vitality, and cellular repair. They're ideal for smoothies, snacks, or as a topping for salads.
- **Apples**: Apples contain fiber, particularly in the skin, which supports digestion and helps remove toxins from the body. They can be enjoyed on their own, sliced into salads, or added to juices.
- **Citrus Fruits (Limes and Lemons)**: While acidic in taste, limes and lemons have an alkalizing effect on the body once metabolized. They're high in vitamin C, promoting immune health, and can be used to flavor water, dress salads, or enhance the taste of many dishes.
- **Melons (Watermelon, Cantaloupe)**: Melons are hydrating, full of natural enzymes, and help detoxify the kidneys. They are refreshing as a snack, in fruit salads, or blended into smoothies.

Including fruits in daily meals, whether as a snack or part of a larger dish, is an easy way to infuse the diet with alkaline-supporting nutrients and hydration.

3. VEGETABLES

Vegetables provide essential vitamins, minerals, and fiber to support digestive health, reduce acidity, and promote detoxification. Dr. Sebi's recommended vegetables are low in starch and high in water content, making them both alkalizing and hydrating:

- **Cucumbers**: Known for their high water content, cucumbers help hydrate the body and support skin health. They can be added to salads, blended into smoothies, or enjoyed as a refreshing snack.
- **Zucchini**: Zucchini is rich in potassium and vitamin C, supporting heart health and immune function. It can be grilled, sautéed, or spiralized as a pasta substitute.
- **Bell Peppers**: These colorful vegetables are packed with antioxidants, particularly vitamin C, which aids immune health. They add flavor and texture to salads, stir-fries, and roasted dishes.
- **Squash (Chayote)**: Chayote squash has a mild flavor and is high in vitamin C and potassium, essential for cardiovascular and muscular health. It can be roasted, steamed, or used in soups and stews.

Incorporating a variety of vegetables into daily meals provides essential nutrients and makes it easier to maintain a balanced pH while enjoying a range of flavors and textures.

4. HERBS AND SPICES

Herbs and spices add flavor to food while offering potent health benefits. Many herbs are anti-inflammatory, antioxidant-rich, and support digestive health. Dr. Sebi recommended several key herbs for their alkalizing and medicinal properties:

- **Basil**: Basil is high in vitamin K and antioxidants, supporting bone health and reducing oxidative stress. It's an excellent addition to sauces, salads, and vegetable dishes.
- **Oregano**: Known for its antibacterial properties, oregano also provides antioxidants and supports digestive health. It can be used in teas, as a seasoning for meals, or infused into oils.
- **Thyme**: Thyme is a powerful herb for respiratory health and immune support. It pairs well with roasted vegetables, soups, and teas.
- **Cilantro**: Cilantro is detoxifying, helping to remove heavy metals from the body, and it's rich in vitamin K, supporting blood health. It works well in salads, salsas, and as a garnish for cooked dishes.

These herbs can be used fresh or dried, allowing for versatile and flavorful additions to meals while supporting health and pH balance.

5. NUTS AND SEEDS

Nuts and seeds provide healthy fats, protein, and minerals, making them an excellent addition to the alkaline diet. They're also satisfying and can help curb hunger between meals. Key alkaline nuts and seeds include:

- **Almonds**: Almonds are a good source of healthy fats, fiber, and vitamin E, which supports skin health and immune function. They can be eaten as a snack, added to salads, or blended into almond milk.
- **Hemp Seeds**: These seeds are rich in omega-3 and omega-6 fatty acids, promoting brain and heart health. They're easy to sprinkle on salads, smoothies, or yogurt.
- **Chia Seeds**: Chia seeds are packed with fiber and omega-3 fatty acids, supporting digestion and cardiovascular health. They can be soaked to create a pudding, added to smoothies, or sprinkled on fruit.
- **Brazil Nuts**: Brazil nuts are an excellent source of selenium, a mineral important for thyroid health and immune function. A few nuts a day are sufficient due to their high selenium content.

Incorporating nuts and seeds as snacks or toppings provides healthy fats, protein, and essential minerals to support overall health and balance.

6. SEA VEGETABLES

Sea vegetables are a unique addition to the alkaline diet, offering high mineral content and a variety of nutrients that support thyroid function, immunity, and detoxification. Dr. Sebi emphasized their importance due to their nutrient density and bioavailability:

- **Sea Moss**: Sea moss is rich in minerals like iodine, potassium, and magnesium, supporting thyroid health and detoxification. It can be added to smoothies or used as a thickener in recipes.
- **Bladderwrack**: Bladderwrack is another sea vegetable high in iodine, which is essential for metabolic health. It's often used in supplement form or can be added to soups and broths.
- **Nori**: Nori is a type of seaweed used in sushi and as a seasoning. It provides iodine, protein, and vitamin C, supporting immune function and skin health.

Sea vegetables can be incorporated into meals, added to soups, or used as snacks, providing a concentrated source of minerals essential for maintaining alkalinity.

This comprehensive guide to Dr. Sebi's approved alkaline foods provides a foundation for those looking to create balanced, nutritious meals that support health and pH balance. By incorporating a variety of these foods daily, individuals can experience the benefits of an alkaline lifestyle, including improved energy, digestion, immunity, and overall vitality.

CHAPTER 2
FOODS TO AVOID

Dr. Sebi's alkaline lifestyle is as much about avoiding harmful foods as it is about consuming beneficial ones. He believed that certain foods contribute to an acidic environment in the body, causing inflammation, mucus buildup, and disrupting the body's natural balance. Avoiding these foods is crucial for anyone seeking to maintain an alkaline state and achieve the health benefits associated with this lifestyle. In this chapter, we'll explore the specific foods Dr. Sebi advised against, why they're considered harmful, and how they impact the body.

1. PROCESSED FOODS AND ADDITIVES

Processed foods are widely recognized for their negative health effects. They're often packed with additives, preservatives, and artificial ingredients that disrupt the body's pH and add to its toxic load. Examples include:

- **Sugary Snacks and Beverages**: Foods high in refined sugars, such as candy, soda, and packaged snacks, can lead to rapid spikes in blood sugar, inflammation, and acidity. These foods lack nutritional value and can strain the body's insulin production, contributing to blood sugar imbalances and fatigue.
- **Packaged Meats**: Deli meats, sausages, and other processed meats contain nitrates, sodium, and preservatives that can increase acidity, stress the liver, and increase inflammation. Many of these foods are also high in unhealthy fats that burden the digestive system and disrupt metabolic balance.
- **Artificial Sweeteners**: While often marketed as low-calorie alternatives, artificial sweeteners like aspartame, saccharin, and sucralose have been linked to inflammation and gut microbiome disruption. These chemicals are foreign to the body, making them difficult to metabolize and increasing acidity.

Processed foods often undergo manufacturing processes that strip them of their natural nutrients, making them "empty" calories that leave the body depleted of essential vitamins and minerals. Avoiding these foods helps prevent unnecessary strain on the digestive and detoxification systems, supporting a balanced, alkaline environment.

2. DAIRY PRODUCTS

Dairy products, including milk, cheese, and yogurt, are a significant source of acidity in the diet. According to Dr. Sebi, dairy also leads to mucus production, which can obstruct respiratory health and create an environment where pathogens can thrive. Common dairy products to avoid include:

- **Milk**: Although often promoted for its calcium content, milk is acidic and can interfere with calcium absorption in the body. It can also contribute to digestive discomfort, particularly for those who are lactose intolerant.
- **Cheese**: Cheese is high in saturated fats and sodium, contributing to acidity and inflammation. Many cheeses also contain additives and preservatives, which can further stress the digestive system.
- **Yogurt**: While some believe yogurt's probiotics benefit gut health, its acidity, along with added sugars and flavorings, can negate these benefits, especially for individuals sensitive to lactose.

By avoiding dairy products, individuals can reduce mucus buildup and inflammation, making it easier for the body to maintain an alkaline state. Alternatives like almond or coconut milk can provide similar textures and flavors without contributing to acidity.

3. MEAT AND ANIMAL PRODUCTS

Meat and other animal products are highly acidic and contribute to mucus production and inflammation. Dr. Sebi recommended avoiding animal-based foods as they often require a more extended digestion process and can lead to a buildup of waste and toxins in the digestive tract. Key foods to avoid include:

- **Red Meat**: Beef and lamb are high in saturated fats and take longer to digest, leading to increased acidity and strain on the liver. Red meat can also be a source of hormones and antibiotics, which can disrupt the body's hormonal balance.
- **Poultry**: While leaner than red meat, chicken and turkey are still acidic and can contribute to inflammation. Most poultry also undergoes processing that involves additives and preservatives, further increasing its acidity.
- **Eggs**: Eggs, especially the yolk, are acidic and contribute to cholesterol buildup. While eggs are a source of protein, Dr. Sebi recommended plant-based protein sources instead to maintain an alkaline state.

Avoiding animal products allows the digestive system to process food more efficiently and reduces the overall acid load in the body, supporting clearer digestion and a healthier gut.

4. REFINED GRAINS

Refined grains, including white flour and white rice, are stripped of their natural fiber and nutrients, making them high-glycemic foods that contribute to blood sugar spikes and acidity. Refined grains lack the minerals and vitamins needed to sustain energy and support digestion. Foods to avoid include:

- **White Bread**: White bread is made from refined flour, which lacks fiber and nutrients, leading to rapid digestion, blood sugar spikes, and increased acidity.
- **White Rice**: White rice has a high glycemic index, contributing to blood sugar imbalances and insulin resistance. Brown rice or wild rice can be more nutrient-dense alternatives.
- **Pasta**: Made from refined wheat, pasta is often highly processed and has limited nutritional value. Pasta alternatives made from vegetables, like zucchini noodles, can be a more alkaline-friendly option.

Switching to whole grains, such as quinoa and amaranth, provides more fiber and essential nutrients, supporting digestion and helping to maintain an alkaline environment.

5. REFINED SUGARS AND ARTIFICIAL SWEETENERS

Refined sugars are highly acidic and have no nutritional value, contributing to rapid blood sugar fluctuations and promoting an acidic environment. Sugary foods can lead to insulin resistance, weight gain, and fatigue. Common sources of refined sugars include:

- **White Sugar**: White sugar is refined, devoid of nutrients, and has been linked to inflammation and blood sugar imbalances.
- **Corn Syrup**: Corn syrup, found in many processed foods, is high in fructose and has been associated with increased risk of metabolic diseases.
- **Artificial Sweeteners**: Aspartame, sucralose, and saccharin are common artificial sweeteners that are difficult for the body to process and disrupt the natural pH balance.

Instead of refined sugars, natural sweeteners like dates, agave nectar, or pure maple syrup offer sweetness without the same acidic load and come with additional vitamins and minerals.

CHAPTER 3

SOURCING AND PREPARING ALKALINE INGREDIENTS

Transitioning to an alkaline lifestyle involves selecting high-quality ingredients that are minimally processed and rich in nutrients. Sourcing fresh, organic, and natural ingredients not only supports alkalinity but also enhances the flavors and textures of meals, making it easier to sustain this lifestyle. In this chapter, we'll explore practical tips on sourcing alkaline foods, preserving their nutrient content, and preparing them to maximize their health benefits.

1. CHOOSING ORGANIC AND LOCALLY GROWN PRODUCE

One of the best ways to source alkaline ingredients is by choosing organic and locally grown produce. Organic produce is grown without synthetic pesticides, herbicides, or fertilizers, which helps reduce the body's toxic load and keeps foods as close to their natural state as possible. Locally grown produce is often fresher and more nutrient-dense, as it doesn't require long transportation times, which can degrade nutrient quality.

- **Farmers' Markets**: Farmers' markets offer seasonal, locally grown produce that is often organic or grown with minimal pesticides. Shopping at farmers' markets supports local agriculture and allows consumers to speak directly with growers about their farming practices.
- **Community-Supported Agriculture (CSA)**: CSA programs allow individuals to purchase shares in local farms and receive fresh produce regularly. This option is convenient and provides access to a variety of seasonal vegetables and fruits.
- **Organic Sections in Grocery Stores**: Many grocery stores offer organic sections where individuals can find fresh, chemical-free produce. Look for certification labels, such as USDA Organic, to ensure quality.

Choosing organic and locally grown produce ensures that ingredients are not only more alkaline-friendly but also better for the environment.

2. STORING AND PRESERVING ALKALINE FOODS

Proper storage is essential for preserving the nutritional quality of alkaline foods. Here are a few tips for maintaining the freshness of key alkaline ingredients:

- **Leafy Greens**: Store leafy greens in the refrigerator, ideally in a damp paper towel or cloth within a perforated bag to maintain moisture. Greens can also be washed and dried before storage to reduce spoilage.
- **Fruits**: Some fruits, such as berries, should be stored in the refrigerator to extend freshness, while others, like bananas and apples, can be kept at room temperature.
- **Herbs**: Fresh herbs can be stored in a glass of water in the refrigerator, with a plastic bag loosely placed over the top to maintain humidity. Herbs can also be chopped and frozen in olive oil or water to preserve flavor and nutrients.

By storing alkaline foods correctly, individuals can reduce waste and maintain the quality of their ingredients.

3. PREPARATION TECHNIQUES TO MAXIMIZE NUTRIENT RETENTION

The way food is prepared can affect its nutritional content. Minimizing heat exposure and using gentle cooking methods helps preserve vitamins, minerals, and enzymes in alkaline foods.

- **Raw and Lightly Steamed**: Consuming vegetables raw or lightly steamed helps retain their nutrients and enzymes. Steaming is preferable to boiling, as it preserves more vitamins and minerals.
- **Blanching**: Blanching involves briefly cooking vegetables in boiling water, then cooling them quickly in ice water. This method retains color, texture, and nutrients while making certain vegetables easier to digest.
- **Low-Heat Cooking**: Cooking at lower temperatures, such as baking at 300°F or using a slow cooker, reduces nutrient degradation. Olive oil or coconut oil are excellent choices for low-heat cooking, as they maintain stability at moderate temperatures.

Preparing food with care helps preserve the nutritional value of alkaline ingredients, enhancing their health benefits and making the diet more enjoyable.

4. SIMPLE ALKALINE RECIPES FOR DAILY USE

Here are a few easy ways to incorporate alkaline foods into daily meals:

DR. SEBI HERBAL BIBLE [30 BOOKS IN 1] 33

- **Green Smoothie**: Blend kale, watercress, cucumber, and a handful of berries with alkaline water or coconut water. This nutrient-packed smoothie is hydrating and easy to digest.
- **Vegetable Stir-Fry**: Lightly stir-fry zucchini, bell peppers, and broccoli in olive oil with a sprinkle of sea salt, garlic, and fresh basil for flavor.
- **Herbal Salad Dressing**: Mix fresh herbs like basil and oregano with olive oil, lemon juice, and a dash of sea salt for a simple, alkaline-friendly dressing.
- **Fruit and Nut Snack**: Slice an apple and sprinkle it with chia seeds and a handful of almonds for a satisfying, nutrient-rich snack.

Incorporating alkaline foods into meals can be simple, flavorful, and convenient, supporting a lifestyle that fosters long-term health and vitality.

This detailed overview of Dr. Sebi's recommendations for foods to avoid and practical guidance on sourcing and preparing alkaline ingredients provides the tools needed to maintain an alkaline lifestyle. By focusing on high-quality ingredients and using gentle preparation methods, individuals can maximize the benefits of an alkaline diet and enjoy a healthful, balanced way of eating.

BOOK 4
Integrating Electric Foods Daily

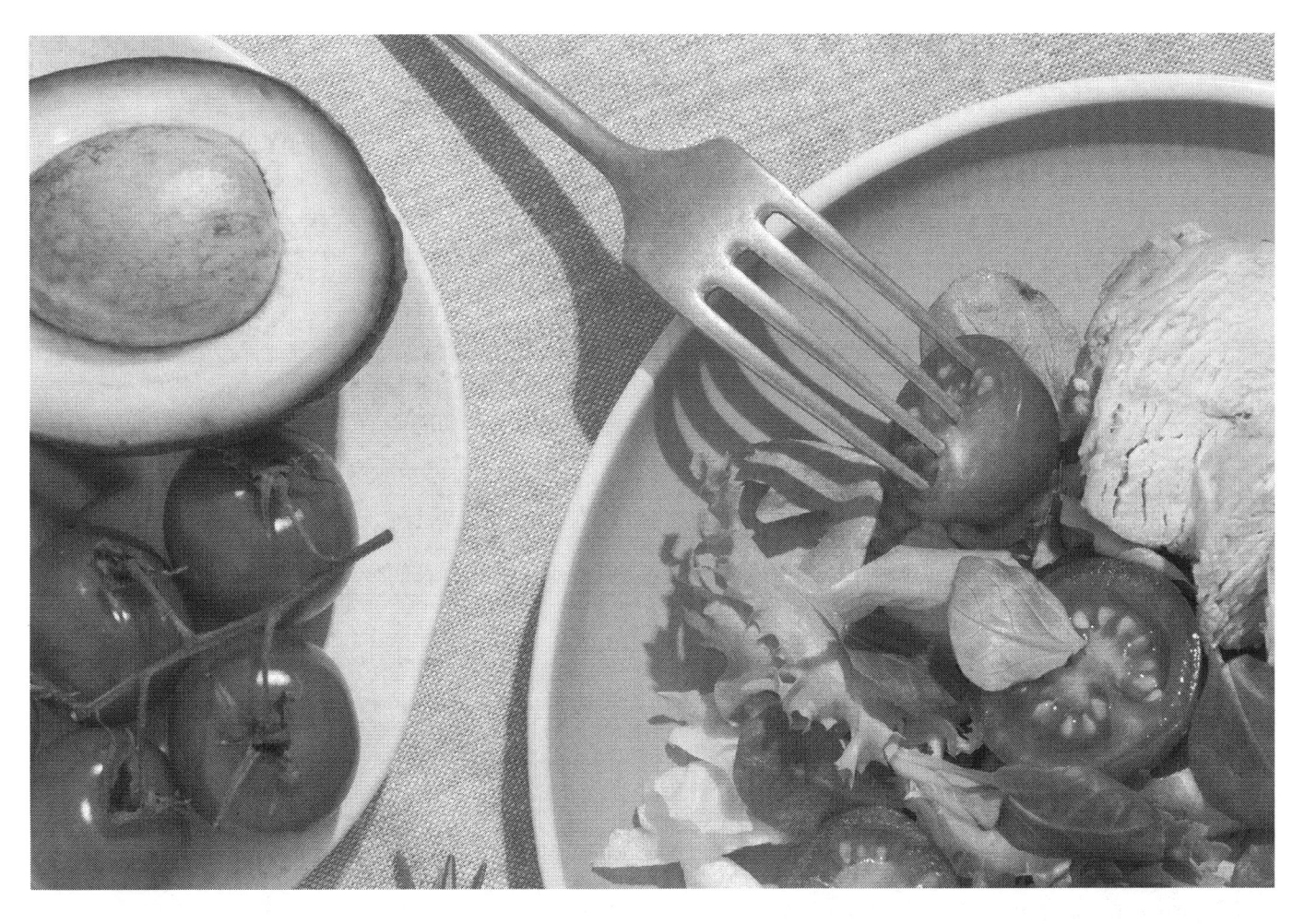

Incorporating Dr. Sebi's recommended electric foods into daily meals is essential for maintaining a balanced, alkaline environment that supports vitality, energy, and overall wellness. An alkaline-focused diet emphasizes fresh, plant-based, and nutrient-dense foods that harmonize with the body's natural processes, aiding in detoxification, cellular health, and energy production. This book provides practical guidance on incorporating electric foods into everyday life, creating satisfying meals that support the alkaline lifestyle without sacrificing flavor or variety.

CHAPTER 1
BUILDING AN ALKALINE PLATE

Creating an "alkaline plate" involves selecting foods that promote an alkaline state in the body, balancing nutrient groups to meet daily needs, and using fresh, whole ingredients to maximize flavor and health benefits. Dr. Sebi's philosophy of building an alkaline plate centers on plant-based foods that are rich in essential minerals, vitamins, and antioxidants to support cellular health, reduce inflammation, and prevent disease. In this chapter, we'll explore the essential components of an alkaline plate, practical guidelines for meal planning, and sample ideas for building nutrient-rich, alkaline meals.

1. THE CORE COMPONENTS OF AN ALKALINE PLATE

An alkaline plate typically includes a balance of leafy greens, vegetables, fruits, herbs, nuts, seeds, and a small amount of healthy fats. The focus is on whole, natural ingredients that are minimally processed to retain their nutrients and vitality. Here's a breakdown of the main components of an alkaline plate:

- **Leafy Greens**: Leafy greens, such as kale, watercress, and dandelion greens, are the foundation of an alkaline plate. These greens provide essential minerals like calcium, magnesium, and potassium, which are important for maintaining pH balance, supporting bone health, and promoting detoxification. Greens are also high in fiber, which aids digestion and helps regulate blood sugar.
- **Vegetables**: Vegetables like cucumbers, zucchini, bell peppers, and squash offer hydration, fiber, and antioxidants. They add bulk to meals and are versatile, allowing for various preparations, including steaming, sautéing, and roasting.
- **Fruits**: Fresh fruits, such as berries, apples, and melons, provide natural sweetness, vitamins, and antioxidants. Fruits are hydrating and support the immune system with their high vitamin C content. They also make meals more flavorful and satisfying without relying on refined sugars.
- **Herbs and Spices**: Herbs like basil, oregano, and thyme add flavor to dishes and are packed with antioxidants and anti-inflammatory compounds. They support digestion, respiratory health, and immune function.
- **Nuts and Seeds**: Nuts like almonds and seeds like chia provide healthy fats, protein, and fiber, which help maintain satiety and stabilize blood sugar levels. They are also rich in omega-3 fatty acids, which support brain and heart health.
- **Healthy Fats**: Small amounts of olive oil, coconut oil, and avocado provide necessary fats that support cellular health, hormone production, and nutrient absorption. These fats are also anti-inflammatory, making them ideal for an alkaline-focused diet.

These components can be adjusted in different proportions based on individual needs, meal preferences, and availability. The goal is to create a balanced plate that is not only alkaline but also enjoyable and varied.

2. BUILDING BALANCED ALKALINE MEALS

To build a balanced alkaline meal, consider dividing the plate into sections to ensure a variety of nutrients and flavors. Here's a basic approach:

- **Half the Plate: Leafy Greens and Vegetables**

Fill half of the plate with a mix of leafy greens and colorful vegetables. The diversity in color often reflects a diversity in nutrients, so including a variety of greens and vegetables ensures a broad range of vitamins, minerals, and antioxidants. For example, a meal might include a bed of kale topped with sliced cucumbers, bell peppers, and a sprinkle of dandelion greens.

- **One-Quarter of the Plate: Fruits and Nuts**

Use a quarter of the plate for fruits, which provide natural sweetness, fiber, and hydration. Berries, apple slices, or a few melon chunks can brighten a meal, adding both flavor and visual appeal. Nuts or seeds, such as almonds or hemp seeds, can be added to provide healthy fats and protein. This section helps balance flavors and textures while supporting nutrient diversity.

- **One-Quarter of the Plate: Protein and Healthy Fats**

The remaining quarter of the plate can be dedicated to plant-based protein sources and healthy fats. While the alkaline diet isn't protein-heavy, options like hemp seeds, chia seeds, and a drizzle of olive oil or coconut oil provide the necessary fats and proteins for satiety and metabolic support.

This plate structure is flexible and can be adapted to different meals throughout the day. For instance, breakfast might include a smoothie packed with leafy greens, fruits, and a spoonful of chia seeds, while dinner could consist of a large salad with leafy greens, roasted vegetables, and a handful of nuts.

3. MEAL PLANNING TIPS FOR THE ALKALINE LIFESTYLE

Meal planning helps ensure a consistent intake of alkaline foods, reduces time spent on daily meal preparation, and supports balanced nutrition. Here are some practical tips for planning alkaline-focused meals:

- **Plan Ahead for Each Meal**: Aim to include a variety of electric foods at each meal. For instance, breakfast might focus on fruits and seeds, lunch on leafy greens and vegetables, and dinner on a mix of greens, vegetables, and healthy fats.
- **Batch Cook Key Ingredients**: Pre-cooking and storing ingredients like steamed vegetables, roasted squash, or quinoa can make meal preparation faster and easier. Store these items in the fridge, so they're ready to add to salads, stir-fries, or bowls throughout the week.
- **Prep Snacks and Smoothies**: Preparing snacks like pre-chopped fruits, nuts, and seeds, or making smoothie packs with fruits and greens can simplify snacks and breakfasts. When hunger strikes, these items are convenient, nutritious, and aligned with the alkaline lifestyle.
- **Include Hydrating and Detoxifying Foods**: To support the body's natural detoxification processes, include hydrating foods like cucumbers, melons, and leafy greens regularly. Drinking herbal teas, such as dandelion or ginger, can also support digestion and detox.

Meal planning ensures that each meal includes a balance of alkaline foods, making it easier to sustain the lifestyle while enjoying diverse flavors and nutrients.

4. ALKALINE MEAL IDEAS FOR BREAKFAST, LUNCH, AND DINNER

Creating a variety of meals that align with Dr. Sebi's principles can help keep the diet enjoyable and sustainable. Here are some sample meal ideas for each part of the day:

Breakfast Ideas

1. **Green Smoothie Bowl**: Blend kale, spinach, berries, a banana, and coconut water. Top with chia seeds, hemp seeds, and sliced fruit.
2. **Chia Pudding with Berries**: Combine chia seeds with almond milk and let it sit overnight. In the morning, add fresh berries, a few almonds, and a sprinkle of cinnamon.
3. **Fruit Salad with Nuts**: Mix a variety of fruits like apples, melons, and berries. Add a handful of almonds or hemp seeds for protein and healthy fats.

Lunch Ideas

1. **Massaged Kale Salad**: Massage kale with olive oil and lemon juice. Add sliced bell peppers, cucumber, avocado, and a handful of dandelion greens. Top with pumpkin seeds for crunch.
2. **Zucchini Noodle Bowl**: Use a spiralizer to make zucchini noodles. Add cherry tomatoes, basil, and sliced cucumber, drizzling with olive oil and a touch of sea salt.
3. **Stuffed Bell Peppers**: Roast a bell pepper and fill it with a mixture of quinoa, diced zucchini, and fresh herbs. Serve with a side of greens and avocado slices.

Dinner Ideas

1. **Roasted Vegetable Bowl**: Roast a mix of vegetables like sweet potato, zucchini, and bell peppers. Serve over a bed of arugula or watercress with a sprinkle of hemp seeds and a drizzle of tahini.
2. **Steamed Greens with Almond Sauce**: Steam greens like kale and dandelion. Make a sauce with almond butter, garlic, lemon juice, and a touch of water, drizzling it over the greens for a flavorful meal.
3. **Herbed Quinoa Salad**: Prepare quinoa and toss it with fresh parsley, cilantro, cucumber, and sliced bell peppers. Add olive oil, lemon juice, and a handful of sunflower seeds.

These meal ideas use simple ingredients and preparation methods to ensure that meals are quick, nutritious, and satisfying.

5. SEASONAL AND LOCAL INGREDIENTS FOR FRESHNESS AND FLAVOR

Using seasonal, locally sourced ingredients not only enhances the flavor of meals but also supports the body's natural cycles and needs. For instance, in the warmer months, fruits like berries, melons, and leafy greens are abundant and offer hydration, while in cooler months, root vegetables and hearty greens like kale are ideal for nourishing warmth.

Shopping seasonally also ensures that ingredients are fresher, often more nutrient-dense, and better for the environment. Visiting farmers' markets or joining a Community-Supported

Agriculture (CSA) program can be great ways to access fresh, seasonal ingredients.

6. HYDRATION AND HERBAL TEAS TO SUPPORT AN ALKALINE STATE

Proper hydration is a vital component of the alkaline lifestyle. Water supports all bodily functions, including digestion, detoxification, and cellular energy production. Dr. Sebi emphasized the importance of drinking alkaline water and herbal teas to maintain pH balance and support the body's natural processes.

- **Alkaline Water**: Drinking alkaline water (pH above 7) can help neutralize acidity and support hydration. Add lemon slices or a pinch of baking soda to regular water to increase its alkalinity.
- **Herbal Teas**: Teas made from herbs like dandelion, ginger, and peppermint support digestion and detoxification. These teas also offer gentle hydration and can be soothing additions to daily meals.

7. FLAVORFUL AND NUTRITIOUS DRESSINGS AND SAUCES

Dressings and sauces are an excellent way to add flavor to alkaline meals without relying on acidic or processed condiments. Using herbs, oils, and citrus can elevate the taste of salads, vegetables, and grains.

- **Lemon Herb Dressing**: Combine olive oil, lemon juice, minced garlic, fresh herbs (like basil and parsley), and a pinch of sea salt for a bright, alkaline-friendly dressing.
- **Tahini Sauce**: Mix tahini with a bit of water, lemon juice, and fresh garlic. This creamy, nutrient-rich sauce is perfect for salads, roasted vegetables, or grain bowls.
- **Avocado-Cilantro Dressing**: Blend avocado, cilantro, a touch of olive oil, and lime juice for a creamy, flavorful dressing.

Adding nutrient-dense dressings and sauces not only makes meals more enjoyable but also provides healthy fats and antioxidants that support the body's health.

By building an alkaline plate with a balance of leafy greens, vegetables, fruits, and healthy fats, you can support your body's natural pH balance, energy levels, and cellular health. These foundational principles make it easy to integrate Dr. Sebi's alkaline recommendations into daily meals, providing a sustainable approach to vitality and wellness.

CHAPTER 2
ALKALINE FOODS FOR ENERGY

A diet rich in alkaline foods provides a natural energy boost, supporting physical vitality and mental clarity. Unlike foods high in refined sugars and processed ingredients, which lead to energy crashes, alkaline foods offer sustained energy by nourishing the body at a cellular level. This chapter explores some of the most effective alkaline foods for energy, explains why they work so well, and offers tips for incorporating them into daily meals for optimal stamina and endurance.

1. LEAFY GREENS: FUEL FOR CELLULAR HEALTH

Leafy greens are some of the most nutrient-dense foods and are rich in vitamins, minerals, and chlorophyll, all of which support energy production at the cellular level. The chlorophyll in greens such as kale, spinach, and watercress helps oxygenate the blood, which in turn promotes cellular energy production and mental clarity.

- **Kale**: Kale is a powerhouse of vitamin C, iron, and calcium, all of which are crucial for sustaining energy levels. Iron supports red blood cell production, which helps transport oxygen to cells and prevents fatigue.
- **Spinach**: Spinach is high in magnesium, which aids in muscle relaxation and supports enzyme reactions that produce cellular energy.
- **Watercress**: This green is particularly rich in antioxidants, which help reduce oxidative stress, preserving the cells' energy and overall vitality.

Add leafy greens to smoothies, salads, and stir-fries to maintain high energy levels throughout the day.

2. SEA VEGETABLES: MINERAL-RICH ENERGY SOURCES

Sea vegetables, including sea moss, bladderwrack, and nori, provide essential minerals like iodine, potassium, and magnesium, all of which are critical for energy metabolism and thyroid function. Proper thyroid function is key for sustaining energy levels and supporting a balanced metabolism.

- **Sea Moss**: Known for its high mineral content, sea moss contains over 90 trace minerals, including potassium and magnesium, which help reduce fatigue and support nerve function.
- **Bladderwrack**: This sea vegetable is rich in iodine, a mineral essential for thyroid health, which plays a vital role in regulating energy levels.
- **Nori**: Often used in sushi, nori provides protein and essential amino acids, which are building blocks for muscle and tissue repair, supporting endurance and recovery.

Sea vegetables can be added to smoothies, soups, or as supplements to keep energy levels stable throughout the day.

3. BERRIES: ANTIOXIDANT-RICH FRUITS FOR ENDURANCE

Berries, including blueberries, strawberries, and blackberries, are high in antioxidants and natural sugars, offering a quick energy boost without the blood sugar spikes that come from refined sugars. The antioxidants in berries also help combat oxidative stress, which can otherwise lead to cellular fatigue.

- **Blueberries**: Rich in vitamin C and antioxidants, blueberries support immune health and reduce inflammation, allowing the body to maintain energy and stamina.
- **Strawberries**: Strawberries contain natural sugars, fiber, and vitamin C, providing an energy boost while supporting immune function.
- **Blackberries**: Blackberries are high in fiber and vitamin K, which support digestion and energy regulation, providing a steady release of energy.

Berries make an excellent snack or addition to breakfast bowls, smoothies, and salads, offering a sweet burst of energy that's both satisfying and nutritious.

4. NUTS AND SEEDS: ENERGY-DENSE SOURCES OF HEALTHY FATS

Nuts and seeds are packed with healthy fats, protein, and minerals, providing sustained energy and promoting satiety. These nutrient-dense foods are ideal for keeping blood sugar stable, preventing energy crashes, and supporting mental clarity.

- **Almonds**: Almonds are rich in vitamin E, magnesium, and healthy fats, which help stabilize blood sugar and prevent mid-day fatigue.
- **Chia Seeds**: Known for their high fiber and omega-3 content, chia seeds help regulate blood sugar and maintain steady energy levels. They also expand when mixed with liquid, helping to keep you feeling full.

- **Hemp Seeds**: With a high protein content and balanced omega-3 to omega-6 ratio, hemp seeds provide energy for both physical and mental activities.

Add nuts and seeds to smoothies, sprinkle them on salads, or mix them into chia pudding for a nutrient-packed snack that promotes lasting energy.

5. FRUITS: NATURAL SOURCES OF HYDRATION AND QUICK ENERGY

Fruits like apples, oranges, and melons provide natural sugars, fiber, and water, making them ideal for a quick energy boost and hydration. The fiber in these fruits helps regulate blood sugar, preventing the energy spikes and crashes associated with refined sugars.

- **Apples**: Apples are high in fiber and water, which support digestion and hydration, offering a steady source of energy. They're ideal for an on-the-go snack.
- **Oranges**: Oranges provide vitamin C and natural sugars, supporting immune health and providing a burst of natural energy.
- **Watermelon**: With a high water content, watermelon keeps the body hydrated and provides natural sugars that fuel both mental and physical activities.

These fruits can be eaten alone, added to salads, or blended into smoothies to keep you hydrated and energized.

6. ROOT VEGETABLES: SUSTAINED ENERGY FROM COMPLEX CARBOHYDRATES

Root vegetables, such as sweet potatoes, beets, and carrots, are rich in complex carbohydrates, which provide a slow release of glucose, the body's primary energy source. Unlike simple carbohydrates, complex carbs sustain energy for a longer period, making them ideal for maintaining endurance.

- **Sweet Potatoes**: These root vegetables are high in fiber, vitamin C, and potassium, helping to stabilize blood sugar and support muscle function, which is essential for physical stamina.
- **Beets**: Known for their high nitrate content, beets help improve blood flow, increasing oxygen supply to the muscles and enhancing physical performance.
- **Carrots**: Carrots are high in beta-carotene and fiber, supporting eye health and providing sustained energy without blood sugar spikes.

Root vegetables can be roasted, steamed, or added to soups and stews, offering a delicious and energy-boosting addition to meals.

7. ALKALINE WATER AND HERBAL TEAS FOR HYDRATION AND ENERGY

Hydration is crucial for maintaining energy levels, as even mild dehydration can lead to fatigue. Drinking alkaline water, which has a pH above 7, supports the body's pH balance and helps prevent acid buildup that can lead to fatigue. Herbal teas also offer hydration and energy support.

- **Alkaline Water**: Alkaline water helps neutralize acidity in the body and supports hydration, enhancing mental clarity and physical energy.
- **Dandelion Tea**: Dandelion tea supports liver health and detoxification, helping to eliminate toxins that can lead to energy depletion.
- **Peppermint Tea**: Known for its refreshing properties, peppermint tea aids digestion and mental alertness, offering a caffeine-free way to boost energy.

Drinking alkaline water and herbal teas throughout the day can keep you hydrated, support digestion, and help maintain optimal energy levels.

Incorporating these alkaline foods into daily meals provides a foundation for sustained energy, mental clarity, and overall vitality. By focusing on nutrient-dense, whole foods that naturally energize the body, you can avoid the energy dips and crashes associated with refined sugars and processed foods. Building meals around these foods ensures that you're fueling your body in a way that aligns with Dr. Sebi's alkaline philosophy, empowering you to feel energized and resilient throughout the day.

CHAPTER 3
ADAPTING RECIPES FOR FAMILY

Adopting an alkaline lifestyle as a family can foster a supportive environment for healthy eating, but it may require some adjustments to meet the diverse tastes and nutritional needs of family members, especially if there are children or teens involved. In this chapter, we'll explore practical ways to adapt alkaline recipes for the whole family, focusing on nutritious and appealing meals that can win over even the pickiest eaters. From balanced breakfasts to family-friendly dinners and snacks, here are strategies to make alkaline eating enjoyable for everyone at the table.

1. MAKE BREAKFAST FUN AND NUTRIENT-PACKED

Starting the day with an alkaline breakfast can set a positive tone for the family's energy and mood. Instead of sugary cereals or processed breakfasts, try these easy and delicious alkaline options that provide lasting energy and nutrition:

- **Smoothie Bowls**: Smoothie bowls are colorful, fun to eat, and customizable, making them ideal for kids and adults alike. Blend kale, spinach, berries, a banana, and almond milk for the base, then let each family member add their own toppings, like sliced fruits, chia seeds, or shredded coconut. This approach lets everyone add their favorite flavors while maintaining the alkaline foundation.
- **Chia Pudding Parfaits**: Combine chia seeds with almond or coconut milk and let it sit overnight in the refrigerator. In the morning, layer the chia pudding with fresh berries, banana slices, and a drizzle of agave syrup for sweetness. This creamy, pudding-like breakfast is rich in omega-3s and fiber, supporting energy and digestion.
- **Veggie-Packed Breakfast Wraps**: For a savory option, wrap scrambled tofu, avocado, and chopped vegetables (like bell peppers and zucchini) in a collard green or nori sheet. Add a sprinkle of sea salt and a dash of lemon for flavor. This protein-rich breakfast is filling and can be customized based on family preferences.

Involving children in preparing these breakfast options can make the meal more engaging and help them feel invested in trying new foods.

2. FAMILY-FRIENDLY LUNCHES AND SCHOOL-READY SNACKS

Lunchtime and snacks present opportunities to keep family members energized without relying on processed foods. Alkaline-friendly lunch ideas are easy to pack for school or work, and snacks can be prepped in advance to simplify busy days:

- **Rainbow Salad Jars**: Prepare salads in mason jars with layers of colorful vegetables, like shredded carrots, bell peppers, cucumber, and leafy greens. Top with a handful of pumpkin seeds and a simple dressing of olive oil and lemon juice. These jars can be made in advance and stored in the fridge, allowing each family member to grab a salad for a nutritious, on-the-go lunch.
- **Alkaline Wraps and Sandwiches**: Using collard greens or nori as a wrap, add fillings like hummus, avocado, shredded carrots, and cucumbers. For a hearty option, spread almond butter on sprouted grain bread and add banana slices. These wraps and sandwiches are flavorful, nutrient-rich, and kid-friendly.
- **Fruit and Nut Snack Packs**: Portion out snack bags with a mix of berries, apple slices, almonds, and a sprinkle of chia seeds. These packs are easy to grab on the way out the door and offer a nutrient boost with natural sweetness and satisfying crunch.

Incorporating these alkaline-friendly lunch and snack ideas into weekly meal prep ensures that the family has nutritious options readily available, reducing the temptation for processed foods.

3. MAKING ALKALINE DINNERS FOR FAMILY MEALS

Dinnertime is an opportunity to bring the family together over a satisfying, balanced meal. Alkaline dinners can be made both flavorful and filling, with options to please everyone at the table. Here are a few family-friendly dinner ideas:

- **Build-Your-Own Veggie Bowl**: Set out a variety of ingredients, like steamed quinoa, roasted sweet potatoes, sautéed zucchini, chopped bell peppers, and leafy greens. Let each family member build their own veggie bowl, adding their favorite toppings like avocado slices, a sprinkle of pumpkin seeds, or a drizzle of tahini dressing. This setup allows everyone to customize their bowl based on personal tastes.
- **Alkaline Pizza Night**: For a family-favorite meal, try making alkaline-friendly pizzas using a spelt or chickpea flour crust. Top with homemade tomato sauce, basil, spinach, bell peppers, and thinly sliced zucchini. Bake until the crust is crispy, and let the kids help add the

toppings. Alkaline pizzas are fun to make and bring a familiar comfort food into the alkaline lifestyle.
- **Stuffed Bell Peppers**: Hollow out bell peppers and stuff them with a mixture of quinoa, diced vegetables, and herbs. Bake until the peppers are tender, and top with a sprinkle of fresh parsley or basil. This dish is visually appealing, nutrient-rich, and can be served with a side salad for a complete family meal.

These dinner ideas encourage family members to explore a variety of textures and flavors while still aligning with Dr. Sebi's alkaline principles.

4. CREATING SWEETS AND TREATS WITH ALKALINE INGREDIENTS

Adapting the alkaline lifestyle doesn't mean giving up on treats! Alkaline-friendly desserts and snacks can satisfy a sweet tooth without relying on refined sugars or processed ingredients. Here are a few ideas for healthier desserts:

- **Frozen Banana Pops**: Slice bananas in half, insert a wooden stick, and dip them in almond butter or melted coconut oil. Roll in shredded coconut or crushed almonds and freeze until firm. These banana pops are naturally sweet and fun to eat, making them a great choice for kids.
- **Fruit and Nut Energy Bites**: Blend dates, almonds, chia seeds, and a dash of cinnamon in a food processor until sticky. Roll into bite-sized balls and refrigerate. These energy bites are portable, delicious, and rich in fiber and healthy fats, making them an ideal post-dinner snack or on-the-go treat.
- **Baked Apple Slices**: Core and slice apples, sprinkle with cinnamon, and bake until soft. Serve with a spoonful of almond butter for added protein. This warm, comforting dessert is easy to make and has the sweetness of apple pie without added sugars.

With these dessert ideas, the whole family can enjoy treats that satisfy cravings while keeping with an alkaline diet.

5. INVOLVE THE FAMILY IN MEAL PREP AND COOKING

One of the most effective ways to encourage a family to embrace an alkaline lifestyle is to involve everyone in meal prep and cooking. Let children help with age-appropriate tasks, like washing vegetables, blending smoothies, or decorating smoothie bowls with fruit toppings. When kids and teens participate in meal preparation, they're more likely to try new foods and enjoy the meals they helped create.

Consider setting aside a specific time for family meal prep, such as Sunday afternoons, where everyone can participate in planning and preparing meals for the week. This can also be a time to talk about the benefits of different foods, helping younger family members understand why alkaline foods are beneficial for their bodies.

6. TIPS FOR TRANSITIONING TO ALKALINE FOODS WITH FAMILY

Switching to an alkaline lifestyle as a family may require some adjustments, but with a few strategies, the transition can be smooth and enjoyable:

- **Start Slowly**: Rather than overhauling every meal at once, start by adding a few alkaline dishes into the weekly menu. Gradually replace processed snacks and sugary treats with alkaline-friendly options.
- **Focus on Familiar Favorites**: Adapting family-favorite meals, like pizza, wraps, and smoothies, makes the transition less intimidating. Familiar foods that are made with alkaline ingredients can help everyone adjust more easily.
- **Keep Snacks Available**: Stock the kitchen with alkaline-friendly snacks, like fruits, nuts, and veggie sticks with hummus. Having these healthy options readily available makes it easy for everyone to choose nutritious foods when hunger strikes.

By making small, consistent changes, the family can adopt an alkaline lifestyle at a comfortable pace, making it a sustainable and enjoyable way to eat and live.

Integrating an alkaline lifestyle into family meals can bring everyone together in a health-focused way. With balanced breakfasts, fun snacks, family-friendly dinners, and healthy treats, this approach encourages everyone to enjoy the benefits of alkaline eating. Involving family members in cooking and meal prep also fosters a shared commitment to wellness, making it easier to sustain a vibrant, alkaline-centered lifestyle.

BOOK 5
Basics of Detoxification

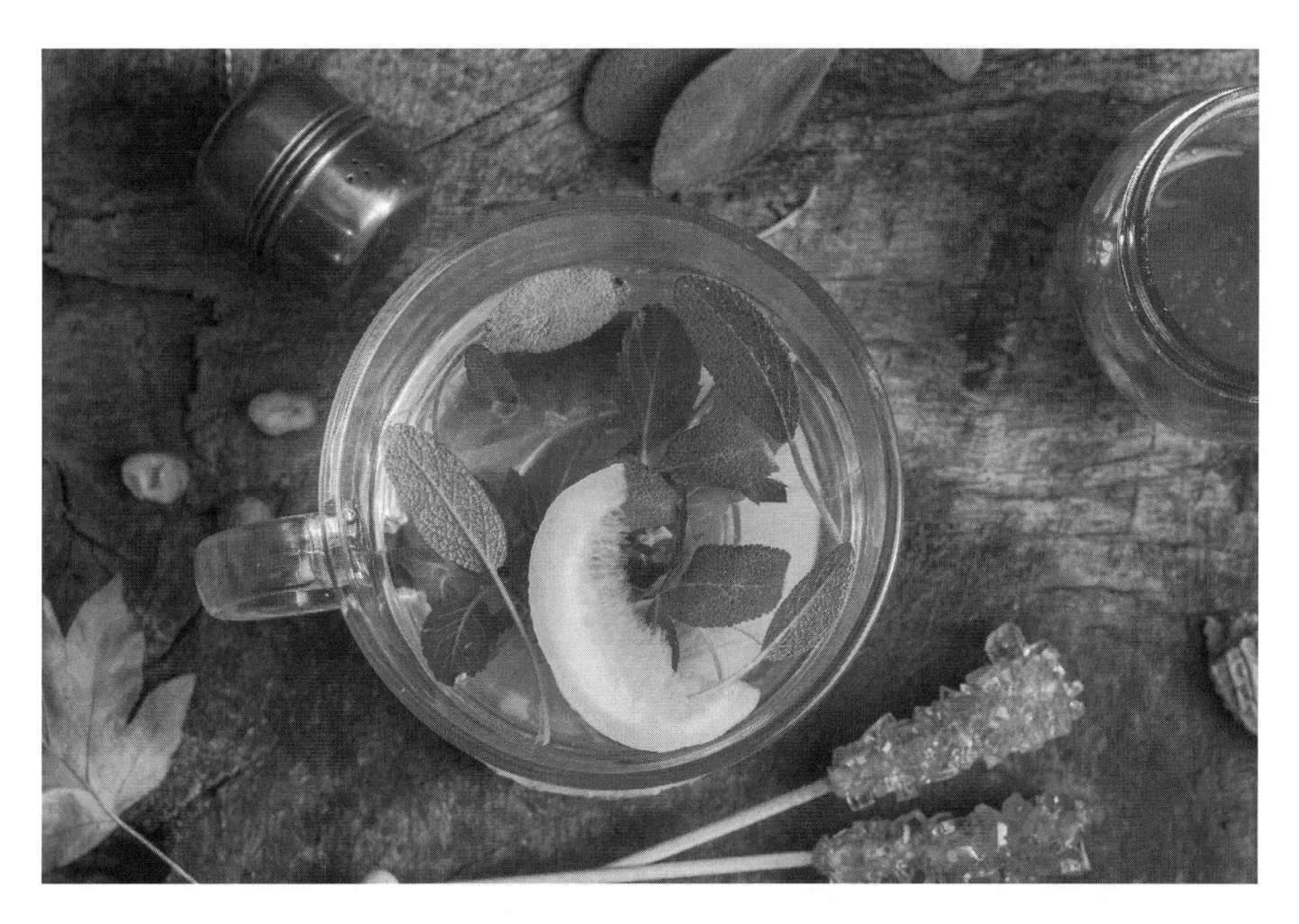

Detoxification is a cornerstone of Dr. Sebi's approach to health and wellness. By removing harmful toxins from the body and creating an environment that supports natural healing, detoxification helps restore balance, improve cellular function, and enhance overall vitality. This book provides a foundational understanding of detoxification, from its importance and benefits to identifying toxins in our daily lives and preparing the body for a detox. Through these chapters, you will gain practical tools and insights to help make detoxification a regular part of a healthy, alkaline lifestyle.

CHAPTER 1
WHY DETOX IS ESSENTIAL

In Dr. Sebi's philosophy, detoxification is essential for achieving and maintaining optimal health. The modern world exposes us to toxins through the air we breathe, the food we eat, and the products we use. Over time, these toxins can build up, burdening our bodies and affecting our energy, immunity, and overall vitality. Detoxification allows us to eliminate these toxins, helping our bodies return to a state of balance where natural healing can occur. In this chapter, we'll explore the importance of detoxification, how it works, and why it's a vital practice for anyone striving for vibrant health.

1. SUPPORTING THE BODY'S NATURAL DETOX SYSTEMS

The human body is equipped with a complex system of organs and processes designed to detoxify itself, including the liver, kidneys, lungs, skin, and lymphatic system. Each of these organs plays a role in identifying, processing, and eliminating waste and toxins:

- **The Liver**: Often called the body's primary detox organ, the liver is responsible for filtering the blood and breaking down toxins into harmless byproducts that can be excreted. It processes everything from environmental pollutants to alcohol and medications.
- **The Kidneys**: The kidneys filter blood, removing waste and excess fluids to form urine. They also help balance the body's electrolytes and pH levels, preventing the buildup of harmful substances.
- **The Lymphatic System**: The lymphatic system transports immune cells throughout the body and removes waste from tissues. It plays a critical role in immune function, ensuring that toxins are carried away from cells and disposed of.
- **The Skin**: As the body's largest organ, the skin helps eliminate toxins through sweat. It also protects the body from external pollutants and UV radiation, acting as a barrier against harmful substances.
- **The Lungs**: The lungs filter the air we breathe, expelling carbon dioxide and other waste gases. They also play a role in defending against airborne toxins and pathogens.

Despite this remarkable system, the body can become overwhelmed due to the high levels of toxins it encounters daily. Environmental pollution, processed foods, pesticides, and household chemicals increase the workload of these organs, sometimes to the point where they can no longer effectively eliminate all harmful substances. Detoxification supports these organs, giving them the "reset" they need to operate efficiently.

2. COUNTERACTING THE EFFECTS OF TOXIN ACCUMULATION

When toxins accumulate faster than the body can eliminate them, they can settle in tissues and organs, leading to inflammation, fatigue, and other health issues. The body often stores toxins in fat cells to protect vital organs, which can lead to weight gain and make it harder to lose excess fat. Toxin accumulation can also affect energy production, hormonal balance, and immunity.

This buildup may initially go unnoticed, but over time it can manifest as symptoms such as:

- **Fatigue**: Chronic fatigue is one of the most common signs of toxin buildup, as the body expends extra energy to manage waste.
- **Brain Fog and Poor Concentration**: Toxins can impair cognitive function, making it difficult to focus and think clearly.
- **Digestive Issues**: Bloating, constipation, and gas can indicate that the digestive system is struggling to process waste.
- **Hormonal Imbalance**: Some toxins, such as endocrine disruptors, mimic hormones, leading to imbalances that can affect mood, metabolism, and reproductive health.
- **Weakened Immunity**: Excessive toxin buildup can weaken immune response, making it harder for the body to fend off infections.

By undergoing detoxification, we help the body clear out these accumulated toxins, restoring balance and alleviating many of these symptoms. Detoxing provides an opportunity to "reboot" the body's natural systems, allowing for better health and resilience.

3. REDUCING INFLAMMATION AND MUCUS

Dr. Sebi emphasized that inflammation and excess mucus are central contributors to disease. Mucus is the body's natural defense mechanism against irritants, but when the body is exposed to too many toxins, it can lead to an overproduction of mucus. This excess mucus can obstruct respiratory pathways, digestive organs, and even blood vessels, hindering the body's ability to function optimally.

Inflammation is another response to toxins. It's a normal immune reaction, but chronic inflammation can lead to tissue damage, joint pain, and increased susceptibility to disease. Foods and substances high in acidity, such as refined sugars, processed meats, and artificial additives, are common culprits of inflammation and mucus buildup.

A detox focused on alkaline foods — like leafy greens, fresh fruits, and herbs — helps break down and remove excess mucus while reducing inflammation. This allows the body to achieve a more balanced state, supporting clearer breathing, smoother digestion, and overall healthier organ function.

4. ENHANCING ENERGY AND MENTAL CLARITY

Many people feel drained because their bodies are working overtime to process and expel toxins. This constant strain depletes energy reserves, leaving individuals feeling fatigued and mentally foggy. When the body undergoes a detox, it can allocate more energy to necessary functions rather than managing a toxic overload.

Detoxing also improves blood flow and oxygenation, which in turn enhances cellular energy production. As toxins are removed and the body's nutrient absorption improves, many people report feeling more energetic, clear-headed, and motivated. This mental clarity comes from the brain's improved access to oxygen and essential nutrients, supporting better focus, memory, and overall cognitive function.

5. BOOSTING IMMUNE SYSTEM FUNCTION

The immune system is highly dependent on the body's overall cleanliness and balance. When overloaded with toxins, the body's ability to fight off infections weakens, leaving it more susceptible to colds, viruses, and other illnesses. Detoxification strengthens immunity by reducing the body's toxic load and providing essential nutrients needed for immune cell function.

Detoxification also improves the balance of beneficial bacteria in the gut, known as the microbiome, which is directly linked to immune health. A detox that emphasizes fiber-rich, whole foods can support the growth of beneficial gut bacteria, enhancing the immune response. By regularly detoxifying, individuals can maintain a strong, resilient immune system capable of defending against pathogens and preventing illness.

6. SUPPORTING WEIGHT LOSS AND METABOLIC HEALTH

Detoxification can also play a valuable role in weight management and metabolic health. Toxins are often stored in fat cells to protect vital organs from their harmful effects. When the body is burdened with toxins, it may retain fat as a defense mechanism, making it difficult to lose weight. By detoxifying, we release these stored toxins, allowing the body to shed excess fat more easily.

Moreover, detoxing helps balance blood sugar and insulin levels by reducing the intake of processed foods and refined sugars. This can be particularly beneficial for individuals struggling with insulin resistance or blood sugar imbalances. As metabolism normalizes, the body can more effectively convert food into energy, preventing cravings and encouraging a balanced appetite.

7. REJUVENATING SKIN, HAIR, AND NAILS

The skin is often a reflection of internal health. When the body is overloaded with toxins, skin issues such as acne, dryness, and premature aging can occur as the body tries to eliminate waste through the skin. Detoxification can lead to clearer, more vibrant skin by reducing the toxic load and enhancing the body's ability to cleanse itself from within.

Improved circulation and hydration, both of which are promoted during a detox, help supply skin cells with nutrients and oxygen, leading to a radiant complexion. Additionally, detoxing can strengthen hair and nails by providing essential minerals and promoting better nutrient absorption, leading to stronger, shinier hair and healthier nails.

8. SUPPORTING LONG-TERM HEALTH AND DISEASE PREVENTION

In addition to providing immediate benefits, detoxification plays a preventive role in long-term health. Chronic exposure to toxins has been linked to diseases such as cancer, diabetes, and cardiovascular disease. By incorporating detoxification into one's lifestyle, individuals can reduce their risk of developing these conditions by minimizing toxic exposure and promoting cellular health.

Detoxification supports the body's natural ability to repair and regenerate itself, fostering a healthier internal environment. When cells are free from toxins, they can divide and replicate without interference, leading to stronger tissues and improved organ function. This foundation of wellness helps prevent disease and enhances the body's resilience to future health challenges.

THE ALKALINE APPROACH TO DETOXIFICATION

In Dr. Sebi's view, detoxification is best supported by an alkaline diet. Alkaline foods, such as leafy greens, fruits, and herbs, neutralize acidity in the body, helping restore a balanced pH. This pH balance is essential because an acidic environment promotes inflammation, weakens immunity, and creates conditions that allow disease to thrive.

Alkaline foods are also naturally detoxifying because they contain high levels of fiber, vitamins, and minerals that support cellular function, digestion, and hydration. Here are some ways an alkaline diet complements the detoxification process:

1. **Hydration and Cellular Health**: Alkaline foods, particularly water-rich fruits and vegetables, provide hydration and essential minerals that support the body's natural filtration systems.
2. **Antioxidant Protection**: Fruits and vegetables are high in antioxidants, which help neutralize free radicals and reduce oxidative stress, preventing cellular damage during the detox.
3. **Fiber-Rich Foods for Digestive Health**: Alkaline foods are often rich in fiber, which aids digestion and helps sweep toxins from the digestive tract, reducing toxic buildup.
4. **Mineral-Rich Support**: Alkaline foods contain minerals like magnesium, potassium, and calcium that play critical roles in maintaining cellular balance and reducing acidity.

MAKING DETOXIFICATION A LIFELONG PRACTICE

For detoxification to have the most significant impact, it's beneficial to make it a regular part of life rather than an occasional cleanse. This doesn't mean constantly undergoing strict detoxes, but instead, incorporating practices that help the body stay clean and balanced.

- **Daily Hydration**: Drinking plenty of alkaline water each day supports the kidneys and prevents dehydration, helping the body expel toxins more effectively.
- **Incorporate Alkaline Foods**: Make alkaline foods a regular part of each meal, ensuring a steady supply of nutrients that promote detoxification.
- **Periodic Detoxes**: Undertaking a focused detox, perhaps once every few months, can give the body the opportunity to reset and recharge.
- **Avoid Toxins Where Possible**: Reducing exposure to known toxins, such as chemicals in food, water, and household products, helps lessen the burden on the body's detox systems.

Detoxification, when approached as an ongoing practice, aligns with Dr. Sebi's vision for a vibrant, resilient life. By supporting the body's natural detox processes, we provide ourselves with the best possible foundation for health, longevity, and well-being.

CHAPTER 2

IDENTIFYING TOXINS AND THEIR EFFECTS

Our environment is filled with toxins that can gradually accumulate in the body, impacting our health, energy, and well-being. These toxins come from the air we breathe, the food we eat, and the products we use. Understanding the sources of toxins and their effects is essential to reducing exposure and supporting the body's natural detoxification process. This chapter covers common toxins, their sources, and the impact they have on the body's systems, laying the groundwork for more effective detoxification.

1. ENVIRONMENTAL TOXINS: AIR, WATER, AND SOIL

Environmental toxins are pervasive and can enter the body through inhalation, ingestion, and skin contact. While we cannot completely avoid exposure to these toxins, understanding their sources helps us minimize our exposure.

- **Air Pollutants**: The air we breathe often contains pollutants from industrial facilities, vehicle emissions, and construction materials. Common airborne toxins include particulate matter, carbon monoxide, sulfur dioxide, and volatile organic compounds (VOCs). These pollutants can impair respiratory health, cause inflammation, and stress the immune system. Long-term exposure to air pollution is linked to conditions such as asthma, cardiovascular disease, and even cognitive decline.
- **Water Contaminants**: Municipal water systems may contain chlorine, fluoride, heavy metals like lead and mercury, and trace amounts of pharmaceuticals and pesticides. While water treatment processes aim to make water safe, these chemicals can still have cumulative effects on health. Heavy metals, in particular, can disrupt cellular function, affect hormone balance, and increase the risk of neurological disorders.
- **Soil Toxins**: The soil where food grows can contain pesticides, herbicides, and other chemicals that end up in the produce we consume. Industrial activities, mining, and improper waste disposal contribute to soil contamination with heavy metals and chemicals. Consuming crops grown in contaminated soil can lead to toxin accumulation in the body, affecting organ function and contributing to inflammation.

While environmental toxins are difficult to avoid completely, reducing exposure through practices like using air purifiers, filtering water, and choosing organic produce can mitigate some of these effects.

2. DIETARY TOXINS: PROCESSED FOODS, ADDITIVES, AND PESTICIDES

The foods we eat play a significant role in our toxic load, especially in diets that include processed, packaged, or non-organic foods. Understanding these dietary sources of toxins can help guide healthier choices.

- **Processed Foods**: Processed and packaged foods are often high in artificial preservatives, colorings, flavorings, and stabilizers. These additives are synthetic chemicals that can disrupt gut health, cause inflammation, and strain the liver as it tries to process these foreign substances. Regular consumption of processed foods has been linked to metabolic issues, cardiovascular disease, and digestive disturbances.
- **Refined Sugars and Artificial Sweeteners**: Refined sugars, found in sugary drinks, candies, and baked goods, cause rapid blood sugar spikes and increase acidity in the body. This acidity can lead to inflammation, fatigue, and insulin resistance. Artificial sweeteners, such as aspartame and sucralose, can interfere with gut bacteria, disrupt metabolism, and are linked to headaches and mood disturbances in some people.
- **Pesticides and Herbicides**: Non-organic fruits and vegetables are frequently treated with pesticides and herbicides to protect against pests and improve crop yield. These chemicals leave residue on produce that cannot always be removed by washing. When ingested, pesticides can disrupt hormone balance, affect the nervous system, and have been linked to conditions such as cancer and autoimmune diseases.

Choosing whole, organic, and minimally processed foods helps reduce exposure to these dietary toxins and supports the body's natural detox processes.

3. HOUSEHOLD TOXINS: CHEMICALS IN CLEANING PRODUCTS AND PERSONAL CARE ITEMS

Household products, including cleaning agents and personal care items, often contain chemicals that can be absorbed through the skin or inhaled. These chemicals are pervasive in daily life but can be replaced with natural alternatives.

- **Cleaning Products**: Many conventional cleaning products contain chemicals like ammonia, bleach, and phthalates, which can emit fumes that irritate the respiratory system and skin. Ammonia can damage the respiratory tract, while phthalates are endocrine disruptors that interfere with hormone function. Long-term exposure to these chemicals has been linked to respiratory conditions and hormonal imbalances.
- **Personal Care Products**: Cosmetics, shampoos, lotions, and deodorants can contain a host of potentially harmful ingredients, including parabens, formaldehyde-releasing preservatives, and synthetic fragrances. Parabens, for example, are endocrine disruptors that mimic estrogen in the body, potentially affecting reproductive health. Synthetic fragrances often contain phthalates, which can further disrupt hormone balance and contribute to conditions like asthma and allergies.
- **Plastics and Packaging**: Many plastic containers and packaging materials contain chemicals like BPA (bisphenol A) and PVC (polyvinyl chloride), which can leach into food and beverages. BPA is a known endocrine disruptor, linked to reproductive health issues, metabolic disorders, and developmental problems in children.

Opting for natural cleaning products, choosing BPA-free containers, and reading labels on personal care products to avoid parabens and phthalates are all strategies for reducing household toxin exposure.

4. HEAVY METALS: HIDDEN TOXINS IN WATER, FOOD, AND PRODUCTS

Heavy metals such as lead, mercury, cadmium, and arsenic are toxic in small amounts and can accumulate in the body over time. These metals are present in water, some foods, and even cosmetics. Heavy metals are particularly harmful because they are difficult for the body to eliminate and can interfere with cellular processes, leading to long-term health issues.

- **Lead**: Lead exposure, often from contaminated water pipes, paints, or soil, can lead to neurological issues, developmental delays in children, and kidney damage. Lead is stored in the bones, where it can remain for years, causing ongoing damage.
- **Mercury**: Found in certain seafood (especially larger fish like tuna), mercury exposure can impair cognitive function and nervous system health. Pregnant women and children are particularly vulnerable to mercury toxicity, which can affect brain development.
- **Cadmium**: Cadmium is commonly found in cigarettes and can accumulate in soils, contaminating crops like leafy greens and root vegetables. Long-term exposure to cadmium can affect kidney function, weaken bones, and contribute to respiratory issues.
- **Arsenic**: Arsenic, a naturally occurring metal, can be found in rice, certain vegetables, and contaminated water. Chronic exposure to arsenic is linked to an increased risk of cancer, skin lesions, and cardiovascular disease.

Reducing exposure to heavy metals includes choosing seafood carefully, using water filters, and opting for products that are certified free from contaminants.

5. PSYCHOLOGICAL AND LIFESTYLE TOXINS

While environmental and dietary toxins are well-known, stress and lifestyle choices can also introduce "toxins" to the body. Chronic stress, negative thought patterns, and sleep deprivation contribute to the body's toxic load by increasing the production of stress hormones, which can affect digestion, immunity, and mental health.

- **Chronic Stress**: Prolonged stress releases cortisol and adrenaline, hormones that prepare the body for "fight or flight." While useful in short bursts, chronic exposure to these hormones can lead to inflammation, reduced immunity, and digestive problems.
- **Negative Thought Patterns**: Negative thinking can affect brain chemistry, leading to increased stress hormones and reduced mental clarity. This mental toxicity can manifest physically, leading to tension, anxiety, and headaches, which can further impact the body's ability to detoxify.
- **Lack of Sleep**: Sleep is crucial for detoxification, as it allows the brain and body to repair and process waste. During sleep, the glymphatic system in the brain removes toxins that accumulate during the day. Chronic sleep deprivation can lead to cognitive decline, increased risk of metabolic disease, and a weakened immune system.

Managing stress through mindfulness, meditation, regular exercise, and ensuring adequate sleep are vital components of a detoxified lifestyle.

6. THE CUMULATIVE EFFECT OF TOXINS AND WHY DETOX IS ESSENTIAL

The body can handle some exposure to toxins; however, the cumulative effect of multiple sources can overwhelm the detoxification system. When the body's ability to eliminate toxins is compromised, these harmful substances can accumulate, leading to a range of symptoms and long-term health problems.

- **Cellular Damage**: Toxins can interfere with cellular processes by damaging DNA, disrupting enzyme function, and impairing nutrient absorption. Over time, this cellular damage can contribute to aging, inflammation, and disease development.
- **Hormonal Imbalance**: Endocrine disruptors in plastics, personal care products, and processed foods mimic hormones, disrupting the body's natural hormonal balance. This can lead to reproductive health issues, mood disorders, and metabolic imbalances.
- **Inflammation and Oxidative Stress**: Many toxins cause inflammation, leading to chronic conditions such as arthritis, cardiovascular disease, and autoimmune disorders. Oxidative stress from toxins contributes to the aging process by damaging cells, tissues, and organs.

The accumulation of toxins, combined with lifestyle factors such as poor diet and stress, makes detoxification essential. By understanding where toxins come from and how they impact the body, we can take proactive steps to reduce exposure and support the body's natural ability to cleanse itself.

PRACTICAL STEPS FOR REDUCING TOXIN EXPOSURE

Here are practical strategies to help limit exposure to various toxins in everyday life:

1. **Choose Organic and Non-GMO Foods**: Organic foods are less likely to contain pesticides, herbicides, and genetically modified organisms (GMOs), reducing dietary toxin intake.
2. **Filter Your Water**: Use a high-quality water filter that removes chlorine, heavy metals, and other contaminants from drinking and cooking water.
3. **Opt for Natural Cleaning Products**: Replace conventional cleaning supplies with plant-based, non-toxic alternatives to avoid inhaling or absorbing harmful chemicals.
4. **Select BPA-Free and Glass Containers**: Replace plastic containers with glass or stainless steel, especially for hot foods and drinks, to prevent leaching of harmful chemicals.
5. **Read Labels on Personal Care Products**: Avoid parabens, phthalates, and synthetic fragrances in cosmetics and hygiene products.
6. **Incorporate Indoor Plants for Air Purification**: Plants such as spider plants, peace lilies, and snake plants naturally filter the air, helping to reduce indoor air pollutants.
7. **Practice Mindfulness and Relaxation Techniques**: Regular mindfulness exercises can reduce stress-related toxins, supporting the body's detox pathways.
8. **Get Quality Sleep**: Prioritize 7–9 hours of sleep each night to allow the brain and body time to detoxify and repair.

By identifying and reducing exposure to common toxins, we support our body's natural detoxification processes. This chapter has laid out the hidden dangers in our environment, diet, and lifestyle that contribute to the toxic load. Understanding these sources empowers us to make cleaner, healthier choices and prepares us for a more effective and sustained detoxification process in alignment with Dr. Sebi's principles.

CHAPTER 3
PREPARING FOR A DETOX

Detoxification is a transformative process that gives the body a "reset" by helping it eliminate harmful toxins, enhance cellular repair, and restore energy levels. However, for the detox to be as effective and comfortable as possible, preparation is key. This chapter outlines the essential steps to take before starting a detox, ensuring that the body is well-supported and that you're mentally and physically ready to achieve the best results.

1. GRADUALLY REDUCE PROCESSED FOODS AND STIMULANTS

Jumping straight into a detox without transitioning away from processed foods, caffeine, alcohol, and sugar can cause withdrawal symptoms, making the experience more difficult. To ease the body into the detox, start eliminating these items gradually a few days before the cleanse begins.

- **Processed Foods**: Processed foods contain preservatives, artificial flavors, and additives that can strain the digestive and detoxification systems. Begin replacing them with whole, natural foods, such as fresh vegetables, fruits, and whole grains.
- **Caffeine**: Cutting back on caffeine reduces the risk of headaches and fatigue during the detox. Start by reducing intake, switching to green tea if needed, and then transitioning to herbal teas.
- **Alcohol and Sugar**: These can cause blood sugar spikes and place strain on the liver, a key organ in detoxification. Cutting back on alcohol and sugary snacks beforehand can make the detox smoother and reduce cravings.

Gradually reducing these items helps the body adjust, minimizes withdrawal effects, and allows it to enter the detox more easily.

2. INCREASE HYDRATION AND ALKALINE WATER INTAKE

Proper hydration is essential to support kidney function and flush toxins from the bloodstream. Drinking plenty of water before beginning a detox ensures that the body is primed to eliminate waste effectively.

- **Alkaline Water**: Alkaline water, with a higher pH than regular water, can help balance the body's pH and reduce acidity. Adding slices of lemon or a pinch of baking soda to water can increase its alkalinity, supporting the body's natural detoxification process.
- **Herbal Teas**: Herbal teas, such as dandelion, peppermint, or ginger, can support the liver, aid digestion, and improve hydration. Replacing caffeinated drinks with herbal teas reduces dependence on stimulants and supports a gentler detox.

Aim for at least 8–10 glasses of water per day. Start each morning with a glass of warm water and lemon juice to kickstart digestion and metabolism.

3. SET CLEAR GOALS AND INTENTIONS

Detoxification is not just a physical journey; it's also mental and emotional. Setting clear goals and intentions helps reinforce motivation and commitment during the detox process. Consider what you hope to achieve, whether it's increased energy, improved digestion, better skin, or a mental reset. Write these goals down and revisit them daily to stay motivated.

- **Journaling**: Start a journal dedicated to your detox experience. Use it to note your goals, track daily progress, and document how you feel. This practice provides a place to reflect and process any emotional or physical shifts that occur during the detox.
- **Visualization and Meditation**: Spend a few minutes each day visualizing yourself reaching your goals. Meditation can also help reduce stress, making the detox experience smoother and helping with mental clarity.

By clarifying your intentions, you can strengthen your resolve, stay motivated, and be better prepared for any challenges that arise.

4. STOCK UP ON DETOX-FRIENDLY FOODS AND HERBS

Having detox-friendly foods readily available makes the process smoother and reduces the temptation to deviate from the detox plan. Stock up on fresh, alkaline foods, including leafy greens, fruits, herbs, and water-rich vegetables.

- **Leafy Greens and Vegetables**: Foods like kale, spinach, cucumbers, and zucchini are high in fiber and water content, helping cleanse the digestive tract and providing essential nutrients.
- **Fruits**: Fruits such as apples, berries, and citrus are rich

in antioxidants and fiber, supporting liver function and aiding in toxin removal.
- **Herbs**: Herbs like cilantro, parsley, and dandelion are known for their detoxifying properties, particularly for liver support. Fresh herbs can be added to salads, smoothies, and teas.

Prepare ingredients in advance by washing and chopping vegetables or pre-making smoothie packs. This helps ensure you have convenient, nourishing options on hand throughout the detox, reducing the temptation to reach for non-detox-friendly foods.

5. PREPARE THE DIGESTIVE SYSTEM WITH FIBER AND PROBIOTICS

A healthy digestive system is essential for effective detoxification, as it's responsible for processing and eliminating waste. Incorporating fiber-rich foods and probiotics before a detox helps "prime" the digestive tract, enhancing its ability to remove toxins.

- **Fiber-Rich Foods**: Foods high in fiber, such as chia seeds, flaxseeds, apples, and leafy greens, support bowel regularity and reduce the buildup of waste in the intestines. Adding these to your meals before a detox encourages smoother digestion during the cleanse.
- **Probiotics**: Probiotics support gut health by promoting beneficial bacteria, which aid digestion and improve nutrient absorption. Natural sources include fermented foods like sauerkraut, kimchi, and coconut yogurt. If preferred, a high-quality probiotic supplement can also be taken to support gut health before detoxing.

Preparing the digestive system with fiber and probiotics ensures that it's ready to handle the increased flow of toxins being eliminated from the body.

6. ADJUST PHYSICAL ACTIVITY TO SUPPORT DETOXIFICATION

Physical activity can help promote circulation, increase oxygen supply, and support the lymphatic system — all essential for detoxification. However, during a detox, it's crucial to balance activity with rest to avoid overburdening the body.

- **Gentle Exercise**: Consider light activities such as yoga, stretching, walking, or tai chi. These exercises help improve circulation and lymphatic flow without placing excess strain on the body. Deep breathing exercises are also beneficial, as they support lung function and oxygenate cells.
- **Avoid High-Intensity Workouts**: During detox, it's best to avoid strenuous activities that can overtax the body and interfere with the detox process. Focus on gentle movement to conserve energy for the body's natural cleansing functions.

Engaging in gentle exercise and focusing on mindfulness during the detox allows the body to function optimally while supporting relaxation and mental clarity.

7. PLAN FOR REST AND SELF-CARE

Detoxification can sometimes lead to temporary fatigue, headaches, or other symptoms as the body adjusts. Giving yourself permission to rest and prioritize self-care is essential for managing these side effects and allowing the body to detoxify efficiently.

- **Schedule Downtime**: Set aside time for rest, naps, or early bedtimes during the detox. The body uses sleep to repair, restore, and eliminate toxins, so prioritizing quality sleep can enhance the detoxification process.
- **Incorporate Self-Care Practices**: Activities like warm baths, dry brushing, and meditation can help manage stress and support the detox process. Dry brushing, in particular, promotes lymphatic drainage and improves circulation, aiding in the removal of toxins through the skin.

Practicing self-care during a detox helps support the body, alleviates symptoms, and fosters a more positive experience.

8. CONSIDER USING DETOXIFYING HERBS AND SUPPLEMENTS

Certain herbs and supplements can provide additional support for the detoxification process by targeting specific organs such as the liver, kidneys, and digestive tract. Dr. Sebi recommended herbs like burdock root, dandelion root, and sea moss for their detoxifying and mineral-rich properties.

- **Burdock Root**: Known for its blood-purifying effects, burdock root supports liver function and helps eliminate toxins from the bloodstream. It can be taken as a tea or in supplement form.
- **Dandelion Root**: Dandelion root promotes bile production, which aids digestion and supports liver detoxification. Dandelion tea is a gentle way to incorporate this herb into a detox regimen.
- **Sea Moss**: Sea moss is rich in essential minerals, including iodine, potassium, and magnesium, which support cellular health and help remove heavy metals and other toxins from the body.

Including these herbs in teas, tinctures, or supplements provides targeted support for detoxification organs, enhancing the overall effectiveness of the detox.

9. MENTALLY PREPARE FOR POTENTIAL DETOX SYMPTOMS

Detoxification can bring about symptoms like fatigue, headaches, and cravings as the body eliminates stored toxins. Mentally preparing for these symptoms can help manage expectations and create a plan for handling them.

- **Headaches**: These are common during the first few days of detox as the body adjusts to eliminating stimulants like caffeine and sugar. Drinking plenty of water, getting rest, and using herbal teas like peppermint can help alleviate headaches.
- **Cravings**: When giving up processed foods and sugars, cravings can occur. Keeping healthy snacks like fresh fruit, herbal tea, or a handful of nuts on hand can help curb cravings without deviating from the detox.
- **Fatigue and Emotional Shifts**: Detoxing can sometimes bring about emotional shifts or low energy. Journaling, meditation, and gentle exercise can help manage these feelings and maintain a positive mindset.

Preparing mentally for these symptoms allows for a smoother detox experience, reducing stress and enhancing resilience.

By following these steps, you create a solid foundation for an effective and safe detox. Preparing both physically and mentally before beginning a detox ensures the body is primed for the cleansing process, supporting a healthier and more rewarding experience. With careful preparation, you can enter the detox period feeling focused, resilient, and ready to embrace the benefits of a toxin-free lifestyle in alignment with Dr. Sebi's principles.

BOOK 6
Dr. Sebi's Detox Protocols

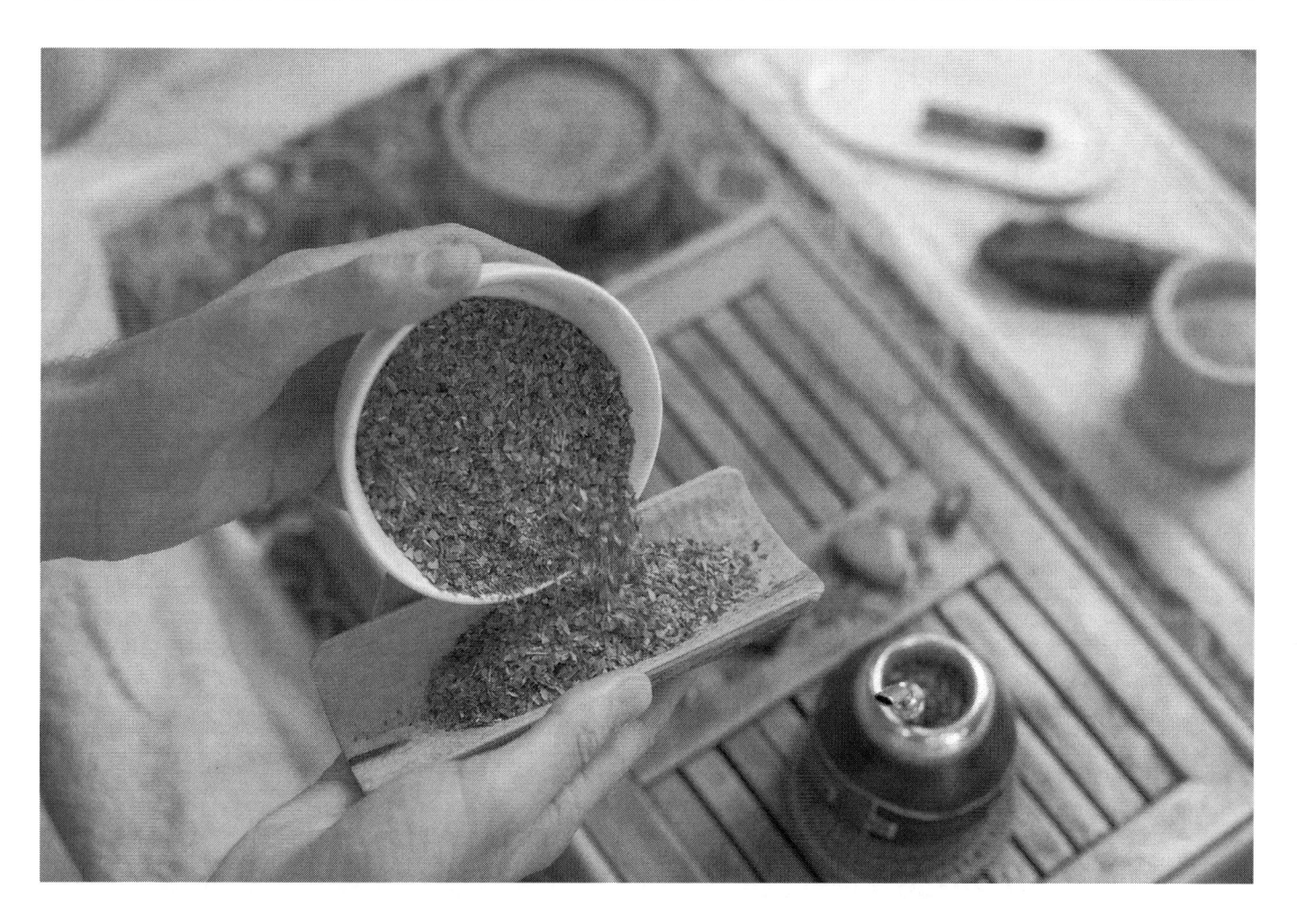

Dr. Sebi's approach to detoxification emphasizes a lifestyle that constantly supports the body's natural ability to cleanse itself. Detoxification is not just a periodic event but an ongoing process that helps maintain a clean internal environment, prevent toxin buildup, and promote overall vitality. This book explores Dr. Sebi's specific protocols for detoxification, from daily habits that enhance wellness to intensive cleanses for deeper cleansing. With these practices, individuals can develop a sustainable approach to detoxification that nurtures long-term health and resilience.

CHAPTER 1
DAILY DETOX HABITS

Daily detox habits form the foundation of a clean and balanced lifestyle, aligning with Dr. Sebi's philosophy of continuous, gentle detoxification. By adopting small yet impactful routines, we can help the body efficiently eliminate toxins, support digestion, and boost overall energy levels. This chapter explores essential daily habits that align with Dr. Sebi's detox principles, offering practical tips for incorporating them into daily life.

1. START THE DAY WITH WARM LEMON WATER

One of the simplest yet most effective daily detox habits is to start the morning with a glass of warm lemon water. Lemons, though acidic outside the body, have an alkalizing effect once metabolized, supporting Dr. Sebi's philosophy of maintaining an alkaline environment.

- **Hydration and Digestion**: Drinking warm lemon water upon waking helps rehydrate the body after hours of sleep and stimulates digestive juices. This gentle hydration kickstarts the liver and supports natural detox processes.
- **Vitamin C Boost**: Lemons are high in vitamin C, an antioxidant that helps neutralize free radicals and reduces oxidative stress on cells. Vitamin C also supports immune function and skin health.
- **pH Balancing**: Lemon water promotes an alkaline pH balance in the body, which Dr. Sebi emphasized as essential for preventing disease and promoting overall wellness.

To make lemon water, simply squeeze the juice of half a lemon into a glass of warm water. Drink it slowly, allowing your body to absorb the nutrients and benefit from its detoxifying properties. This habit is a quick and easy way to prime the body for a day of efficient detoxification.

2. EMBRACE ALKALINE FOODS THROUGHOUT THE DAY

According to Dr. Sebi, alkaline foods are crucial for reducing acidity, preventing inflammation, and supporting the body's detox pathways. Incorporating a variety of alkaline foods into daily meals helps the body maintain a balanced pH, aids digestion, and reduces toxic buildup.

- **Leafy Greens**: Foods like kale, spinach, and watercress are packed with chlorophyll, which helps oxygenate the blood and promote cellular detoxification.
- **Fruits**: Berries, apples, and melons are rich in antioxidants, fiber, and natural sugars, providing energy while supporting liver and kidney function.
- **Vegetables**: Cucumbers, zucchini, and bell peppers are water-rich and help hydrate the body, while their fiber content supports digestion and elimination.

Focus on eating more alkaline foods by filling half of each plate with fruits and vegetables, adding leafy greens to smoothies, and snacking on fresh produce. This habit strengthens the body's natural detox processes and provides vital nutrients.

3. PRACTICE MINDFUL EATING FOR BETTER DIGESTION

The way we eat is just as important as what we eat when it comes to detoxification. Practicing mindful eating can improve digestion and support detoxification by ensuring that nutrients are absorbed efficiently and waste is eliminated smoothly.

- **Eat Slowly and Chew Thoroughly**: Taking time to chew food thoroughly breaks it down into smaller particles, making it easier for the stomach and intestines to digest and absorb nutrients. This also reduces the risk of bloating and indigestion.
- **Listen to Hunger Cues**: Eating only when hungry and stopping when full helps prevent overeating, which can strain the digestive system and slow down detoxification.
- **Avoid Eating Late at Night**: Eating heavy meals late in the evening can interfere with digestion and reduce the quality of sleep, which is essential for cellular repair and detox.

Mindful eating supports the digestive system by reducing stress on the stomach, enhancing nutrient absorption, and preventing the accumulation of undigested food that can lead to toxicity.

4. STAY HYDRATED WITH WATER AND HERBAL TEAS

Hydration is one of the most important aspects of detoxification, as water is needed for nearly every bodily function, including the elimination of waste. Dehydration can lead to sluggish digestion, toxin buildup, and fatigue.

- **Drink Plenty of Water**: Aim to drink at least 8–10 glasses of water daily. This amount may vary based on activity level, climate, and individual needs, but the goal is to keep the body well-hydrated for optimal detox.
- **Incorporate Herbal Teas**: Herbal teas such as dandelion,

ginger, and peppermint can support liver function, digestion, and kidney health. Dandelion tea, for instance, is known to aid liver detoxification and improve bile production, while ginger tea can soothe digestion and reduce inflammation.

Having a water bottle handy throughout the day and drinking herbal teas can keep hydration levels stable, supporting the kidneys and aiding in the natural elimination of toxins.

5. PRACTICE DAILY MOVEMENT AND STRETCHING

Physical movement promotes circulation, stimulates the lymphatic system, and encourages the release of toxins through sweat. Regular activity, whether through walking, stretching, or light exercise, enhances the body's ability to cleanse itself.

- **Walking**: Walking is a low-impact way to stimulate circulation, aid digestion, and support mental clarity. A 20–30 minute walk each day can help improve cardiovascular health and encourage the lymphatic system to eliminate waste.
- **Stretching and Yoga**: Stretching and yoga exercises improve flexibility and circulation, helping to release toxins stored in muscles. Yoga poses such as twists, forward folds, and gentle inversions stimulate the digestive organs, kidneys, and liver, promoting detox.
- **Deep Breathing**: Incorporating deep breathing exercises into physical activity increases oxygen flow to cells, which is essential for cellular energy production and detoxification.

Making movement a daily habit supports physical health, reduces tension, and assists the body in ridding itself of toxins through improved circulation and lymphatic flow.

6. PRIORITIZE FIBER-RICH FOODS FOR DAILY ELIMINATION

Regular elimination is essential to prevent toxins from being reabsorbed into the bloodstream. Fiber-rich foods play a key role in supporting bowel regularity, binding to waste, and facilitating its removal from the body.

- **Soluble Fiber**: Foods like oats, apples, and chia seeds contain soluble fiber, which absorbs water and forms a gel-like substance in the gut. This helps slow digestion, allowing for better nutrient absorption.
- **Insoluble Fiber**: Foods like leafy greens, whole grains, and carrots contain insoluble fiber, which adds bulk to stool and promotes regular bowel movements.
- **Fermented Foods**: Fermented foods like sauerkraut and kimchi contain beneficial bacteria that support gut health and enhance digestion, further aiding elimination.

Incorporating fiber into each meal by adding vegetables, fruits, and whole grains ensures that the digestive system functions optimally and toxins are efficiently eliminated.

7. PRACTICE DRY BRUSHING FOR LYMPHATIC SUPPORT

The lymphatic system is responsible for transporting waste, toxins, and immune cells throughout the body. Dry brushing is a technique that helps stimulate the lymphatic system, promoting the flow of lymph and aiding in the removal of toxins through the skin.

- **How to Dry Brush**: Using a natural-bristle brush, gently brush the skin in circular motions, starting from the feet and moving toward the heart. This method encourages lymphatic flow toward the core, where toxins can be filtered out and eliminated.
- **Benefits of Dry Brushing**: In addition to stimulating lymphatic flow, dry brushing exfoliates the skin, improves circulation, and reduces the appearance of cellulite.

Practicing dry brushing for a few minutes each day before a shower is an easy and effective way to support detoxification through the skin and lymphatic system.

8. GET SUFFICIENT SLEEP FOR CELLULAR REPAIR

Sleep is essential for detoxification because it allows the body to repair itself, process waste, and eliminate toxins from the brain through the glymphatic system. During deep sleep, the body cleanses itself, clears out cellular waste, and restores energy for the next day.

- **Establish a Sleep Routine**: Aim for 7–9 hours of sleep each night to ensure that the body has enough time to rest and repair. Establishing a consistent sleep schedule helps regulate circadian rhythms, promoting better quality sleep.
- **Create a Relaxing Sleep Environment**: Reduce exposure to screens and blue light in the evening, keep the bedroom cool, and practice relaxation techniques like reading or meditation before bed.

Prioritizing sufficient, quality sleep supports the brain's detoxification system and allows the body to cleanse itself of waste and toxins accumulated during the day.

9. LIMIT EXPOSURE TO TOXINS IN HOUSEHOLD PRODUCTS

Toxins in household products, such as cleaning supplies, plastics, and personal care items, can contribute to the body's toxic load. Reducing exposure to these everyday toxins by choosing natural alternatives is a simple yet powerful daily detox habit.

- **Choose Natural Cleaning Products**: Opt for natural, plant-based cleaning products that are free from harsh chemicals. Ingredients like vinegar, baking soda, and essential oils can be used as safe and effective cleaning agents.
- **Use BPA-Free Containers**: Avoid plastic containers and bottles that contain BPA, a chemical known to disrupt hormones. Glass, stainless steel, and silicone are safer alternatives for food storage.
- **Read Personal Care Labels**: Select personal care products that are free from parabens, phthalates, and synthetic fragrances. Many natural brands offer toxin-free options for skincare, shampoo, and deodorant.

Limiting exposure to household toxins reduces the body's overall toxic load, lightening the burden on detox organs and supporting a cleaner, healthier environment.

Daily detox habits are essential for maintaining a healthy and balanced body, ensuring that toxins are continually processed and eliminated. By incorporating simple practices like hydrating with lemon water, eating alkaline foods, and prioritizing sleep, we can gently support the body's natural detox pathways every day. These habits align with Dr. Sebi's principles, creating a lifestyle that sustains wellness and helps prevent toxin buildup. Practiced consistently, these habits form a foundation for long-term health and vitality, empowering you to live in a way that honors the body's natural ability to cleanse and heal itself.

CHAPTER 2
STEP-BY-STEP DETOX PROGRAMS

For those ready to take detoxification to the next level, structured detox programs can provide a deeper cleanse and reset. Dr. Sebi's detox philosophy emphasizes using natural, plant-based, and alkaline foods to support the body's ability to heal itself. This chapter outlines step-by-step detox programs, from a one-day introductory cleanse to more intensive 7-day and 21-day protocols, catering to different experience levels and goals. Each program incorporates Dr. Sebi's principles and includes practical tips to ensure a successful detox.

1. THE ONE-DAY INTRODUCTORY DETOX

The one-day detox is a gentle way to introduce detoxification, perfect for those who are new to cleansing or looking for a quick reset. This short detox focuses on hydrating the body, supporting digestion, and eliminating processed foods, providing a boost without extensive planning.

Goal: Reduce inflammation, hydrate, and give the digestive system a break.

Steps:

- **Morning**: Start the day with a glass of warm lemon water to kickstart digestion and alkalize the body.
- **Breakfast**: Have a green smoothie made with spinach, cucumber, an apple, and a tablespoon of chia seeds. This provides fiber, antioxidants, and hydration.
- **Mid-Morning Snack**: Drink a cup of herbal tea, such as dandelion or ginger tea, to support liver function and aid digestion.
- **Lunch**: Eat a large salad with leafy greens (like kale and arugula), bell peppers, cucumbers, and a sprinkle of hemp seeds. Dress with olive oil and lemon juice for added healthy fats.
- **Afternoon Snack**: Snack on a handful of raw almonds or an apple to provide energy and fiber.
- **Dinner**: Have a bowl of vegetable soup with ingredients like zucchini, carrots, celery, and parsley. This is easy to digest and provides essential vitamins and minerals.
- **Evening**: End the day with a cup of peppermint tea to soothe digestion and support relaxation.

Tips: Avoid caffeine, sugar, and processed foods during the day. Drink plenty of water throughout, aiming for at least 8–10 glasses to support the kidneys in flushing out toxins.

2. THE THREE-DAY DETOX PROGRAM

The three-day detox program offers a more intensive cleanse, giving the body additional time to eliminate toxins and reset. This detox focuses on alkaline juices, smoothies, and soups to provide nourishment while minimizing digestive workload, supporting liver and kidney function.

Goal: Deeper hydration, support for liver and kidney detoxification, and a reduction in inflammation.

Steps:

- **Day 1**: Focus on hydrating with plenty of water and herbal teas. Eat a light, plant-based dinner, such as a vegetable soup or salad, to ease into the detox.
- **Days 2 and 3**:
  - **Morning**: Begin with lemon water followed by a green juice made with cucumber, celery, spinach, and a squeeze of lemon.
  - **Breakfast**: Have a smoothie with berries, almond milk, and a tablespoon of chia seeds for fiber and antioxidants.
  - **Mid-Morning Snack**: Drink a cup of herbal tea (such as dandelion or peppermint) to support liver and digestive health.
  - **Lunch**: Enjoy a blended vegetable soup made with zucchini, carrots, and celery, seasoned with fresh herbs like basil and parsley.
  - **Afternoon Snack**: Have a green juice or smoothie with kale, cucumber, apple, and lemon.
  - **Dinner**: Eat a large salad with leafy greens, bell peppers, cucumbers, and avocado. Add hemp seeds or a sprinkle of chia for extra nutrients.
  - **Evening**: Drink herbal tea (such as chamomile) to aid digestion and relax before bed.

Tips: Avoid caffeine, sugar, alcohol, and processed foods during the three days. Listen to your body, resting as needed, as detox symptoms like mild headaches or fatigue can occur.

3. THE SEVEN-DAY ALKALINE DETOX

The seven-day detox program is a structured cleanse that provides enough time for deeper detoxification, improved digestion, and better energy. This program is designed to support liver, kidney, and gut health through an alkaline, nutrient-dense diet that includes juices, smoothies, and light meals.

Goal: To reset digestion, improve energy levels, and cleanse the liver and kidneys.

Steps:

- **Days 1–2**: Prepare the body for detox by gradually eliminating caffeine, sugar, and processed foods. Focus on whole, plant-based meals.
- **Days 3–7**:
  - » **Morning**: Start each day with lemon water to stimulate digestion and hydrate.
  - » **Breakfast**: Have an alkaline smoothie made with greens, berries, almond milk, and chia or hemp seeds.
  - » **Mid-Morning Snack**: Drink a green juice with cucumber, celery, and apple to increase hydration and alkalinity.
  - » **Lunch**: Eat a large, nutrient-dense salad with a variety of vegetables and a drizzle of olive oil and lemon.
  - » **Afternoon Snack**: Enjoy a cup of herbal tea (such as dandelion, ginger, or peppermint) to support the liver and aid digestion.
  - » **Dinner**: Rotate between vegetable soups, salads, and steamed vegetables with herbs. For example, a light vegetable stew with zucchini, carrots, and celery, or a plate of lightly steamed greens with a sprinkle of sea salt and olive oil.
  - » **Evening**: End each day with a calming tea (such as chamomile or peppermint) and practice light stretching or meditation.

Tips: Maintain hydration by drinking plenty of water throughout the day. The seven-day detox may cause temporary detox symptoms, such as fatigue or mild headaches. Rest as needed and avoid strenuous activities.

4. THE 21-DAY DEEP CLEANSE

The 21-day detox program is an extended cleanse for those seeking a comprehensive reset of body and mind. This longer detox allows for the complete elimination of toxins and the rebuilding of healthy habits, supporting sustained improvements in energy, digestion, and overall health.

Goal: Deep cleansing of the liver, kidneys, and digestive system, reduction in inflammation, and resetting of lifestyle habits.

Steps:

- **Days 1–3**: Begin by transitioning to an alkaline diet, eliminating all processed foods, caffeine, and sugar.
- **Days 4–14**:
  - » **Morning**: Start each day with lemon water followed by a green juice with cucumber, celery, and spinach.
  - » **Breakfast**: Alternate between alkaline smoothies (made with greens, berries, and almond milk) and fruit bowls with chia seeds.
  - » **Lunch**: Have a large salad with a wide variety of vegetables, topped with seeds or nuts for added protein and healthy fats.
  - » **Dinner**: Rotate between alkaline soups, steamed vegetables, and salads with herbs. Incorporate sea vegetables, such as sea moss or kelp, for added minerals.
- **Days 15–21**:
  - » **Morning**: Continue with lemon water and green juice or smoothie.
  - » **Meals**: Focus on lighter meals, such as blended soups, green smoothies, and salads. Reduce dense foods, focusing on foods that are easy to digest, such as steamed greens and water-rich fruits.
  - » **Evening**: End each day with a calming herbal tea and gentle stretches or meditation.

Tips: A 21-day detox requires commitment and may involve more pronounced detox symptoms. Ensure ample rest, stay hydrated, and focus on relaxation practices. Emphasize alkaline foods to maintain pH balance and support the body's detox pathways.

ADDITIONAL TIPS FOR A SUCCESSFUL DETOX

- **Stay Hydrated**: Hydration is key for any detox. Aim to drink water consistently throughout the day and incorporate herbal teas to support liver and kidney function.
- **Listen to Your Body**: Detoxing may bring temporary discomfort, such as fatigue or mild headaches, as the body releases stored toxins. Rest as needed and allow the body to adjust.
- **Practice Mindfulness and Rest**: Detoxification is not just physical; it's also mental and emotional. Incorporate mindfulness practices, such as journaling, meditation, or light stretching, to support mental clarity and emotional balance.
- **Keep Meals Simple**: Avoid complex meals with many ingredients, which can be harder to digest. Simple, nutrient-dense foods reduce digestive workload and support the body's detox pathways.
- **Gradually Return to Regular Eating**: After a detox, reintroduce foods slowly to prevent digestive discomfort. Start with light, plant-based meals and avoid processed foods to maintain the benefits of the detox.

By following these step-by-step detox programs, individuals can experience a deeper cleanse that aligns with Dr. Sebi's principles of natural healing and balance. Whether opting for a short, one-day reset or a comprehensive 21-day cleanse, each detox program supports the body's natural ability to cleanse, reset, and heal. With commitment, these structured detoxes can bring clarity, energy, and a renewed sense of wellness.

CHAPTER 3
BENEFITS OF REGULAR DETOXIFICATION

Regular detoxification brings a multitude of health benefits, supporting physical, mental, and emotional well-being. Detoxing routinely allows the body to clear toxins, improve its resilience, and function at its best, all in line with Dr. Sebi's focus on promoting natural healing. This chapter explores the extensive benefits of maintaining a regular detox regimen and how it can positively impact health, energy, and overall quality of life.

1. ENHANCED ENERGY AND VITALITY

One of the most immediate benefits people notice from regular detoxification is an increase in energy and vitality. When toxins accumulate in the body, they can weigh down metabolic processes, leading to feelings of fatigue and sluggishness. Regular detoxing helps the liver, kidneys, and digestive system eliminate these toxins, freeing up energy that the body can use for essential functions and overall well-being.

- **Boosted Metabolism**: By reducing the toxic load, regular detoxification improves cellular metabolism, helping the body to produce and use energy more efficiently.
- **Improved Sleep Quality**: Detoxing can also lead to better sleep, as it reduces the body's need to work overtime on digestion and elimination, resulting in a more restful and rejuvenating night's sleep.
- **Mental Clarity**: Many people report feeling mentally sharper and more focused after a detox, as removing toxins from the bloodstream and brain reduces "brain fog."

By enhancing energy and vitality, regular detoxification supports a more active lifestyle and improved mental and emotional resilience.

2. STRENGTHENED IMMUNE SYSTEM

The immune system plays a central role in keeping the body healthy, but when overloaded with toxins, it can become compromised. Regular detoxification strengthens the immune system by reducing the workload on the body's organs and freeing up resources to focus on immune defense.

- **Reduced Inflammation**: Chronic inflammation is a common consequence of toxin buildup. Detoxification helps clear inflammatory substances from the body, reducing the risk of autoimmune responses and illnesses that stem from chronic inflammation.
- **Improved Gut Health**: Since a large part of the immune system is located in the gut, regular detoxing supports immune function by maintaining a balanced gut microbiome and reducing harmful bacteria.
- **Increased Resilience Against Infections**: A cleaner, more efficient body can better defend against common infections, viruses, and illnesses.

Regular detoxification helps fortify the immune system, making it more responsive and effective in defending against both acute and chronic health challenges.

3. BETTER DIGESTION AND NUTRIENT ABSORPTION

Detoxing regularly can improve digestion by reducing the buildup of waste, supporting gut health, and enhancing nutrient absorption. The digestive system is the body's primary route for absorbing nutrients, so keeping it clean and well-functioning is essential for overall health.

- **Improved Bowel Regularity**: A detox that includes fiber-rich, whole foods helps clear the intestines of residual waste, promoting regular bowel movements and preventing constipation.
- **Enhanced Enzyme Production**: Detoxing reduces the strain on digestive organs, enabling them to produce the enzymes necessary for efficient digestion and nutrient absorption.
- **Balanced Gut Bacteria**: Regular detoxes can encourage a healthier balance of gut bacteria, as the removal of processed and sugary foods minimizes the growth of harmful bacteria and supports beneficial microbes.

By promoting better digestion and nutrient absorption, regular detoxification helps ensure that the body receives and utilizes essential vitamins, minerals, and nutrients efficiently.

4. WEIGHT MANAGEMENT AND METABOLIC HEALTH

Detoxification can be an effective tool for weight management, especially when combined with Dr. Sebi's alkaline, plant-based dietary principles. Toxins are often stored in fat cells, so detoxing helps the body eliminate these substances and may make it easier to lose or maintain a healthy weight.

- **Reduced Water Retention**: Detoxing can help eliminate excess sodium and reduce water retention, leading to a leaner, less bloated appearance.
- **Regulated Blood Sugar Levels**: Avoiding processed foods and sugars during a detox helps stabilize blood sugar, supporting metabolic health and reducing cravings.
- **Increased Fat-Burning Capacity**: Regular detoxification supports the liver, which plays a critical role in fat metabolism. A well-functioning liver can more effectively break down and use stored fat for energy.

By aiding weight management and metabolic health, regular detoxification helps prevent weight gain and supports healthy body composition.

5. CLEARER, HEALTHIER SKIN

The skin is the body's largest organ and one of its primary detoxification pathways. Toxins in the bloodstream are often excreted through the skin, and when there's a toxic buildup, it can manifest in skin issues like acne, dryness, or inflammation. Regular detoxing can lead to clearer, more radiant skin by supporting the body's ability to cleanse itself.

- **Reduction in Acne and Blemishes**: Detoxing reduces the body's toxic load, preventing the need for it to purge toxins through the skin, which can result in acne and blemishes.
- **Improved Skin Texture and Tone**: By promoting hydration and removing inflammatory substances, regular detoxes can help improve skin elasticity, reduce puffiness, and give the skin a healthier tone.
- **Delayed Aging Signs**: Detoxification helps reduce oxidative stress, which is linked to premature aging. By lowering toxin levels, the body produces fewer free radicals, reducing wrinkles and signs of aging.

Regular detoxification supports skin health from the inside out, promoting a natural glow and resilience against environmental stressors.

6. REDUCED RISK OF CHRONIC ILLNESS

One of the long-term benefits of regular detoxification is a reduced risk of chronic illnesses, many of which are linked to toxin buildup, chronic inflammation, and lifestyle factors. By helping the body cleanse itself regularly, detoxification supports overall health and can prevent the conditions that contribute to chronic disease.

- **Lowered Inflammation Levels**: Inflammation is a root cause of many chronic illnesses, including heart disease, arthritis, and diabetes. Regular detoxes reduce inflammation by removing acidic foods and substances that trigger immune responses.
- **Support for Heart Health**: Detoxing with an alkaline diet can help reduce high cholesterol, blood pressure, and triglycerides, all of which contribute to heart disease. Clearing out toxins also improves blood flow and reduces stress on the cardiovascular system.
- **Improved Liver Function**: A well-functioning liver is essential for maintaining overall health, as it processes everything from food and medication to environmental toxins. Regular detoxing supports liver health, which in turn protects the body from the effects of toxic buildup and improves resilience against chronic disease.

Through regular detoxification, individuals can proactively protect themselves from chronic illnesses, enhancing quality of life and promoting longevity.

7. MENTAL AND EMOTIONAL CLARITY

Regular detoxification benefits not only the body but also the mind, supporting mental clarity, emotional balance, and stress reduction. Many people find that by removing toxins, they experience an improvement in mood, focus, and overall mental well-being.

- **Reduced Brain Fog**: Toxins in the bloodstream and brain can impair cognitive function, leading to brain fog and mental fatigue. Detoxing regularly helps clear out these toxins, allowing for sharper focus and memory.
- **Improved Mood and Emotional Resilience**: Detoxing can help stabilize hormones and reduce inflammation, both of which are linked to mood. A cleaner, healthier body often correlates with a more balanced and positive emotional state.
- **Enhanced Stress Response**: Regular detoxing helps the body handle stress more effectively by reducing the physical strain on the body and enhancing mental clarity. Many people experience greater emotional resilience and mental calm as a result of ongoing detox practices.

Mental and emotional clarity is a valuable benefit of regular detoxification, allowing individuals to engage more fully in daily life and enjoy a balanced, positive outlook.

8. GREATER COMMITMENT TO A HEALTHY LIFESTYLE

Regular detoxing fosters an ongoing commitment to wellness, as it encourages awareness of food, environment, and habits. Detoxing regularly builds mindfulness around the choices that impact health, making it easier to sustain a healthy lifestyle.

- **Building Positive Habits**: By engaging in regular detoxes, individuals develop habits like drinking more water, eating

more whole foods, and avoiding processed ingredients, which promote lasting wellness.
- **Increased Awareness of Body and Mind**: Detoxing encourages tuning into the body's needs and recognizing signs of toxicity, enabling a proactive approach to health.
- **Encouragement to Avoid Toxins**: The benefits experienced from regular detoxing often inspire people to avoid toxins in their daily lives, whether by choosing natural products, organic foods, or a cleaner lifestyle.

The benefits of regular detoxification go beyond physical health, fostering an appreciation for wellness and a lifestyle centered on mindful, balanced living.

Regular detoxification offers numerous benefits, from increased energy and mental clarity to strengthened immunity and reduced chronic illness risk. These benefits align with Dr. Sebi's holistic approach, supporting the body's natural healing processes and helping maintain optimal wellness. Embracing regular detox practices promotes a vibrant, resilient body and mind, contributing to a life filled with vitality and balance.

BOOK 7
Dr. Sebi's Healing Herbs

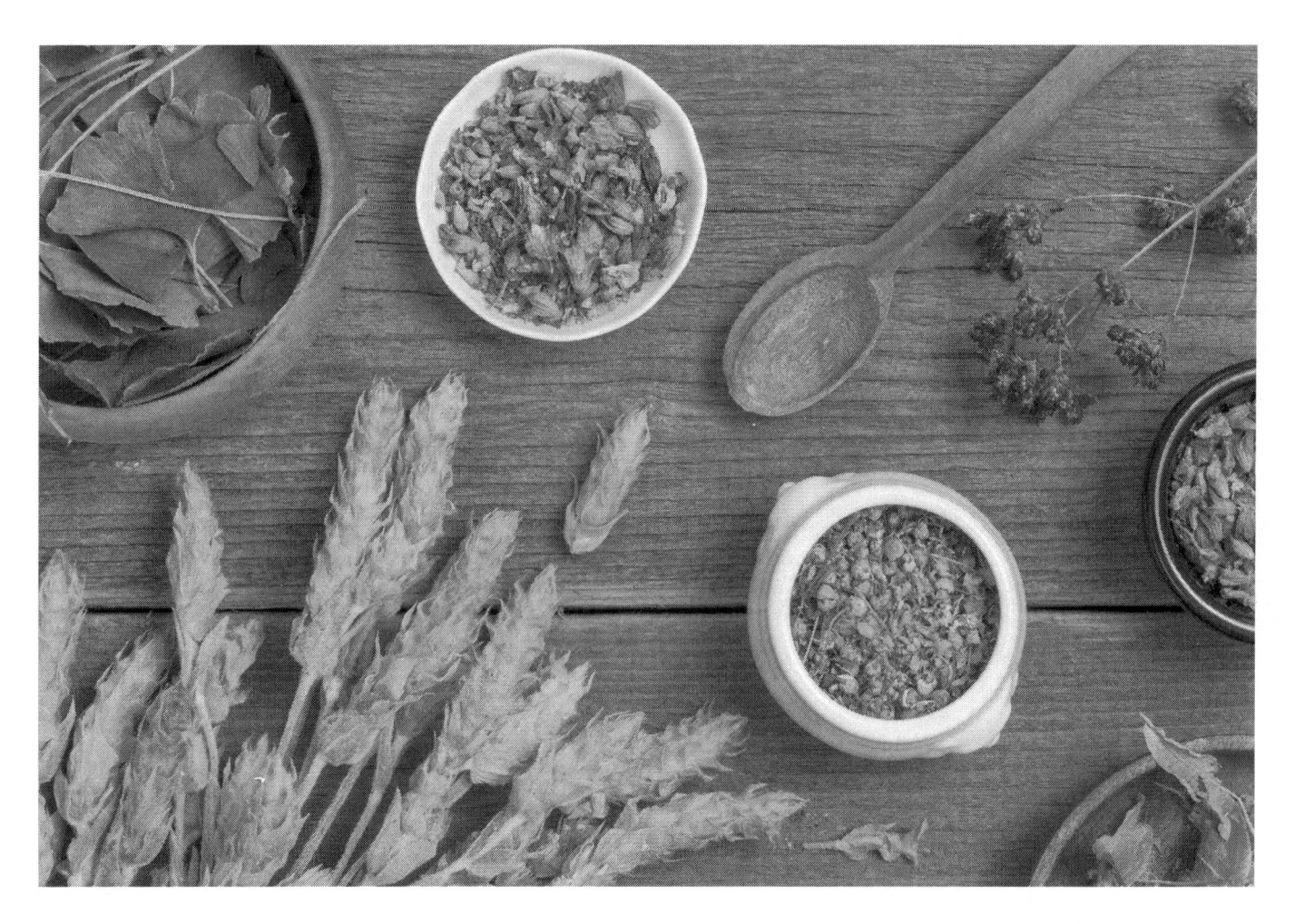

Dr. Sebi's approach to wellness goes beyond detoxification and diet, reaching into the world of natural, plant-based medicine. He emphasized the importance of alkaline herbs for maintaining the body's pH balance, supporting detoxification, and promoting natural healing. This book delves into the use of Dr. Sebi's recommended herbs, each selected for its specific healing properties and alkaline benefits. By incorporating these powerful plants into daily life, individuals can align with Dr. Sebi's vision for health, achieving greater resilience, energy, and balance.

CHAPTER 1
INTRODUCTION TO ALKALINE HERBS

In the realm of natural healing, herbs are revered for their ability to restore balance, ease symptoms, and support overall health. Dr. Sebi recognized the unique potential of alkaline herbs, plants that naturally align with the body's pH and biochemical composition, making them effective in promoting healing without creating an acidic burden. This chapter introduces the core principles of using alkaline herbs in daily life, their benefits, and how they work with the body to foster holistic wellness.

1. THE POWER OF ALKALINE HERBS: A NATURAL PATH TO HEALTH

Dr. Sebi's herbal philosophy is built on the understanding that our bodies are electrical systems requiring "electric" foods and herbs—plants that maintain an alkaline state. Just as processed and acidic foods can disrupt the body's balance, certain herbs can replenish minerals, cleanse toxins, and restore an alkaline environment, essential for optimal health.

- **Alkaline Herbs and pH Balance**: When our bodies are too acidic, we're more prone to inflammation, fatigue, and a host of other issues. Alkaline herbs help counteract acidity, providing a buffer that stabilizes the body's internal environment and allows it to function smoothly. Alkaline herbs, unlike many conventional medications, work synergistically with the body, providing minerals and nutrients in a form that's easily absorbed and utilized.
- **Herbs as Daily Allies**: Alkaline herbs aren't just used in response to illness; they can be incorporated daily to maintain balance and vitality. Whether enjoyed in teas, tinctures, or foods, these herbs serve as daily allies in promoting wellness, ensuring the body remains resilient and prepared to fend off illnesses.

2. KEY ALKALINE HERBS IN DR. SEBI'S PROTOCOL

Dr. Sebi identified several herbs as foundational to his healing philosophy, each chosen for its specific properties and ability to harmonize with the body's natural processes. Here are some of the key alkaline herbs that play central roles in his protocol:

- **Burdock Root**: Known for its blood-purifying properties, burdock root is often recommended for supporting liver health and skin clarity. This root is rich in antioxidants and promotes circulation, helping remove toxins from the bloodstream. Burdock can be taken as a tea or a tincture and is especially helpful for clearing skin issues, supporting the immune system, and aiding in digestion.
- **Dandelion Root**: Dandelion root is a powerhouse for liver detoxification. It encourages bile production, helping the liver break down fats and remove waste from the body. Dandelion also acts as a diuretic, promoting kidney health by facilitating the release of excess water and toxins through urine. It's frequently used as a tea, making it a simple addition to a daily routine.
- **Sarsaparilla**: Known for its high mineral content, particularly iron, sarsaparilla helps combat fatigue and supports immune health. It's also used for cleansing the blood and addressing skin issues. Sarsaparilla is commonly available as a tea, tincture, or powder, making it easy to incorporate into smoothies or drinks for a daily mineral boost.
- **Elderberry**: Elderberry is renowned for its immune-boosting properties, particularly helpful during cold and flu season. Rich in antioxidants and vitamin C, elderberry fights off pathogens and reduces inflammation, making it effective for both prevention and recovery from illness. Elderberry can be consumed as a syrup, tea, or tincture, offering versatile options for daily immune support.
- **Bladderwrack and Sea Moss**: These two sea vegetables are high in essential minerals, including iodine, potassium, and magnesium, which support thyroid health and overall vitality. Bladderwrack and sea moss are especially beneficial for those with mineral deficiencies, providing the body with trace elements crucial for cellular function. These can be taken in powder form, added to smoothies, or used in capsule form.
- **Nettle**: Known for its anti-inflammatory and nutrient-rich profile, nettle is beneficial for supporting joint health, skin, and hair. It's also rich in iron, making it helpful for those needing an energy boost. Nettle is usually consumed as a tea or tincture and can also be added to soups and other dishes.

Each of these herbs serves a specific purpose, working in harmony with the body to encourage balance and natural healing. By understanding these herbs and their properties, individuals can begin using them intentionally, either as daily supplements or as targeted support during illness or periods of stress.

3. BENEFITS OF INCORPORATING ALKALINE HERBS INTO DAILY LIFE

Incorporating alkaline herbs into daily life can offer profound health benefits, from immune support to digestive wellness.

Here are some of the key advantages that regular use of these herbs provides:

- **Enhanced Immune Support**: Herbs like elderberry and sarsaparilla help fortify the immune system, preparing it to ward off pathogens. In times of stress or exposure to illness, these herbs can provide added protection, reducing the likelihood of colds, flu, and infections.
- **Improved Digestion and Detoxification**: Dandelion and burdock root support liver and kidney function, promoting detoxification and digestive health. By using these herbs regularly, the body can more efficiently process and eliminate waste, preventing buildup and reducing digestive discomfort.
- **Increased Energy and Mental Clarity**: Alkaline herbs are mineral-rich, supporting overall energy levels and cognitive function. Sea moss and bladderwrack, in particular, provide essential nutrients that support mental clarity and reduce fatigue, making them valuable for maintaining focus and productivity.
- **Support for Skin Health**: Burdock root, nettle, and sarsaparilla are excellent for promoting clear, healthy skin. They reduce inflammation, cleanse the blood, and combat skin issues from within, addressing the root causes rather than masking symptoms.

The regular use of alkaline herbs encourages a state of balance, allowing the body to remain resilient, energized, and ready to handle life's demands.

4. PRACTICAL WAYS TO USE ALKALINE HERBS DAILY

Incorporating these herbs doesn't have to be complicated; they can be seamlessly added to meals, beverages, and daily routines. Here are practical ways to include alkaline herbs in everyday life:

- **Herbal Teas**: Many alkaline herbs are available as loose-leaf or bagged teas, making them easy to brew and enjoy. Drinking a cup of dandelion, nettle, or burdock tea each day is a simple and effective way to incorporate these herbs into your routine. Herbal teas are also calming, making them ideal for starting or ending the day.
- **Smoothies and Powders**: Alkaline herbs like sea moss, bladderwrack, and sarsaparilla are available in powder form, which can easily be added to smoothies. Blending a spoonful of these powders into your morning smoothie provides a mineral boost without altering the flavor.
- **Herbal Tinctures**: Tinctures are concentrated liquid extracts of herbs, making them convenient for quick use. Just a few drops of sarsaparilla or burdock root tincture in water can provide potent health benefits. Tinctures are particularly useful for individuals who prefer not to drink multiple cups of tea daily but still want the benefits of various herbs.
- **Herbal Capsules**: For those with busy lifestyles, herbal capsules offer a quick and easy way to incorporate alkaline herbs without preparation. Sea moss and bladderwrack are often available in capsule form, providing a ready-to-go option for daily mineral support.
- **Herbal Blends and Syrups**: Pre-mixed herbal syrups, such as elderberry syrup, offer an easy way to support immunity, especially during cold and flu season. These blends often include multiple herbs that work together, making them an effective way to enhance daily wellness.

Integrating these practices into daily life ensures a consistent supply of alkaline herbs, promoting continuous health benefits and supporting the body's natural functions.

5. UNDERSTANDING QUALITY AND SOURCING

When it comes to using alkaline herbs, quality matters. Sourcing herbs from reputable suppliers ensures they are free from pesticides, heavy metals, and other contaminants. Dr. Sebi emphasized the importance of natural, wild-crafted herbs because they retain higher mineral content and are more effective in promoting healing.

- **Organic and Wild-Crafted Herbs**: Organic herbs are grown without synthetic chemicals, while wild-crafted herbs are harvested from their natural habitats, ensuring they have high nutrient density. Both options are ideal for maximizing the potency of alkaline herbs.
- **Avoiding Fillers and Additives**: Many supplements contain fillers and preservatives, which can dilute the effectiveness of the herb. Look for herbs in pure form, whether as teas, tinctures, or powders, to ensure maximum health benefits.
- **Reputable Suppliers**: Choose suppliers that prioritize quality, transparency, and ethical harvesting practices. Companies that provide information about the source and quality of their herbs are more likely to offer products that align with Dr. Sebi's philosophy.

With careful selection, the herbs incorporated into daily life can be trusted allies in the pursuit of health and well-being, each one playing a role in supporting the body's natural healing processes.

Incorporating alkaline herbs is a powerful way to support health in line with Dr. Sebi's vision. These herbs not only provide physical benefits but also align with a philosophy of wellness that nurtures the body, mind, and spirit. By making alkaline herbs a daily habit, you invest in a foundation of wellness that supports resilience, longevity, and vitality.

CHAPTER 2
PROPERTIES AND BENEFITS OF KEY HERBS

Imagine walking into a room filled with herbs, each with its own unique scent, appearance, and history of healing. Each plant offers a different benefit, whether it's purifying the blood, supporting digestion, or boosting immunity. In Dr. Sebi's world, herbs are much more than plants; they're the natural allies of our bodies, grounding us, protecting us, and bringing balance. Let's explore some of these extraordinary herbs in detail, each with its own unique benefits, and see how they might become part of your wellness journey.

1. BURDOCK ROOT: THE BLOOD CLEANSER

If you're looking for a fresh start, burdock root might be the herb that calls to you. Known as a natural "blood cleanser," it works deeply to detoxify the body, almost like a gentle internal sweep. Imagine burdock root as the broom clearing out toxins and making space for healthy cells to flourish. Its rich, earthy flavor is a reminder that true healing starts from deep within.

- **Purifies and Strengthens the Blood**: Burdock root is known for its role in supporting liver function and cleansing the blood. By reducing the toxic load in our bodies, it promotes clearer skin, brighter energy, and a lighter, healthier feeling overall. You can think of it as a "refresh button" for the bloodstream.
- **Supports Healthy Skin**: Because burdock root works at a cellular level, it's also a powerful tool for skin health. Imagine using burdock regularly and watching your skin gradually become clearer, more radiant, and resilient. For anyone dealing with breakouts, eczema, or psoriasis, burdock root's blood-cleansing properties can address some of the root causes that often show up on the skin.
- **Immune Support**: This root is also packed with antioxidants, helping the body fend off infections and reducing inflammation. Using burdock regularly can help ease the strain on your immune system, allowing it to focus on more vital defenses.
- **Incorporate It Into Your Day**: Burdock is commonly used as a tea or tincture. It's a grounding, warming herb, so sipping a cup of burdock tea each morning can set a steady, calming tone for the day. You can also add powdered burdock root to smoothies, bringing a nourishing, earthy touch to your routine.

2. DANDELION ROOT: THE LIVER AND DIGESTION HEALER

Dandelion might be the humble weed we often overlook, but its roots hold powerful healing properties, especially when it comes to liver health. Picture dandelion root as a gentle yet persistent "scrubber" for the liver, helping it function at its peak. This is the herb you turn to when you need to give your digestion a helping hand and your liver a chance to breathe.

- **Liver Detox and Bile Production**: Dandelion root supports the liver by promoting bile production, which plays a crucial role in digestion. Think of bile as a "dish detergent" for fats, breaking them down and helping the liver eliminate waste more efficiently. By supporting bile production, dandelion root helps keep digestion smooth and regular, especially after heavier meals.
- **Gentle Diuretic and Kidney Support**: One of the unique things about dandelion root is its diuretic effect, which encourages the kidneys to flush out excess water and sodium. This can be particularly refreshing if you're feeling bloated or retaining water. Imagine dandelion root as the friend who brings clarity and lightness, especially after days when you might feel sluggish.
- **Easy Ways to Enjoy Dandelion Root**: Dandelion root tea is a popular option and has a slightly bitter, earthy taste that can feel grounding. A cup in the morning or before bed offers a gentle, consistent way to support the liver and digestion. If you're not a tea drinker, you can find dandelion root tinctures or capsules that provide similar benefits.

3. SARSAPARILLA: IRON-RICH AND ENERGY-BOOSTING

If you're ever feeling low on energy, sarsaparilla could be the answer you're looking for. With its high iron content, it's an herbal powerhouse for those seeking a natural energy boost. Picture sarsaparilla as your go-to herb when you need to lift your spirits and revitalize your body from the inside out.

- **Iron-Rich for Blood Health**: Sarsaparilla is rich in bioavailable iron, making it a natural choice for anyone needing to support their blood health. Iron is essential for creating hemoglobin, the molecule that carries oxygen throughout the body. Regularly using sarsaparilla can help boost your energy naturally, especially if you're prone to feeling fatigued or rundown.

- **Hormonal and Immune Support**: Sarsaparilla is not only rich in iron but also contains plant compounds that can help balance hormones. This makes it particularly valuable for women seeking natural support for menstrual health or those looking for gentle hormonal balance.
- **Simple Ways to Incorporate Sarsaparilla**: Try sarsaparilla tea, or if you're on the go, a tincture may be a quick and convenient option. For an extra iron boost, you could add sarsaparilla powder to a morning smoothie alongside fruits like berries or greens like spinach. It's a practical way to start your day with a burst of energy and iron.

4. ELDERBERRY: IMMUNE PROTECTION IN A BERRY

Elderberry is one of the best natural allies for immune support. Known for its rich purple-black color and tart flavor, elderberry has become a staple during cold and flu season. Picture elderberry as a protective layer that keeps your immune system strong and ready to fend off invaders.

- **Immune Boosting and Antiviral Properties**: Elderberries are loaded with antioxidants, particularly anthocyanins, which give them their deep color. These compounds help shield cells from damage and make the immune system more robust. Elderberry is particularly well-suited for reducing the severity of colds and flu, acting like a "coat of armor" for your immune health.
- **Anti-Inflammatory Benefits**: Beyond immunity, elderberry also has anti-inflammatory properties, soothing sore throats, easing congestion, and reducing the aches and pains that come with colds. Think of it as a natural, comforting remedy that nurtures you through cold symptoms.
- **Practical Uses**: Elderberry syrup is a popular way to take this herb and is particularly loved by kids. You can find elderberry syrup recipes online if you prefer to make your own. If syrup isn't your thing, try elderberry tea, tinctures, or capsules for a convenient dose of immune support, especially during high-risk seasons.

5. SEA MOSS AND BLADDERWRACK: MINERAL BOOST FOR THYROID HEALTH

Imagine two sea vegetables—sea moss and bladderwrack—that offer over 90 essential minerals, feeding your body what it needs for peak performance. These two herbs work especially well for thyroid health and are a valuable addition for anyone seeking mineral support.

- **Thyroid Support and Hormonal Balance**: Sea moss and bladderwrack are naturally rich in iodine, which is vital for thyroid health. A well-functioning thyroid regulates energy, metabolism, and hormonal balance. These sea vegetables provide the raw materials your body needs to support your thyroid without synthetic supplements.
- **Packed with Essential Minerals**: Sea moss and bladderwrack contain calcium, potassium, and magnesium, helping replenish the body with minerals it needs daily. Imagine them as your natural multivitamin, supporting not only the thyroid but also joint health, immunity, and skin vitality.
- **How to Use Sea Moss and Bladderwrack**: These herbs can be taken in powder or capsule form. Sea moss gel is another popular method and can be added to smoothies, soups, or even taken alone. Sea moss and bladderwrack can also be mixed in powdered form into morning smoothies for a mineral-rich start to the day.

6. NETTLE: NATURE'S NUTRIENT POWERHOUSE

Nettle might surprise you; it's known for its high nutrient content and anti-inflammatory properties. This herb is like a multi-purpose nutrient boost in plant form, providing iron, calcium, magnesium, and vitamin C. Nettle is the herb you reach for if you want an all-around strengthener that supports immunity, energy, and even skin health.

- **Anti-Inflammatory and Skin Support**: Nettle is well-regarded for its anti-inflammatory properties, making it an excellent choice for soothing skin issues like eczema, psoriasis, or even mild rashes. Nettle's high vitamin C content also supports collagen production, giving skin a youthful glow.
- **Bone and Joint Health**: With its high calcium and magnesium content, nettle is fantastic for bone health. It's an ideal herb to include if you're looking to support joint health or prevent bone loss as you age.
- **Enjoy Nettle Daily**: Nettle is delicious as a tea, and its mild, grassy flavor is both nourishing and refreshing. You can also use nettle tincture if you're short on time or add dried nettle to soups and stews as a nutrient booster.

Each of these herbs offers unique, powerful benefits that align with Dr. Sebi's vision of healing through nature. By incorporating these plants into your daily life, you tap into the earth's natural pharmacy, helping your body cleanse, energize, and thrive. Imagine each herb as a partner in wellness, offering not just immediate benefits but a path toward long-term health and resilience.

CHAPTER 3
ESSENTIAL HERBAL BLENDS

One of the most powerful ways to experience the benefits of herbs is through thoughtfully crafted blends. Each herb brings its own unique properties, but when combined, they can create a synergistic effect that amplifies their healing potential. Whether you're looking to boost your immune system, improve digestion, or reduce stress, herbal blends offer a practical and potent way to incorporate the healing properties of multiple plants into daily life. This chapter introduces a selection of essential herbal blends based on Dr. Sebi's principles, each designed to support specific aspects of health.

1. IMMUNE BOOSTING BLEND

In today's world, where we're constantly exposed to environmental toxins and pathogens, a strong immune system is more important than ever. This immune-boosting blend combines elderberry, echinacea, ginger, and burdock root to create a natural shield against infections and colds. Each of these herbs brings a unique quality to the blend, supporting the body in fending off illness.

- **Ingredients**:
  - **Elderberry**: Packed with antioxidants and vitamin C, elderberry boosts immune response and is known for its antiviral properties.
  - **Echinacea**: Often used in traditional medicine, echinacea strengthens the immune system and reduces the severity of colds and flu.
  - **Ginger**: Ginger adds warmth to the blend, aiding circulation and supporting immune health by reducing inflammation.
  - **Burdock Root**: Burdock purifies the blood and supports the liver, helping to clear toxins and enhance immunity.
- **Preparation**:
  - Combine equal parts of each dried herb in a jar.
  - For a tea, add 1 tablespoon of the blend to 8 ounces of boiling water. Steep for 10–15 minutes, strain, and drink. Take 1–2 cups daily, especially during cold and flu season, to keep immunity strong.
- **Practical Tip**: To make a larger batch, prepare the blend as a tea concentrate. Boil a pot of water with a handful of the blend, simmer for 20 minutes, strain, and store in the refrigerator. Drink a small cup daily as a preventive measure or increase the amount during times of illness.

2. DIGESTIVE HARMONY BLEND

Digestive health is central to overall wellness, and this blend is designed to soothe and support the digestive system. The combination of dandelion root, peppermint, fennel, and ginger works together to relieve bloating, improve digestion, and promote regularity.

- **Ingredients**:
  - **Dandelion Root**: Dandelion root stimulates bile production, aiding digestion and liver function.
  - **Peppermint**: Known for its cooling and soothing effect, peppermint relaxes the digestive tract, easing gas and bloating.
  - **Fennel**: Fennel seeds have long been used to reduce bloating and support digestion by relaxing the smooth muscles in the gastrointestinal tract.
  - **Ginger**: Ginger improves digestion by reducing inflammation and stimulating digestive enzymes.
- **Preparation**:
  - Mix equal parts of each herb in a jar.
  - To make a tea, add 1 teaspoon of the blend to a cup of hot water. Steep for 5–10 minutes, strain, and sip slowly. Drink before or after meals to support digestion and relieve discomfort.
- **Practical Tip**: This blend can also be prepared as a digestive tonic by adding the herbs to an apple cider vinegar base. Steep the blend in apple cider vinegar for two weeks, strain, and take 1–2 teaspoons before meals to stimulate digestion.

3. STRESS RELIEF AND RELAXATION BLEND

Incorporating herbs to manage stress and promote relaxation can be a simple yet profound addition to your routine. This blend includes chamomile, lemon balm, lavender, and passionflower, all of which are known for their calming effects on the nervous system. This blend is ideal for unwinding in the evening or finding calm during a busy day.

- **Ingredients**:
  - **Chamomile**: Known for its mild sedative effects, chamomile promotes relaxation and helps reduce anxiety.
  - **Lemon Balm**: This gentle herb calms the mind and

is particularly helpful for relieving mild stress and anxiety.
- » **Lavender**: Lavender supports relaxation, helping to ease tension and promote restful sleep.
- » **Passionflower**: Passionflower is a natural tranquilizer that reduces nervousness and improves sleep quality.
- **Preparation**:
  - » Combine equal parts of each herb.
  - » To prepare, add 1–2 teaspoons of the blend to a cup of hot water, steep for 10 minutes, strain, and enjoy before bed or whenever stress relief is needed.
- **Practical Tip**: This blend can also be infused in oil for a relaxing bath or massage oil. Place the blend in a jar, cover it with almond or jojoba oil, and let it steep for 2–4 weeks. Strain and add a few drops to bath water for a calming soak.

4. BLOOD CLEANSING AND DETOX BLEND

Detoxification is essential for overall health, helping to clear the body of accumulated toxins. This blend of burdock root, nettle, red clover, and dandelion root works gently to purify the blood, support the liver and kidneys, and promote clear skin.

- **Ingredients**:
  - » **Burdock Root**: Burdock root purifies the blood and supports liver function, essential for detoxification.
  - » **Nettle**: Nettle is rich in nutrients and supports kidney health, helping the body flush out toxins through urine.
  - » **Red Clover**: Red clover helps cleanse the blood and supports healthy skin.
  - » **Dandelion Root**: Dandelion root aids liver detoxification, making it easier for the body to eliminate waste.
- **Preparation**:
  - » Mix equal parts of each dried herb.
  - » For a detox tea, add 1 tablespoon of the blend to a cup of boiling water, steep for 10–15 minutes, and strain. Drink 1–2 cups daily as part of a detox routine.
- **Practical Tip**: This blend can be simmered with water for 20 minutes to create a stronger decoction, which can then be stored in the refrigerator and consumed daily as part of a gentle, ongoing detox program.

5. RESPIRATORY SUPPORT BLEND

Respiratory health is essential, especially during times of seasonal allergies or respiratory challenges. This blend combines mullein, eucalyptus, peppermint, and thyme to clear airways, reduce inflammation, and support lung health.

- **Ingredients**:
  - » **Mullein**: Mullein soothes the respiratory tract and reduces inflammation, making it easier to breathe.
  - » **Eucalyptus**: Known for its strong aroma, eucalyptus opens up nasal passages and helps clear congestion.
  - » **Peppermint**: Peppermint's menthol content cools and clears the sinuses, supporting respiratory comfort.
  - » **Thyme**: Thyme acts as a natural antiseptic, fighting off respiratory infections and easing coughs.
- **Preparation**:
  - » Combine equal parts of each herb in a jar.
  - » To make a tea, add 1 teaspoon of the blend to a cup of hot water, steep for 5–10 minutes, and drink. Alternatively, create a steam inhalation by adding 1–2 tablespoons to a bowl of hot water and inhaling the steam to clear nasal passages.
- **Practical Tip**: For those with chronic respiratory issues, consider making a larger batch of this blend and keeping it on hand for inhalation or tea during seasonal changes.

6. FEMALE BALANCE BLEND

For those seeking to support hormonal balance and female reproductive health, this blend combines red raspberry leaf, nettle, motherwort, and chamomile. These herbs work together to ease menstrual discomfort, support hormonal balance, and provide nourishment.

- **Ingredients**:
  - » **Red Raspberry Leaf**: Known as the "woman's herb," red raspberry leaf strengthens the uterus and provides vitamins and minerals.
  - » **Nettle**: Nettle supports blood health and provides essential nutrients, helping to replenish the body during menstruation.
  - » **Motherwort**: This herb balances hormones and helps relieve menstrual cramps and stress.
  - » **Chamomile**: Chamomile offers a calming effect, helping to ease tension and pain.
- **Preparation**:
  - » Combine equal parts of each herb in a jar.
  - » For tea, add 1 tablespoon to 8 ounces of boiling water, steep for 10–15 minutes, strain, and enjoy. Drinking 1–2 cups per day, especially leading up to menstruation, can support a smoother cycle.
- **Practical Tip**: This blend can also be used as a herbal infusion in a bath to ease menstrual cramps and promote relaxation. Simply add a handful of the blend to warm bath water and soak for 20–30 minutes.

7. ENERGIZING BLEND

When you need a natural boost without relying on caffeine, an energizing blend of green tea, ginseng, rosemary, and peppermint can be revitalizing. This blend supports mental clarity, alertness, and sustained energy throughout the day.

- **Ingredients**:
  - **Green Tea**: Green tea contains a mild amount of caffeine and antioxidants, promoting mental focus and calm energy.
  - **Ginseng**: Known for its adaptogenic properties, ginseng supports energy and endurance, especially during times of stress.
  - **Rosemary**: Rosemary improves circulation and mental clarity, providing a subtle pick-me-up.
  - **Peppermint**: Peppermint refreshes the mind and body, enhancing alertness and focus.
- **Preparation**:
  - Combine equal parts of each herb.
  - To make a tea, add 1 tablespoon of the blend to a cup of hot water, steep for 5–10 minutes, strain, and enjoy. Drink in the morning or early afternoon for sustained energy.
- **Practical Tip**: If you're sensitive to caffeine, you can make this blend caffeine-free by omitting green tea. Ginseng, rosemary, and peppermint alone still provide a significant boost without caffeine.

These herbal blends offer a natural, accessible approach to addressing specific health needs, from immunity to energy and hormonal balance. Integrating these blends into daily routines not only enhances wellness but also provides a moment to pause, breathe, and connect with nature's healing properties. Each blend serves as a reminder of the body's ability to heal and thrive when supported by the right herbs in the right combination.

BOOK 8
Dr. Sebi's Herbal Apothecary

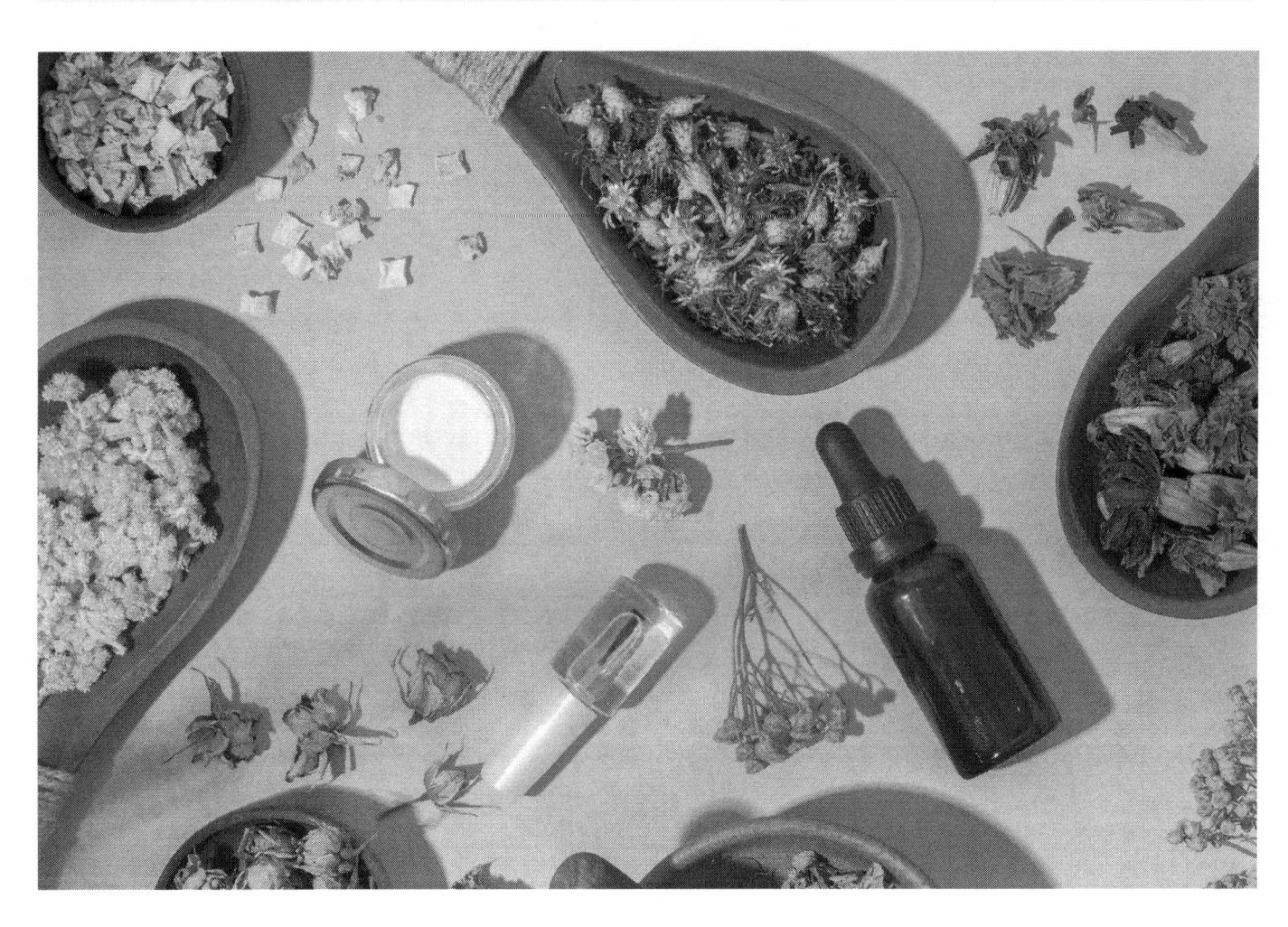

Dr. Sebi's approach to healing emphasizes the use of nature's gifts to maintain and restore health. His herbal apothecary includes powerful plant-based remedies for various everyday health issues, from headaches and digestive discomfort to fatigue and immunity. These remedies are designed to be accessible and easy to incorporate into daily life, offering natural solutions that align with the body's need for balance and healing. This chapter focuses on simple herbal remedies for common health concerns, providing practical methods to support well-being.

CHAPTER 1
HERBAL REMEDIES FOR EVERYDAY HEALTH

Whether it's a mild headache, digestive upset, or low energy, everyday health issues can impact quality of life and productivity. Having natural remedies on hand can make a big difference, allowing us to address these concerns without turning to synthetic medications. Here, we explore effective, easy-to-make herbal remedies for some of the most common health issues. These recipes use herbs aligned with Dr. Sebi's teachings, each selected for its healing properties and compatibility with the body's natural functions.

1. HEADACHE RELIEF TEA

Headaches can be caused by various factors, including stress, dehydration, and tension. Instead of reaching for over-the-counter painkillers, a blend of peppermint, chamomile, and lavender can help alleviate the pain naturally. Each of these herbs provides unique properties to soothe headaches and ease tension.

- **Ingredients**:
  - » 1 teaspoon dried peppermint
  - » 1 teaspoon dried chamomile
  - » 1/2 teaspoon dried lavender
- **Instructions**:
  - » Combine the herbs in a cup of boiling water.
  - » Steep for 10 minutes, then strain and sip slowly.
  - » Drink 1–2 cups as needed until the headache eases.
- **How It Works**: Peppermint relaxes muscles and improves blood flow, while chamomile calms the nervous system, reducing tension-related pain. Lavender is known for its relaxing properties, which can ease stress and promote calmness.

2. DIGESTIVE SOOTHING TONIC

Indigestion and bloating are common issues, often due to dietary choices or stress. For a gentle, effective remedy, a blend of fennel, ginger, and dandelion root can help improve digestion, reduce bloating, and soothe the stomach.

- **Ingredients**:
  - » 1 teaspoon fennel seeds
  - » 1/2 teaspoon dried ginger
  - » 1 teaspoon dried dandelion root
- **Instructions**:
  - » Combine the herbs in a cup of boiling water.
  - » Steep for 10–15 minutes, strain, and sip slowly.
  - » Drink 1 cup after meals as needed to relieve discomfort.
- **How It Works**: Fennel seeds relieve bloating by relaxing the gastrointestinal tract, while ginger reduces inflammation and aids digestion. Dandelion root supports liver function, helping the body process food more efficiently.

3. ENERGY-BOOSTING SMOOTHIE

For those days when you feel sluggish or mentally foggy, a nutrient-rich smoothie with sea moss, spirulina, and berries can provide a natural energy boost. This blend offers essential minerals and antioxidants, supporting sustained energy and mental clarity.

- **Ingredients**:
  - » 1 tablespoon sea moss gel
  - » 1 teaspoon spirulina powder
  - » 1/2 cup mixed berries (like blueberries, strawberries, or blackberries)
  - » 1 cup almond or coconut milk
  - » 1 teaspoon chia seeds (optional)
- **Instructions**:
  - » Blend all ingredients until smooth.
  - » Drink as a morning or midday snack for a natural energy lift.
- **How It Works**: Sea moss is rich in minerals like potassium, magnesium, and iodine, which support thyroid function and energy levels. Spirulina offers plant-based protein and antioxidants that reduce fatigue and promote focus, while berries provide natural sugars and vitamins to keep you energized.

4. IMMUNE-STRENGTHENING SYRUP

For boosting immunity, especially during cold and flu season, an elderberry syrup infused with ginger and cinnamon offers a delicious, effective remedy. This syrup can be taken daily as a preventive measure or at the onset of cold symptoms.

- **Ingredients**:
  - » 1 cup dried elderberries
  - » 1 tablespoon grated ginger
  - » 1 cinnamon stick

- 2 cups water
- 1/2 cup raw honey (optional)

- **Instructions**:
  - In a saucepan, combine elderberries, ginger, cinnamon, and water.
  - Bring to a boil, then simmer for 30 minutes.
  - Strain the mixture, pressing the berries to extract as much liquid as possible.
  - Add honey (if desired) once the syrup has cooled slightly, and stir well.
  - Store in a glass jar in the refrigerator for up to two weeks.
  - Take 1 tablespoon daily for immune support or up to three times daily when experiencing cold symptoms.
- **How It Works**: Elderberries are known for their antiviral properties and high vitamin C content. Ginger boosts circulation and immunity, while cinnamon helps stabilize blood sugar and enhances the immune response.

5. CALMING TEA FOR STRESS AND ANXIETY

Stress and anxiety can take a toll on both mental and physical health. A tea made with lemon balm, chamomile, and passionflower can promote relaxation, reduce tension, and support restful sleep.

- **Ingredients**:
  - 1 teaspoon dried lemon balm
  - 1 teaspoon dried chamomile
  - 1/2 teaspoon passionflower
- **Instructions**:
  - Combine herbs in a cup of boiling water.
  - Steep for 10 minutes, strain, and drink.
  - Enjoy 1–2 cups in the evening or whenever you need to unwind.
- **How It Works**: Lemon balm is known for its calming effects on the nervous system, while chamomile reduces anxiety and promotes relaxation. Passionflower acts as a natural tranquilizer, helping to ease mental tension and improve sleep quality.

6. SKIN-SOOTHING HERBAL STEAM

For glowing skin and respiratory relief, a facial steam with rosemary, thyme, and lavender can be a soothing remedy. This blend cleanses pores, improves circulation, and provides gentle relief for the respiratory system, especially during seasonal allergies or colds.

- **Ingredients**:
  - 1 tablespoon dried rosemary
  - 1 tablespoon dried thyme
  - 1 tablespoon dried lavender
- **Instructions**:
  - Add herbs to a large bowl and pour in boiling water.
  - Place your face over the bowl, covering your head with a towel to trap the steam.
  - Inhale deeply for 5–10 minutes, allowing the steam to open your pores and soothe your respiratory system.
- **How It Works**: Rosemary and thyme are antimicrobial, cleansing the skin and sinuses, while lavender relaxes and soothes both skin and nerves. This steam can improve complexion, open sinuses, and provide a moment of calm.

7. MUSCLE SOOTHING BATH FOR PAIN RELIEF

After a long day or intense workout, a warm bath infused with arnica, chamomile, and Epsom salts can provide relief from muscle soreness and tension. This bath soothes muscles, reduces inflammation, and promotes relaxation.

- **Ingredients**:
  - 1 tablespoon dried arnica (for external use only)
  - 1 tablespoon dried chamomile
  - 1/2 cup Epsom salts
- **Instructions**:
  - Place the dried herbs in a cloth bag or tea infuser and add to warm bath water.
  - Add Epsom salts and soak for at least 20 minutes.
- **How It Works**: Arnica is an anti-inflammatory herb that relieves pain and swelling, while chamomile provides relaxation. Epsom salts offer magnesium, which helps relax muscles and alleviate cramps or soreness.

8. COLD SORE RELIEF WITH LICORICE AND LEMON BALM

Cold sores are not only uncomfortable but also can be persistent. Licorice root and lemon balm both have antiviral properties that can help reduce the duration and severity of cold sores.

- **Ingredients**:
  - 1 teaspoon powdered licorice root
  - 1 teaspoon dried lemon balm
  - Coconut oil (enough to make a paste)
- **Instructions**:

- » Mix the licorice root and lemon balm with a small amount of coconut oil to create a paste.
- » Apply the paste directly to the cold sore and leave it on for 15–20 minutes.
- » Rinse and repeat twice daily until the sore heals.
- **How It Works**: Licorice root contains glycyrrhizic acid, which is known for its antiviral properties, while lemon balm reduces the virus's activity, helping to shorten the cold sore's life.

9. NATURAL SLEEP AID BLEND

If you're struggling with sleep, a simple blend of valerian root, chamomile, and hops can act as a natural sleep aid, promoting restful and restorative sleep without the side effects of synthetic sleep medications.

- **Ingredients**:
  - » 1 teaspoon dried valerian root
  - » 1 teaspoon dried chamomile
  - » 1/2 teaspoon dried hops
- **Instructions**:
  - » Add herbs to a cup of boiling water, steep for 10–15 minutes, then strain.
  - » Drink 30 minutes before bed to help induce sleep.
- **How It Works**: Valerian root is a natural sedative that calms the nervous system, while chamomile relaxes and promotes sleep. Hops enhance valerian's effects, providing a gentle yet effective remedy for insomnia.

These herbal remedies serve as a foundational toolkit for everyday health issues, allowing you to approach common concerns with natural, effective solutions. By incorporating these simple, accessible recipes, you can align with Dr. Sebi's philosophy of health through nature, creating a lifestyle that is gentle, supportive, and in harmony with the body's own healing potential.

CHAPTER 2
STORAGE AND PREPARATION TECHNIQUES

Storing and preparing herbs may seem like a simple task, but there's an art to it that brings out their full healing potential. Like any ingredient in our lives, herbs benefit from mindful handling, which not only preserves their potency but also respects their origin and purpose. This chapter guides you through best practices for storing and preparing herbs, ensuring they remain effective, fresh, and ready to provide their benefits when needed. Let's explore how to treat these natural treasures, making each step a part of the healing process.

1. THE IMPORTANCE OF PROPER STORAGE

Imagine storing herbs as preserving the "life" within them. Just as food can spoil if left out, herbs need specific conditions to maintain their potency and avoid degradation. Factors like light, temperature, and humidity can drastically affect herbal quality. Proper storage can keep them effective for months or even years.

- **Light Sensitivity**: Herbs are sensitive to sunlight and artificial light, which can cause their colors and active compounds to fade. To prevent this, store dried herbs in opaque containers, like amber glass jars, or in dark cabinets away from windows.
- **Humidity Control**: Moisture is an enemy of dried herbs, encouraging mold growth and spoiling the herbs' effectiveness. For this reason, it's best to keep herbs in a cool, dry place, away from areas like the bathroom or kitchen sink, where humidity levels fluctuate.
- **Temperature Stability**: Heat can degrade herbs over time, so avoid storing them near heat sources, like stoves or direct sunlight. A stable, moderate temperature is ideal—think of a pantry or a dedicated storage shelf.
- **Airtight Containers**: Glass jars with airtight lids are your best option for storage, as they don't absorb odors or chemicals, and they help keep herbs fresh. Plastic containers may leach chemicals into the herbs, especially if exposed to sunlight or heat, so it's best to avoid them when possible.

2. CHOOSING THE RIGHT CONTAINER FOR YOUR HERBS

Imagine walking into an apothecary filled with glass jars labeled with the names of herbs; each jar preserves the life and healing energy of its contents. Choosing the right containers for your herbs not only keeps them fresh but also creates a practical, beautiful setup that respects the herbs' value.

- **Glass Jars for Dried Herbs**: Glass jars are ideal for dried herbs because they are impermeable and won't absorb odors or oils from the herbs. If you use glass jars, select ones with tight-sealing lids to keep out moisture and air.
- **Metal Containers for Small Quantities**: Some people prefer small metal tins for herbs they use frequently. These are especially useful for travel or on-the-go storage, as they are durable and lightweight.
- **Paper Bags for Short-Term Storage**: For herbs you'll use quickly, paper bags can work well, but they don't provide as much protection from light and humidity. These are suitable for fresh herbs that you might dry yourself or for making a quick tea blend.

3. BASIC PREPARATION TECHNIQUES

Preparing herbs for use brings you closer to the natural healing process. From teas to tinctures, each method has its own steps, transforming dried leaves, roots, and flowers into forms your body can easily absorb. Here are the most common preparation techniques for various purposes.

- **Infusions (Teas)**: Infusions are the simplest form of herbal preparation, typically made with soft plant parts like leaves and flowers. To make an infusion, add 1–2 teaspoons of dried herbs to a cup of boiling water, cover, and steep for 5–15 minutes. Strain and enjoy. Infusions are best consumed immediately but can be refrigerated for up to 24 hours.
- **Decoctions**: Decoctions are more robust than infusions, used primarily for roots, barks, and seeds. These denser plant parts need longer to release their medicinal compounds. To make a decoction, add the herb to a pot of water, bring it to a boil, then simmer for 20–30 minutes. Strain and drink, storing any extra in the refrigerator for up to two days.
- **Tinctures**: Tinctures are potent, alcohol-based herbal extracts that preserve herbs for years. Combine dried or fresh herbs with a high-proof alcohol like vodka or brandy, usually in a 1:4 or 1:5 herb-to-alcohol ratio. Seal in a glass jar, shake daily, and let it steep in a dark place for 4–6 weeks. After straining, the tincture is ready for use and should be stored in a dark glass bottle to preserve its potency.

- **Herbal Oils**: Infused oils are typically used for external applications, such as massage oils or balms. To make an herbal oil, place dried herbs in a jar, cover them with a carrier oil (like olive or coconut), and let the mixture sit in a sunny window for 2–4 weeks. Strain the oil and store it in a dark glass bottle. Oils are sensitive to light and should be stored in a cool place to prevent them from going rancid.

4. FRESH HERB PREPARATIONS

Sometimes, fresh herbs are readily available, especially if you grow them or buy them fresh from a local market. Fresh herbs bring a different quality to preparations, often being more potent due to their moisture content. Here's how to use fresh herbs in various ways:

- **Herbal Poultices**: For direct application on the skin, fresh herbs like plantain or comfrey can be crushed into a paste and applied to the affected area. Poultices are commonly used for wounds, bruises, or sore muscles and work by delivering active compounds directly through the skin.
- **Fresh Herb Juices**: Certain fresh herbs, like dandelion greens or burdock, can be juiced and consumed for a concentrated dose of nutrients. A juicer or blender can help extract the liquid, which can be added to smoothies or enjoyed alone in small doses.
- **Freeze Fresh Herbs for Longevity**: Freezing is a great way to preserve fresh herbs for future use. Chop fresh herbs like basil, cilantro, or parsley, place them in ice cube trays, and cover with water or oil before freezing. These frozen cubes can be added to teas, infusions, or recipes as needed.

5. HERBAL PRESERVATION FOR LONG-TERM USE

If you plan to store herbs for more than a few months, consider additional preservation techniques to retain potency over time. Properly preserved herbs last longer and are more effective when needed.

- **Drying Fresh Herbs**: For herbs you harvest yourself, drying them properly is crucial. Hang them in small bundles in a well-ventilated, dark space, or use a dehydrator set at a low temperature. Once fully dried, store in airtight containers.
- **Freezing Dried Herbs**: For long-term storage, especially for herbs sensitive to oxidation, consider freezing dried herbs in an airtight bag or container. This method can preserve their color, flavor, and potency for up to a year.

CHAPTER 3
SAFETY AND DOSAGE TIPS

Working with herbs is deeply rewarding, but it requires mindfulness and respect for their potency. Knowing how to measure, dose, and use herbs safely helps you achieve the best outcomes while minimizing risks. This chapter offers guidelines on dosages, safe practices, and how to avoid potential adverse effects, ensuring that herbs can be integrated into daily life effectively and responsibly.

1. UNDERSTANDING DOSAGES FOR DIFFERENT FORMS

Herbal dosages vary significantly depending on the form—teas, tinctures, capsules, or oils. Each preparation method extracts different concentrations of the herb's active compounds, making dosage guidance essential.

- **Teas and Infusions**: Generally, teas are gentle, and adults can drink 1–3 cups per day, depending on the herb. For example, chamomile tea is safe to drink multiple times daily, while stronger herbs like valerian root should be limited to one cup per day.
- **Tinctures**: Tinctures are concentrated and usually dosed by drops. A typical adult dosage is 20–30 drops, or 1–2 dropperfuls, taken 2–3 times per day. Always start with a smaller dose and gradually increase to assess tolerance, as tinctures are powerful.
- **Capsules and Powders**: For herbal powders, a common dose is 1/2–1 teaspoon, mixed with water or juice. Capsules are pre-dosed but should still be used according to product instructions or herbalist recommendations, typically ranging from 1–3 capsules per day.

2. SAFETY CONSIDERATIONS FOR SPECIFIC HERBS

Not all herbs are suitable for everyone, and certain herbs require special caution. Some may be unsuitable for children, pregnant women, or those with specific health conditions.

- **Pregnancy and Breastfeeding**: Herbs like red raspberry leaf can support pregnancy, but others, such as licorice root or sage, may be harmful. Always consult with a healthcare provider or herbalist before using herbs during pregnancy or breastfeeding.
- **Allergies and Sensitivities**: People with plant allergies should be cautious with new herbs. For instance, individuals allergic to ragweed may react to chamomile. Conduct a patch test by applying a small amount of the herb to your skin to check for irritation before ingesting it.

3. UNDERSTANDING HERB INTERACTIONS WITH MEDICATIONS

Some herbs interact with medications, amplifying or diminishing their effects. It's important to be aware of potential interactions, especially if you're taking prescription medications.

- **St. John's Wort and Antidepressants**: St. John's Wort is known to interact with antidepressants and can increase serotonin levels, potentially leading to serotonin syndrome. Those on antidepressants should avoid using this herb or consult a healthcare provider.
- **Ginkgo Biloba and Blood Thinners**: Ginkgo has blood-thinning properties and should be used cautiously with blood-thinning medications to prevent bleeding risks.

4. TIPS FOR SAFE USAGE

Following best practices for safe herbal use helps prevent adverse reactions and ensures that you receive the full benefit from each herb.

- **Start Small and Increase Gradually**: When trying a new herb, start with a small dose and observe how your body reacts. Increase the dose gradually, if needed, to reach the desired effect.
- **Stay Hydrated**: Herbal preparations, especially teas, may have diuretic effects, which can lead to dehydration. Drinking plenty of water alongside herbal remedies helps maintain hydration.
- **Keep a Health Journal**: Tracking your herbal usage, dosages, and any effects you experience helps you understand how herbs work with your body over time. A journal can also help identify which combinations work best and highlight any potential adverse reactions.

These guidelines on storage, preparation, safety, and dosage create a framework for responsible, effective herbal use, ensuring herbs provide their healing properties safely and effectively. By approaching herbalism with care and respect, you can incorporate Dr. Sebi's principles of natural healing into everyday life, benefiting from the powerful and balanced support that herbs have to offer.

BOOK 9
Remedies for Detoxification

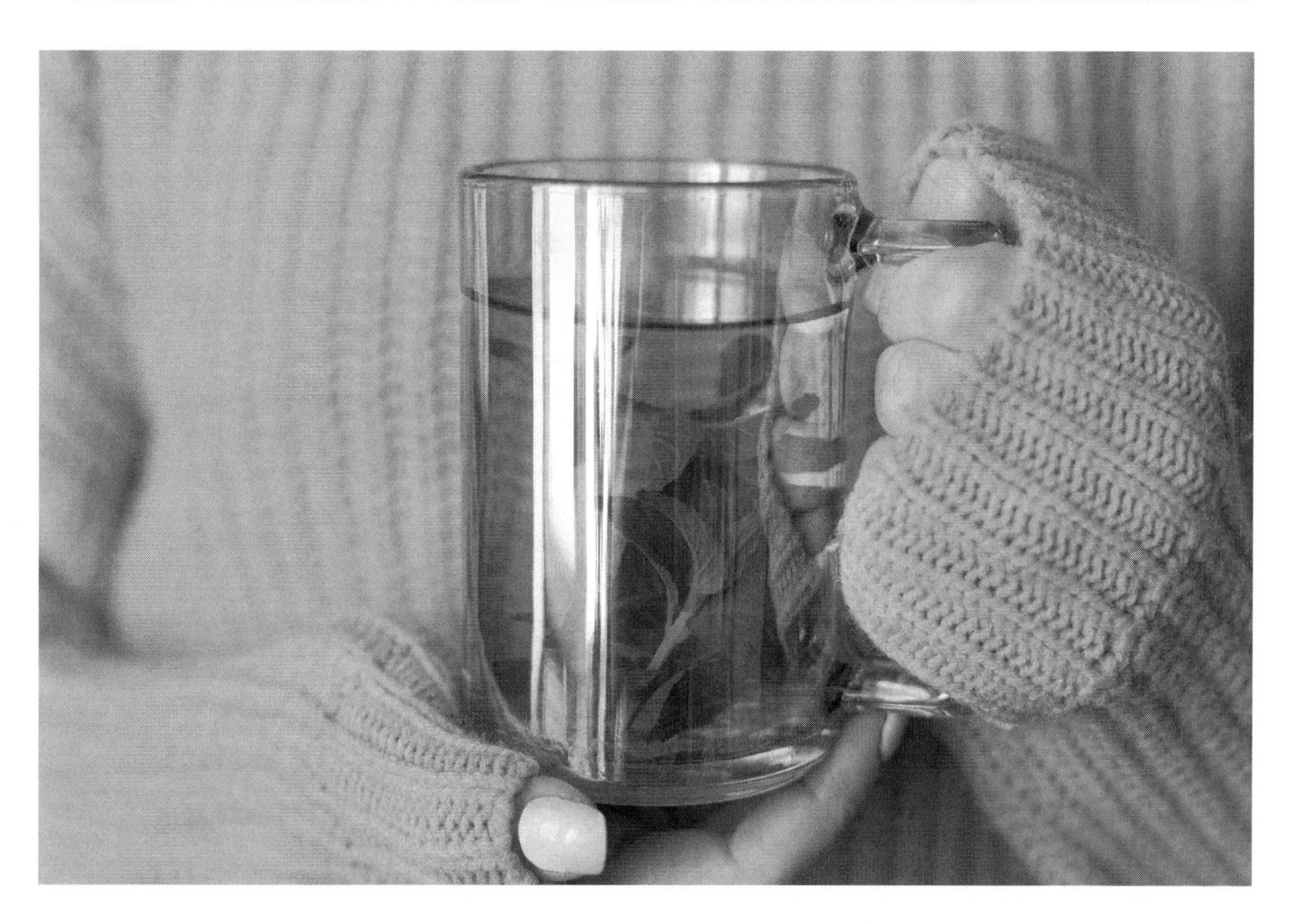

Dr. Sebi's approach to detoxification is rooted in the idea of natural and consistent cleansing. Regular detoxification supports the body's ability to flush out toxins and maintain a balanced internal environment, which is essential for long-term health. In this book, we explore herbal remedies crafted to assist with detoxification, from teas and decoctions to more complex detox protocols. By incorporating these simple yet powerful remedies, you can help your body stay resilient and vibrant, naturally eliminating toxins while nourishing the cells.

CHAPTER 1
DETOX TEAS AND DECOCTIONS

Detoxification doesn't need to be complicated. In fact, some of the most effective detox remedies come in the form of teas and decoctions. These gentle preparations use heat to extract beneficial compounds from herbs, delivering nutrients directly into the bloodstream and supporting organs involved in cleansing. This chapter introduces you to a variety of detox teas and decoctions that align with Dr. Sebi's philosophy, offering a natural, daily approach to detoxification.

1. THE POWER OF DETOX TEAS

Drinking herbal detox teas can be a simple yet powerful way to support the body's natural cleansing systems. Teas are typically gentle and can be consumed daily to support various detox functions, from liver health to kidney support.

Why Detox Teas Work: Teas allow herbs to be absorbed gradually, giving the body consistent access to healing compounds. Unlike intense detoxes, which may shock the system, teas provide a steady, gentle cleanse that the body can easily handle.

Key Benefits:

- **Hydration**: Many detox teas encourage hydration, which is crucial for flushing out toxins.
- **Liver Support**: Herbs like dandelion and milk thistle are renowned for supporting liver function, helping the body process and eliminate toxins.
- **Kidney Health**: Herbs like nettle and parsley act as gentle diuretics, encouraging the kidneys to release excess water and waste.
- **Digestive Aid**: Teas with ginger or fennel aid digestion, supporting efficient waste elimination and reducing toxin buildup.

2. HERBAL DETOX TEAS

Here are a few detox teas you can prepare easily at home. Each blend has a specific function in the body, allowing you to tailor your detox routine according to your needs.

Dandelion and Burdock Root Tea

This tea is perfect for liver and blood detoxification. Both dandelion and burdock root are powerful blood purifiers and liver-supportive herbs, working to reduce inflammation and remove waste.

- **Ingredients**:
  - » 1 teaspoon dried dandelion root
  - » 1 teaspoon dried burdock root
  - » 2 cups of water
- **Instructions**:
  - » Combine the herbs in a pot with water.
  - » Bring to a boil, then reduce heat and simmer for 15–20 minutes.
  - » Strain and enjoy. Drink 1–2 cups daily for a gentle, ongoing detox.
- **Benefits**: Dandelion stimulates bile production, enhancing liver function, while burdock root cleanses the blood, reducing toxin buildup in the skin and organs. This combination helps to clear out toxins from the liver and bloodstream, supporting skin clarity and energy levels.

Nettle and Peppermint Detox Tea

This refreshing tea supports kidney function and digestion, making it ideal for those needing a gentle detox. Nettle is rich in minerals and acts as a diuretic, while peppermint soothes the digestive tract, reducing bloating and aiding nutrient absorption.

- **Ingredients**:
  - » 1 teaspoon dried nettle leaves
  - » 1 teaspoon dried peppermint leaves
  - » 1 cup of boiling water
- **Instructions**:
  - » Combine herbs in a cup and pour boiling water over them.
  - » Cover and steep for 10 minutes.
  - » Strain and drink. Enjoy 1–2 cups per day for kidney support.
- **Benefits**: Nettle promotes urination, flushing toxins out of the kidneys, while peppermint relaxes the digestive system. This tea is particularly beneficial for those who experience water retention or sluggish digestion.

Ginger and Lemon Detox Tea

Ginger and lemon are classic detoxifiers, each with its own cleansing properties. Ginger stimulates circulation and digestion, while lemon alkalizes the body and supports liver function.

- **Ingredients**:
  - » 1 inch of fresh ginger root, sliced
  - » Juice of half a lemon
  - » 2 cups of water
- **Instructions**:

- Bring water to a boil, add ginger, and simmer for 10–15 minutes.
- Strain, add lemon juice, and drink while warm.
- Enjoy 1–2 cups daily, ideally in the morning, to kick-start detoxification.

- **Benefits**: Ginger's warming properties stimulate blood flow and digestion, helping to break down toxins, while lemon provides a dose of vitamin C, which supports the liver in processing toxins. Drinking this tea in the morning can set a detoxifying tone for the day.

3. DEEP CLEANSING DECOCTIONS

Decoctions are stronger than teas, extracting more potent compounds from dense plant parts like roots and barks. They're often used in short-term detox regimens or for a deeper cleanse. Here are a few powerful decoctions that support specific detox organs.

Milk Thistle and Dandelion Root Liver Decoction

Milk thistle is one of the most revered herbs for liver health. Combined with dandelion root, this decoction provides a potent liver detox.

- **Ingredients**:
  - 1 tablespoon milk thistle seeds (crushed)
  - 1 tablespoon dried dandelion root
  - 3 cups of water
- **Instructions**:
  - Add the herbs to a pot with water and bring to a boil.
  - Reduce heat and simmer for 20–30 minutes.
  - Strain and drink 1 cup daily, storing any leftovers in the fridge.
- **Benefits**: Milk thistle contains silymarin, a compound that helps repair liver cells and protect the liver from toxins, while dandelion root promotes bile flow. This decoction is ideal for deep liver detoxification, especially after exposure to environmental pollutants or processed foods.

Burdock Root and Red Clover Blood Purifier Decoction

This blend is particularly effective for blood purification, helping to eliminate toxins that can affect the skin, energy levels, and overall health.

- **Ingredients**:
  - 1 tablespoon dried burdock root
  - 1 tablespoon dried red clover flowers
  - 3 cups of water
- **Instructions**:
  - Combine the herbs in a pot with water.
  - Bring to a boil, then reduce to a simmer for 20–25 minutes.
  - Strain and drink 1–2 cups over the course of the day. This can be stored in the refrigerator for up to two days.
- **Benefits**: Burdock root purifies the blood and reduces inflammation, while red clover aids in lymphatic drainage and cleanses the blood. This decoction supports skin clarity and can be particularly helpful for individuals experiencing fatigue, acne, or other signs of toxin buildup.

Parsley and Horsetail Kidney Cleanse Decoction

Both parsley and horsetail are excellent for supporting kidney health, as they encourage the elimination of excess water and reduce the burden on the kidneys.

- **Ingredients**:
  - 1 tablespoon fresh parsley (chopped)
  - 1 tablespoon dried horsetail
  - 3 cups of water
- **Instructions**:
  - Add parsley and horsetail to water, bring to a boil, then simmer for 15–20 minutes.
  - Strain and drink 1 cup per day, storing the rest in the refrigerator.
- **Benefits**: Parsley acts as a natural diuretic, flushing out toxins, while horsetail provides silica, which strengthens connective tissues and aids kidney function. This decoction is ideal for people with mild edema, bloating, or kidney concerns.

4. CREATING YOUR OWN DETOX ROUTINE WITH TEAS AND DECOCTIONS

Incorporating detox teas and decoctions into your routine is a simple, effective way to maintain a gentle, ongoing cleanse. Here's a sample schedule to help you get started, adapting it to fit your unique health goals:

- **Morning**: Begin with a ginger and lemon tea to stimulate digestion and wake up the liver.
- **Mid-Morning**: Have a cup of dandelion and burdock root tea to support liver health and blood purification.
- **Afternoon**: Drink a nettle and peppermint tea to support the kidneys and keep energy steady.
- **Evening**: Opt for a milk thistle and dandelion root decoction for a final dose of liver support before bed.

Adjust the schedule based on your personal needs, choosing the teas or decoctions that align with your detox goals.

5. TIPS FOR EFFECTIVE DETOX TEA AND DECOCTION USE

For the best results, follow these guidelines when using detox teas and decoctions:

- **Stay Consistent**: Consistency is key for gentle detoxification. Drinking detox teas regularly provides a steady supply of healing compounds, which can gradually eliminate toxins without overwhelming the body.
- **Listen to Your Body**: Herbs affect people differently, so pay attention to how your body responds. If you feel overly fatigued or experience digestive discomfort, reduce the quantity or frequency.
- **Hydrate**: Herbal teas can have a mild diuretic effect, so it's essential to drink plenty of water alongside detox teas to stay hydrated and facilitate toxin elimination.
- **Cycle Teas and Decoctions**: While some teas can be used daily, stronger decoctions are best taken in cycles. A common practice is to use a particular decoction for one or two weeks, then take a break before starting again.

6. INTEGRATING DETOX TEAS AND DECOCTIONS INTO DAILY LIFE

Rather than seeing detox teas and decoctions as temporary cleanses, consider them part of a holistic wellness routine. Each time you prepare and drink these teas, you're taking a small step toward better health, supporting the organs that do the hard work of detoxifying the body.

To make this a seamless part of your day:

- Set a specific time to enjoy a detox tea, whether it's a morning ritual, a post-lunch digestive aid, or an evening wind-down.
- Consider creating a weekly tea preparation session, where you make larger batches to refrigerate and drink throughout the week.

Drinking detox teas and decoctions is more than a habit; it's a practice of self-care that brings you closer to the healing power of plants. By incorporating these herbal allies into your daily life, you can provide continuous support for the organs that keep you healthy and resilient. These teas offer a gentle, natural way to maintain balance, cleanse the body, and promote long-term vitality, all in alignment with Dr. Sebi's principles of natural wellness.

CHAPTER 2
PREPARATION TECHNIQUES

The journey to effective detoxification begins with the way we prepare our herbs. Knowing how to properly prepare detox teas, decoctions, infusions, and tinctures can make a world of difference in the potency and effectiveness of these remedies. This chapter offers practical, step-by-step techniques for each preparation method, allowing you to make the most of the herbs you're using. Think of it as a guide to unlocking the full power of natural remedies, enhancing their effects, and making your detox practice more enjoyable and sustainable.

1. INFUSIONS: SIMPLE YET EFFECTIVE

Infusions are one of the easiest ways to prepare herbs, making them a great starting point for beginners. When you're working with delicate herbs, like flowers and leaves, an infusion is ideal for extracting their benefits. By pouring hot water over the herbs, you allow their natural compounds to blend into the water.

- **How to Prepare an Infusion**:
    - » Choose a glass or ceramic teapot, or a heat-safe cup.
    - » Place 1–2 teaspoons of dried herbs (or 1 tablespoon of fresh herbs) into the pot.
    - » Pour boiling water over the herbs and cover to retain the beneficial oils.
    - » Let steep for 10–15 minutes, then strain and drink while warm.
- **Best Herbs for Infusions**: Chamomile, peppermint, nettle, lemon balm, and dandelion leaf.

Infusions are ideal for daily use, allowing you to enjoy the detox benefits of herbs without any intense preparation. They're perfect for gentle cleansing and can be taken several times a day, especially when using herbs like chamomile or peppermint, which are mild yet effective.

2. DECOCTIONS: FOR DEEP AND ROBUST EXTRACTION

Decoctions are designed for harder plant parts, like roots and barks, which require a longer time to release their medicinal compounds. A decoction is essentially a "long brew," allowing tough plant material to break down and release its benefits into the water.

- **How to Prepare a Decoction**:
    - » Place 1 tablespoon of dried roots or bark in a pot with 2 cups of water.
    - » Bring to a boil, then reduce to a simmer for 20–30 minutes.
    - » Allow the decoction to cool slightly, strain, and drink warm.
- **Best Herbs for Decoctions**: Burdock root, dandelion root, ginger, milk thistle, and reishi mushroom.

Decoctions are best when you need a stronger preparation, especially for liver and kidney support. The longer simmering time ensures that the potent compounds are extracted thoroughly, making decoctions a great option for those days when you want a deeper cleanse.

3. TINCTURES: POTENT AND LONG-LASTING

Tinctures are concentrated extracts typically made with alcohol, which acts as a preservative and solvent, pulling out compounds that water cannot extract. They're particularly useful if you need a stronger dose or a portable option for daily detox support.

- **How to Prepare a Tincture**:
    - » Fill a glass jar about halfway with dried or fresh herbs.
    - » Pour alcohol (vodka or brandy, 40% alcohol by volume) over the herbs until fully submerged.
    - » Seal the jar tightly and store it in a cool, dark place for 4–6 weeks, shaking daily.
    - » After steeping, strain the herbs, bottle the liquid in a dark glass dropper bottle, and store it away from light.
- **Best Herbs for Tinctures**: Milk thistle, echinacea, burdock, and ginseng.

Tinctures are particularly potent and should be taken in small doses, usually around 20–30 drops. They're ideal for liver support and immune boosting, as they offer a quick way to ingest highly concentrated herbal benefits.

4. HERBAL VINEGARS: AN ALTERNATIVE TO ALCOHOL-BASED TINCTURES

If you prefer to avoid alcohol, herbal vinegars are a great alternative. Apple cider vinegar works well as a solvent, extracting both the water-soluble and acetic compounds from the herbs, while offering its own health benefits, like supporting digestion and pH balance.

- **How to Prepare an Herbal Vinegar**:
  - » Place dried or fresh herbs in a glass jar and fill with apple cider vinegar, ensuring the herbs are completely covered.
  - » Seal the jar and store in a dark place for 2–4 weeks, shaking occasionally.
  - » After steeping, strain the vinegar and store it in a glass bottle.
- **Best Herbs for Herbal Vinegars**: Dandelion, nettle, rosemary, and garlic.

Herbal vinegars can be used in salad dressings, added to water, or taken by the teaspoon as part of a detox regimen. They provide a gentle detox effect while also helping to support digestion.

5. POWDERS AND CAPSULES: CONVENIENT FOR ON-THE-GO

Powdered herbs can be mixed into smoothies, water, or juices for a convenient, quick way to ingest detoxifying herbs. Capsules are also an excellent option for busy days when you may not have time to prepare a tea or decoction.

- **Using Powdered Herbs**:
  - » Add 1/2–1 teaspoon of powdered herb to a smoothie, water, or juice, stirring well.
  - » For digestive ease, pair powdered herbs with a meal or blend with fibrous ingredients.
- **Using Capsules**: Capsules are typically pre-dosed, making them easy to take on a consistent schedule. Follow recommended dosages on the bottle, as dosages vary by herb.
- **Best Herbs for Powders and Capsules**: Sea moss, spirulina, chlorella, and ginger.

Powders and capsules are particularly useful for those looking to add detoxifying greens to their diet, as they're easy to mix and offer a high dose of nutrients.

CHAPTER 3
USING REMEDIES FOR REGULAR DETOX

Regular detoxification doesn't have to be a major event; it can be a gentle, daily practice that aligns with the body's natural rhythms. When we incorporate herbs and other natural detox aids into our daily lives, we provide ongoing support for our liver, kidneys, and digestive system, making it easier for the body to process and eliminate toxins. This chapter will walk you through a step-by-step approach to creating a regular detox routine, showing you how to use herbal teas, decoctions, and supplements in a way that's sustainable and manageable.

1. WHY REGULAR DETOXIFICATION MATTERS

Our bodies are constantly exposed to pollutants, processed foods, and environmental toxins that can accumulate over time. Regular detoxification supports the body's natural cleansing processes, giving a boost to organs like the liver, kidneys, and lymphatic system. By integrating gentle detox practices into daily life, you're helping your body stay balanced and resilient.

Key Benefits of Regular Detoxification:

- **Improved Digestion and Nutrient Absorption**: Detoxifying the digestive system can lead to better digestion and absorption of nutrients, which in turn supports energy and immunity.
- **Enhanced Skin Health**: Regular detoxification supports clearer skin by addressing toxins that may lead to skin issues like acne or inflammation.
- **Balanced Energy Levels**: A steady detox routine can help maintain stable energy levels by preventing toxin buildup, which often contributes to fatigue.

2. DESIGNING YOUR DAILY DETOX ROUTINE

A regular detox routine doesn't need to be complicated. By setting aside a few minutes each day to prepare herbal teas, powders, or tinctures, you can create a detox plan that's easy to follow and fits seamlessly into your lifestyle.

Sample Daily Detox Schedule:

- **Morning**: Start with a warm lemon and ginger tea or an infusion of nettle for kidney support and hydration.
- **Mid-Morning**: Add a dropperful of a liver-supporting tincture like milk thistle to water for a gentle liver cleanse.
- **Afternoon**: Blend chlorella or spirulina powder into a smoothie to add a dose of greens that aid detoxification.
- **Evening**: Sip on a burdock root and dandelion tea to support digestion and blood cleansing overnight.

You can adjust this routine based on your own preferences, using herbs that target the organs you feel need the most support.

3. WEEKLY DETOX BOOSTERS

In addition to a daily routine, adding a weekly detox boost can be particularly beneficial. For instance, choosing one day each week to focus on deeper detox practices, like a stronger decoction or a 24-hour herbal tea cleanse, can provide an extra layer of support.

Sample Weekly Detox Booster:

- **Detox Day**: Choose a day each week to focus on cleansing. You might start with a large pot of burdock root and dandelion decoction, sipping on it throughout the day. For meals, focus on light, plant-based foods that are easy to digest.

By committing to a weekly detox booster, you give your body a consistent opportunity to release built-up toxins and reset, reinforcing the benefits of your daily detox practices.

4. SEASONAL DETOX RITUALS

Our bodies often go through natural cycles with the changing seasons, and supporting these cycles with seasonal detox practices can enhance health and balance. A seasonal detox doesn't need to be restrictive; instead, it's about aligning with the body's needs during different times of the year.

Spring and Fall Detox Suggestions:

- **Spring**: Focus on liver-supporting herbs, like dandelion and milk thistle, to prepare the body for increased energy and renewal. Consider a week of liver-supporting teas and light, fresh meals.
- **Fall**: Emphasize immune-boosting herbs, like elderberry and echinacea, while supporting lung health with mullein or thyme. Incorporate warming teas to prepare the body for colder months.

Each season presents an opportunity to fine-tune your detox routine, ensuring that your body has the support it needs to transition smoothly.

5. TIPS FOR SUCCESS IN REGULAR DETOXIFICATION

To keep your detox routine effective and sustainable, it's important to establish habits that align with your lifestyle. Here are some tips to ensure success in regular detoxification:

- **Listen to Your Body**: Every person's detox needs are unique, so observe how you feel and adjust your routine accordingly.
- **Stay Hydrated**: Herbal teas and detox practices can have diuretic effects, so drinking enough water helps flush out toxins and keeps the body balanced.
- **Incorporate Movement**: Physical activity, like yoga or a brisk walk, helps stimulate lymphatic drainage and supports the body's detox processes.
- **Limit Processed Foods**: By reducing processed foods and incorporating whole, plant-based options, you enhance the benefits of your detox routine.

6. AVOIDING DETOX PITFALLS

While regular detox practices are beneficial, there are a few pitfalls to watch for. Over-detoxing or using overly strong preparations too often can stress the body, so it's important to keep your routine gentle and consistent.

- **Avoid Excessive Use of Strong Decoctions**: Decoctions are potent, and daily use of strong decoctions can strain the body. Reserve stronger preparations for weekly or monthly detox boosts.
- **Don't Overdo Diuretics**: While diuretic herbs are helpful, using them in excess can lead to dehydration. Balance diuretic teas with plenty of water or hydrating herbal teas.

Regular detoxification is a gentle way to keep your body's systems functioning optimally, creating a foundation for resilience and wellness. By integrating these practices into your daily life, you're supporting long-term health in a way that's sustainable and deeply aligned with Dr. Sebi's philosophy.

BOOK 10
Herbal Remedies for Common Conditions

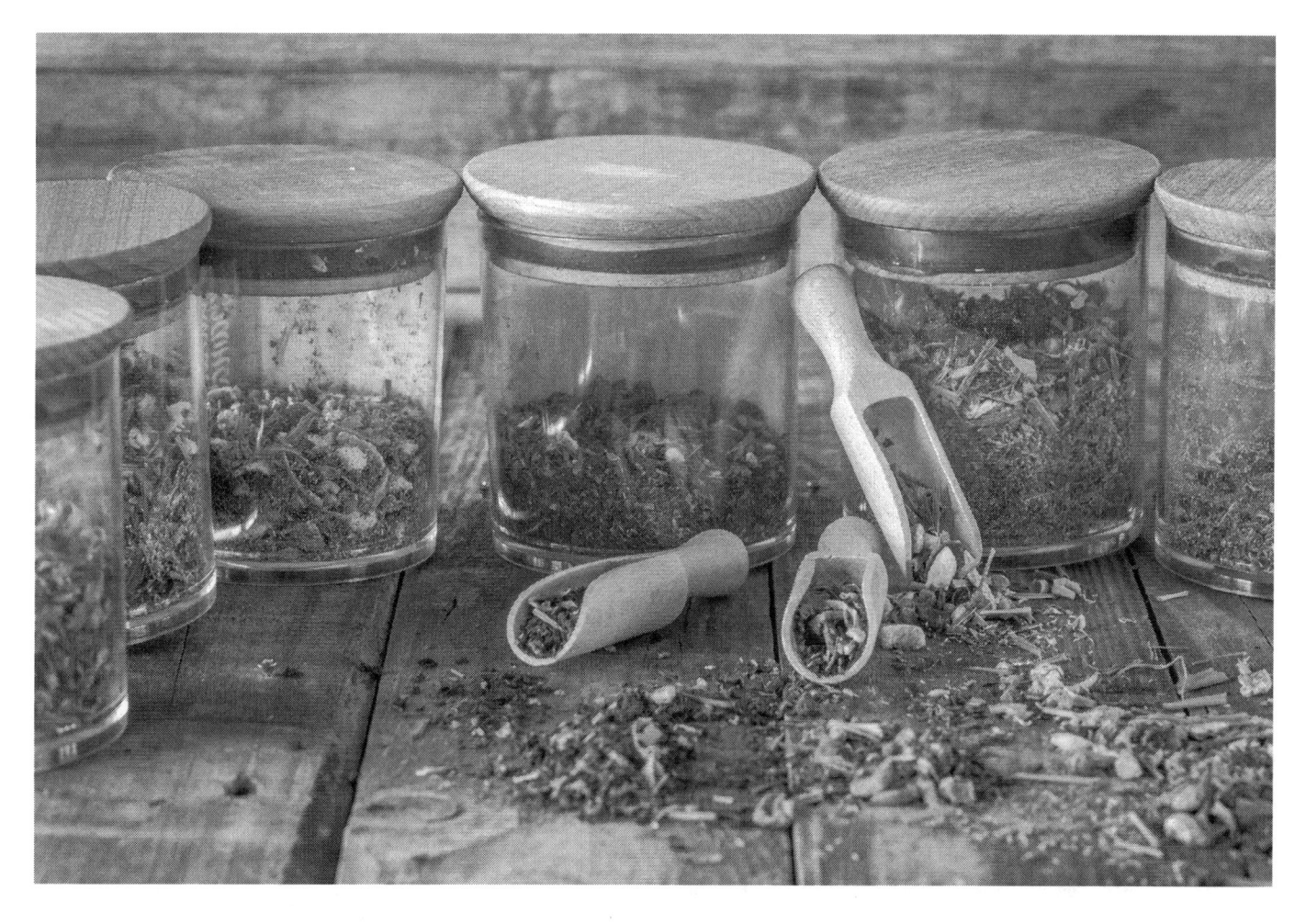

In Dr. Sebi's philosophy, healing often begins with nature's simplest remedies. Herbal blends offer a powerful yet gentle way to address everyday health issues, providing relief and support through carefully chosen combinations of herbs. This book explores the art of creating herbal blends for common conditions, from respiratory issues and digestive discomfort to stress relief and immune support. By learning how to make your own blends, you gain the flexibility to personalize your remedies, adjusting them to meet your unique needs.

CHAPTER 1
CREATING HEALING BLENDS

Creating healing blends is a deeply personal and rewarding process. Each blend brings together the properties of various herbs, allowing them to work in harmony to support the body. In this chapter, we'll dive into the essentials of blending herbs effectively, covering the basics of choosing herbs, balancing flavors, and preparing remedies for specific health concerns. With this knowledge, you can start crafting herbal blends that not only meet your needs but also provide a nurturing experience, inviting you to engage with the healing process in a holistic way.

1. THE ART OF SELECTING HERBS

Choosing the right herbs is the first step in creating effective healing blends. Each herb has unique properties that can address different aspects of health. When selecting herbs for a blend, it's essential to consider both the primary health concern and any supportive actions the blend should provide.

- **Identify the Primary Issue**: Begin by identifying the main health concern. For example, if you're creating a blend for respiratory health, your primary herbs might include mullein, thyme, and eucalyptus, which directly support lung function.
- **Choose Supporting Herbs**: Once you've identified your primary herbs, select additional herbs that support the body's overall wellness. For instance, licorice root may be added to a respiratory blend as it soothes irritation and adds sweetness, enhancing the blend's effectiveness and taste.
- **Consider Individual Properties**: Some herbs, like ginger, have warming properties, while others, like peppermint, are cooling. Balancing these properties ensures the blend is both effective and gentle on the body.

2. BASIC BLENDING TECHNIQUES

Creating an herbal blend is similar to crafting a balanced meal. You want a combination of primary herbs that address the main concern, secondary herbs to support those effects, and optional herbs for flavor and balance. Here's a look at some basic techniques to help you create effective and enjoyable blends.

- **The 3-3-1 Rule**: A simple rule to follow is the 3-3-1 ratio: three parts of a primary herb, three parts of a supportive herb, and one part of a flavoring or balancing herb. This structure creates a well-rounded blend that's easy to adjust for different conditions.
  - » **Example**: For an immune-boosting tea, you might use three parts echinacea (primary), three parts elderberry (supportive), and one part ginger (balancing and warming).
- **Balancing Flavors**: Taste is a key part of herbal blending. Bitter herbs, like dandelion, are highly beneficial but may need a sweeter or spicier herb, like licorice or cinnamon, to balance the flavor. Blending herbs that vary in flavor makes your remedy enjoyable and more likely to be used consistently.
- **Creating Synergy**: Synergy refers to the way herbs enhance each other's effects when combined. For instance, chamomile and lemon balm both have calming properties, but when blended, they create a more potent remedy for relaxation than either herb alone.

3. CRAFTING HEALING BLENDS FOR COMMON CONDITIONS

Now that we've covered the basics of selecting and balancing herbs, let's look at specific blends for common conditions. Each of these blends is designed to address a particular health issue, using Dr. Sebi's principles of natural healing.

Respiratory Support Blend

This blend helps open the airways, reduce inflammation, and support the respiratory system. It's perfect for cold and flu season or for people dealing with respiratory issues, such as asthma or seasonal allergies.

- **Ingredients**:
  - » 3 parts mullein (primary, to open airways)
  - » 3 parts thyme (supportive, to reduce mucus)
  - » 1 part licorice root (balancing, to soothe irritation)
- **Preparation**:
  - » Mix the herbs and store them in an airtight jar.
  - » Use 1 tablespoon of the blend per cup of hot water. Steep for 10–15 minutes, then strain and drink. Take 1–2 cups daily when respiratory support is needed.
- **How It Works**: Mullein supports lung health by opening the airways and soothing the respiratory tract, while thyme is a natural antimicrobial that helps break down mucus. Licorice root adds a sweet flavor and soothes the throat, reducing irritation.

Digestive Ease Blend

Designed to ease bloating, gas, and mild digestive discomfort, this blend combines warming and soothing herbs to support healthy digestion.

- **Ingredients**:
  - » 3 parts peppermint (primary, for soothing digestion)
  - » 3 parts fennel seeds (supportive, to reduce gas)
  - » 1 part ginger (balancing, to stimulate digestion)
- **Preparation**:
  - » Combine the herbs and store in an airtight container.
  - » Use 1 teaspoon per cup of hot water, steeping for 5–10 minutes. Drink before or after meals to support digestion.
- **How It Works**: Peppermint relaxes the digestive tract, reducing bloating, while fennel seeds relieve gas and promote smooth digestion. Ginger stimulates digestive enzymes, making this blend effective for a variety of digestive complaints.

Calming Blend for Stress and Anxiety

This soothing blend is ideal for winding down in the evening or anytime you need relief from stress. It combines calming herbs that support the nervous system and promote relaxation.

- **Ingredients**:
  - » 3 parts chamomile (primary, for calming effects)
  - » 3 parts lemon balm (supportive, to relieve anxiety)
  - » 1 part lavender (balancing, to enhance relaxation)
- **Preparation**:
  - » Blend the herbs and store in a sealed container.
  - » Use 1 tablespoon of the blend per cup of hot water. Steep for 10 minutes, strain, and drink in the evening or whenever stress relief is needed.
- **How It Works**: Chamomile gently calms the nerves, while lemon balm relieves anxiety and tension. Lavender adds a pleasant aroma and enhances relaxation, making this blend a perfect choice for unwinding.

Immune Booster Blend

Strengthening the immune system is crucial, especially during cold and flu season. This blend combines immune-boosting and antiviral herbs to support the body's natural defenses.

- **Ingredients**:
  - » 3 parts echinacea (primary, for immune support)
  - » 3 parts elderberry (supportive, with antiviral properties)
  - » 1 part ginger (balancing, for warming and enhancing immunity)
- **Preparation**:
  - » Combine herbs and store in an airtight jar.
  - » Use 1 tablespoon per cup of boiling water, steeping for 15 minutes. Drink 1–2 cups daily during flu season or at the onset of cold symptoms.
- **How It Works**: Echinacea strengthens immune response, while elderberry has antiviral properties, helping to fight off infections. Ginger's warming effect supports circulation, making the immune-boosting properties of the other herbs more effective.

Sleep and Relaxation Blend

If you have trouble falling or staying asleep, this blend is designed to relax the nervous system and promote restful sleep without any groggy side effects.

- **Ingredients**:
  - » 3 parts valerian root (primary, for sleep support)
  - » 3 parts passionflower (supportive, to calm the mind)
  - » 1 part chamomile (balancing, to ease tension)
- **Preparation**:
  - » Blend the herbs and store in a container.
  - » Use 1 tablespoon of the mix per cup of hot water, steeping for 10 minutes. Drink 30 minutes before bed.
- **How It Works**: Valerian root is a natural sedative, helping to induce sleep, while passionflower calms the mind and reduces anxiety. Chamomile eases tension, making this blend effective for those who struggle to relax before bedtime.

Energy-Boosting Blend

This blend is ideal for a natural energy lift without the jitters of caffeine. It combines adaptogenic and energizing herbs to improve focus and mental clarity.

- **Ingredients**:
  - » 3 parts ginseng (primary, for energy and endurance)
  - » 3 parts rosemary (supportive, for mental clarity)
  - » 1 part peppermint (balancing, to refresh and revitalize)
- **Preparation**:
  - » Mix herbs and store in an airtight jar.
  - » Use 1 tablespoon per cup of hot water, steep for 10 minutes, and drink in the morning or early afternoon.
- **How It Works**: Ginseng provides sustained energy and supports adrenal health, rosemary improves focus and memory, and peppermint adds a refreshing taste and enhances alertness.

4. CUSTOMIZING BLENDS FOR INDIVIDUAL NEEDS

Creating your own blends allows you to customize each remedy based on your unique needs and preferences. For example, if you find certain herbs too strong, you can reduce their amounts or add a sweeter herb, like licorice, to balance the flavor.

- **Experiment with Ratios**: The 3-3-1 rule is a guideline, but you can adjust the ratios based on your preferences. If you prefer a stronger flavor, increase the primary herb; for a gentler effect, add more of the balancing herb.
- **Adjust Based on Season**: In colder months, add warming herbs like ginger or cinnamon to your blends, while in warmer months, consider cooling herbs like peppermint or hibiscus.
- **Track Your Responses**: Keep a health journal to note how each blend makes you feel, adjusting recipes as needed to match your body's responses.

5. STORING AND USING YOUR HEALING BLENDS

Storing your blends properly helps maintain their potency and freshness. Use airtight containers, preferably glass jars, and keep them in a cool, dark place. Label each jar with the date and name of the blend so you can track freshness.

- **Shelf Life**: Most dried herbal blends will stay fresh for 6–12 months if stored correctly. However, potency decreases over time, so it's best to make smaller batches and use them within six months.
- **Daily Use**: Incorporate your healing blends into your daily routine. For example, an immune-boosting tea can become part of your morning ritual, while a sleep blend may be your go-to for winding down at night.

6. CREATING RITUALS WITH HEALING BLENDS

Using herbal blends goes beyond physical health—it can also be a calming ritual that centers the mind. Take a moment each day to prepare your blend mindfully, setting an intention for healing and well-being.

- **Make It Personal**: Add a favorite mug or candle to your tea ritual, creating a comforting atmosphere that enhances the effects of the herbs.
- **Practice Gratitude**: As you blend and drink your teas, reflect on the healing properties of each herb, and consider the benefits they bring to your life.

Creating healing blends empowers you to take charge of your wellness. With the knowledge of herbs and their properties, you can craft remedies that provide natural relief and nurturing support, aligning with Dr. Sebi's vision of a plant-based approach to health. By developing a personal routine with these blends, you're setting the foundation for a lifestyle that honors nature's healing power and cultivates lasting vitality.

CHAPTER 2

HERBAL SOLUTIONS FOR EVERYDAY ILLNESSES

Each remedy in this chapter is crafted to address a specific health issue, using herbs that align with Dr. Sebi's philosophy. These natural solutions are gentle yet effective, providing relief without the side effects associated with many conventional treatments. Let's explore these ten herbal remedies for common ailments, from respiratory issues to stress.

1. COLD AND FLU RELIEF TEA

Colds and flu can leave you feeling congested and fatigued. This soothing tea combines elderberry, echinacea, and ginger to boost immunity and ease symptoms.

- **Ingredients**:
  - » 1 teaspoon dried elderberries
  - » 1 teaspoon dried echinacea
  - » 1/2 teaspoon grated ginger
  - » 1 cup boiling water
- **Instructions**:
  - » Combine the herbs in a mug and pour boiling water over them.
  - » Cover and steep for 10–15 minutes.
  - » Strain and drink up to three times daily during cold or flu symptoms.
- **How It Works**: Elderberry and echinacea are powerful immune boosters with antiviral properties, while ginger warms the body and improves circulation, helping to relieve congestion and reduce inflammation.

2. HEADACHE SOOTHING TEA

For headaches due to tension or mild stress, this tea with peppermint, chamomile, and lavender can provide natural relief. It's a calming blend that relaxes the mind and eases muscle tension.

- **Ingredients**:
  - » 1 teaspoon dried peppermint
  - » 1 teaspoon dried chamomile
  - » 1/2 teaspoon dried lavender
- **Instructions**:
  - » Combine the herbs in a cup and add boiling water.
  - » Cover and let steep for 10 minutes.
  - » Strain and sip slowly, breathing deeply.
- **How It Works**: Peppermint relaxes muscles and improves blood flow, chamomile calms the nervous system, and lavender promotes relaxation, reducing stress-related headaches.

3. DIGESTIVE AID TEA FOR BLOATING AND GAS

This tea, with fennel, ginger, and peppermint, is designed to reduce bloating, gas, and mild digestive discomfort. It's best taken after meals to support smooth digestion.

- **Ingredients**:
  - » 1 teaspoon fennel seeds
  - » 1/2 teaspoon grated fresh ginger
  - » 1 teaspoon dried peppermint
- **Instructions**:
  - » Place the herbs in a pot, cover with boiling water, and steep for 10 minutes.
  - » Strain and drink after meals.
- **How It Works**: Fennel helps relax the digestive tract and reduce gas, while ginger stimulates digestive enzymes and peppermint soothes the stomach, relieving bloating and aiding digestion.

4. IMMUNE-BOOSTING ELDERBERRY SYRUP

This elderberry syrup can be taken daily during cold and flu season to strengthen immunity or at the first sign of illness to shorten recovery time.

- **Ingredients**:
  - » 1 cup dried elderberries
  - » 1 tablespoon grated ginger
  - » 1 cinnamon stick
  - » 3 cups water
  - » 1/2 cup raw honey (optional)
- **Instructions**:
  - » Combine elderberries, ginger, and cinnamon with water in a saucepan.
  - » Bring to a boil, then simmer for 30 minutes.
  - » Strain, let cool, and stir in honey. Store in a glass jar in the fridge.
  - » Take 1 tablespoon daily for immune support or 3 times daily when sick.
- **How It Works**: Elderberries are packed with antioxidants

and vitamins that support immune function, ginger improves circulation, and cinnamon adds warmth, enhancing the immune system's response.

5. SORE THROAT GARGLE WITH SAGE AND SALT

This simple gargle helps soothe a sore throat with the antibacterial properties of sage and the cleansing effect of salt.

- **Ingredients:**
    - » 1 teaspoon dried sage leaves
    - » 1/2 teaspoon sea salt
    - » 1 cup boiling water
- **Instructions:**
    - » Combine sage and salt in a cup, add boiling water, and let cool slightly.
    - » Gargle with the mixture for 30 seconds, then spit it out.
    - » Repeat 2–3 times daily as needed.
- **How It Works:** Sage has antimicrobial properties that help kill germs in the throat, while salt cleanses and reduces inflammation, providing relief for sore throats.

6. NATURAL SLEEP AID TEA

For a restful night, this blend of valerian root, chamomile, and lemon balm promotes relaxation and helps calm the mind for sleep.

- **Ingredients:**
    - » 1 teaspoon dried valerian root
    - » 1 teaspoon dried chamomile
    - » 1 teaspoon dried lemon balm
- **Instructions:**
    - » Add the herbs to a cup, pour boiling water over them, and cover.
    - » Let steep for 10–15 minutes, strain, and drink 30 minutes before bed.
- **How It Works:** Valerian root is a natural sedative, while chamomile and lemon balm relax the mind, helping to ease anxiety and promote deeper, more restful sleep.

7. ALLERGY RELIEF TEA WITH NETTLE AND PEPPERMINT

Nettle and peppermint are a powerful combination for reducing seasonal allergy symptoms. This tea can help reduce inflammation, clear sinuses, and relieve itchiness.

- **Ingredients:**
    - » 1 teaspoon dried nettle
    - » 1 teaspoon dried peppermint
    - » 1 cup boiling water
- **Instructions:**
    - » Combine the herbs in a cup and cover with boiling water.
    - » Steep for 10 minutes, strain, and drink twice daily during allergy season.
- **How It Works:** Nettle acts as a natural antihistamine, reducing allergic reactions, while peppermint opens the sinuses and provides relief from congestion and itchiness.

8. SKIN-CLEARING TEA FOR ACNE

For clearer skin, this tea combines burdock root, dandelion root, and red clover, which work together to purify the blood and support skin health.

- **Ingredients:**
    - » 1 teaspoon burdock root
    - » 1 teaspoon dandelion root
    - » 1 teaspoon red clover
- **Instructions:**
    - » Place the herbs in a pot with 2 cups of water, bring to a boil, and simmer for 15 minutes.
    - » Strain and drink 1–2 cups daily for clearer skin.
- **How It Works:** Burdock root purifies the blood and reduces inflammation, while dandelion supports liver detoxification, and red clover aids in cleansing the skin, reducing acne and other skin issues.

9. MUSCLE SOOTHING BATH FOR PAIN RELIEF

This herbal bath is ideal for easing muscle pain and soreness. It uses arnica, chamomile, and Epsom salts to relax muscles, reduce inflammation, and promote recovery.

- **Ingredients:**
    - » 1 tablespoon dried arnica flowers
    - » 1 tablespoon dried chamomile
    - » 1/2 cup Epsom salts
- **Instructions:**
    - » Place the arnica and chamomile in a cloth bag or tea infuser, and add to a warm bath along with Epsom salts.
    - » Soak for at least 20 minutes to allow the herbs to relieve soreness and tension.
- **How It Works:** Arnica reduces inflammation and pain in

muscles, chamomile provides relaxation, and Epsom salts add magnesium, which helps relieve cramps and soreness.

10. ENERGY-BOOSTING SMOOTHIE WITH SEA MOSS AND SPIRULINA

This smoothie is perfect for natural energy support, providing essential minerals and nutrients that boost vitality without caffeine.

- **Ingredients**:
  - 1 tablespoon sea moss gel
  - 1 teaspoon spirulina powder
  - 1/2 cup spinach
  - 1 cup coconut water or almond milk
  - 1/2 cup mixed berries
- **Instructions**:
  - Blend all ingredients until smooth.
  - Enjoy as a morning or midday energy boost.
- **How It Works**: Sea moss provides a range of minerals, including iodine and potassium, which support thyroid health and energy. Spirulina offers plant-based protein and antioxidants, while spinach and berries add fiber and vitamins for sustained vitality.

These herbal remedies bring the healing power of plants into your daily routine, offering natural, effective relief for common conditions. Each blend is carefully crafted to support specific body systems and align with the body's natural healing processes. With these easy-to-make remedies, you can embrace a holistic approach to wellness and find gentle yet powerful solutions for everyday health challenges.

CHAPTER 3
DR. SEBI'S FAVORITE REMEDIES

These five remedies represent Dr. Sebi's core healing philosophy. They address a range of health concerns, from cleansing the body and strengthening immunity to restoring vital nutrients. Each remedy can be easily prepared and incorporated into your daily routine, offering a gentle yet effective way to support your wellness journey.

1. IRON-RICH TONIC FOR VITALITY AND ENERGY

One of Dr. Sebi's cornerstone teachings was the importance of bioavailable iron for energy and cellular health. This tonic combines iron-rich herbs that support blood health and increase vitality, making it ideal for those feeling fatigued or depleted.

- **Ingredients**:
  - 1 tablespoon dried sarsaparilla root
  - 1 tablespoon burdock root
  - 1 tablespoon yellow dock root
  - 3 cups water
- **Instructions**:
  - Place the roots in a pot with water, bring to a boil, then reduce to a simmer for 20–30 minutes.
  - Strain and drink 1 cup per day. Store any remaining tonic in the refrigerator for up to three days.
- **How It Works**: Sarsaparilla, burdock, and yellow dock are high in bioavailable iron and other essential minerals, supporting blood health and energy production. This tonic enhances oxygen transport in the blood, making it a go-to remedy for sustained energy and overall vitality.

2. SEA MOSS AND BLADDERWRACK MINERAL BOOST

Dr. Sebi frequently recommended sea moss and bladderwrack as a powerful combination to replenish the body with essential minerals. This blend provides over 90 trace minerals, making it an excellent daily tonic for cellular health and immunity.

- **Ingredients**:
  - 1 tablespoon dried sea moss
  - 1 tablespoon dried bladderwrack
  - 2 cups water
- **Instructions**:
  - Soak sea moss and bladderwrack in water for 1–2 hours.
  - After soaking, blend with fresh water until smooth. If you prefer, simmer the mixture for 10 minutes before blending.
  - Take 1–2 tablespoons daily, either alone or added to smoothies.
- **How It Works**: Sea moss and bladderwrack contain iodine, potassium, calcium, and other essential minerals that support thyroid health, immunity, and overall cellular function. This remedy helps maintain electrolyte balance, which is key for energy and resilience.

3. DETOXIFYING BURDOCK AND DANDELION ROOT TEA

Burdock and dandelion root tea is one of Dr. Sebi's preferred remedies for detoxifying the liver and blood. This tea acts as a gentle cleanse, supporting the body's natural elimination processes and helping to reduce the toxin load on organs.

- **Ingredients**:
  - 1 teaspoon dried burdock root
  - 1 teaspoon dried dandelion root
  - 2 cups water
- **Instructions**:
  - Add the herbs to a pot with water and bring to a boil.
  - Reduce the heat and simmer for 15–20 minutes, then strain.
  - Drink 1 cup daily, either in the morning or evening, to support ongoing detoxification.
- **How It Works**: Burdock root cleanses the blood by removing impurities, while dandelion root supports liver function and bile production. Together, they provide a full-body detox that aids digestion, clears the skin, and promotes better energy levels by reducing toxin buildup.

4. IMMUNE-SUPPORTING ELDERBERRY AND ECHINACEA SYRUP

Dr. Sebi was a proponent of natural immunity, and elderberry and echinacea were two herbs he frequently recommended for strengthening the immune system. This syrup is ideal for taking during cold and flu season or at the onset of symptoms.

- **Ingredients**:
  - 1 cup dried elderberries
  - 1 tablespoon dried echinacea
  - 2 cups water
  - 1/2 cup raw honey (optional, for sweetness)
- **Instructions**:
  - In a saucepan, combine elderberries, echinacea, and water.
  - Bring to a boil, then reduce heat and simmer for 30–40 minutes.
  - Strain and let cool, then add honey if desired. Store in a glass jar in the refrigerator for up to two weeks.
  - Take 1 tablespoon daily for immune support or 3 times daily at the first sign of illness.
- **How It Works**: Elderberries are rich in antioxidants and vitamin C, providing a natural defense against infections, while echinacea boosts immune cell activity, helping the body ward off viruses and bacteria. This syrup can reduce the severity and duration of colds and flu, making it a staple for seasonal health.

5. HERBAL LAXATIVE FOR DIGESTIVE HEALTH

Dr. Sebi emphasized the importance of regular bowel movements for overall health and detoxification. This gentle herbal laxative blend combines cascara sagrada, senna, and licorice root to promote regularity without harsh effects.

- **Ingredients**:
  - 1/2 teaspoon cascara sagrada bark
  - 1/2 teaspoon senna leaves
  - 1/2 teaspoon licorice root
- **Instructions**:
  - Place herbs in a cup and cover with boiling water.
  - Steep for 10 minutes, then strain and sip slowly. Drink only once a day and not for more than a week at a time.
- **How It Works**: Cascara sagrada and senna are natural laxatives that encourage gentle bowel movements, while licorice root soothes the digestive tract. This blend helps the body eliminate waste effectively, reducing the buildup of toxins that can occur with constipation.

INCORPORATING DR. SEBI'S FAVORITE REMEDIES INTO DAILY LIFE

These remedies can be rotated or used as needed, depending on your health goals. Here are a few tips for making them a regular part of your wellness routine:

- **Morning Start**: Begin your day with a cup of burdock and dandelion tea or the iron-rich tonic to support energy and detoxification.
- **Immune Boost**: Keep a batch of elderberry and echinacea syrup in the refrigerator during cold and flu season, taking it daily as a preventive measure.
- **Daily Mineral Support**: Add a spoonful of sea moss and bladderwrack to your morning smoothie to ensure your body is getting essential minerals.
- **Gentle Detox**: Use the herbal laxative blend once a week or as needed to support digestive health, ensuring your body can eliminate waste efficiently.

Dr. Sebi's favorite remedies offer a simple, effective approach to everyday health concerns. By incorporating these natural solutions into your life, you're aligning with a philosophy that prioritizes cellular health, balance, and the body's natural ability to heal itself. These remedies empower you to take charge of your wellness journey, using nature's gifts to restore and maintain vitality.

BOOK 11
Cultivating Your Own Healing Herbs

Dr. Sebi's philosophy promotes a lifestyle grounded in nature and self-sufficiency. One of the best ways to embody this approach is by growing your own herbs. Cultivating alkaline herbs at home not only brings you closer to the healing process but also ensures a fresh, reliable source of herbs for teas, remedies, and everyday use. This book introduces you to the basics of growing your own healing herbs, including choosing the right plants, setting up your garden, and harvesting with care.

CHAPTER 1
GROWING ALKALINE HERBS

Growing alkaline herbs at home can be a deeply rewarding practice. Many of the herbs Dr. Sebi recommended, such as dandelion, burdock, and nettle, are resilient and relatively easy to grow with the right care. Whether you have a large garden or a small indoor space, you can cultivate a variety of healing herbs that align with Dr. Sebi's principles. This chapter covers the essentials of growing alkaline herbs, offering practical advice on how to create a thriving herb garden tailored to your space and lifestyle.

1. SELECTING ALKALINE HERBS FOR YOUR GARDEN

The first step in creating an alkaline herb garden is selecting the herbs you want to grow. Dr. Sebi often emphasized herbs that support detoxification, immunity, and cellular health. When choosing your herbs, consider their medicinal properties as well as their compatibility with your growing environment.

- **Key Alkaline Herbs to Grow**:
  - **Dandelion**: Known for its liver-detoxifying properties, dandelion is easy to grow and can be used for teas and salads.
  - **Burdock**: Another powerful detoxifier, burdock root is excellent for supporting skin health and blood purification.
  - **Nettle**: Rich in iron and minerals, nettle is valuable for energy and cellular health.
  - **Lemon Balm**: A calming herb, lemon balm supports relaxation and is also suitable for teas and tinctures.
  - **Chamomile**: This gentle, calming herb supports digestion and sleep and is ideal for herbal teas.

These herbs thrive in various conditions and can be grown in containers, garden beds, or even indoors, making them versatile choices for any space.

2. SETTING UP YOUR ALKALINE HERB GARDEN

Creating an alkaline herb garden starts with choosing the right location, soil, and containers for your plants. Herbs generally require plenty of sunlight, good drainage, and nutrient-rich soil, so setting up the garden with these elements in mind will ensure your herbs grow strong and healthy.

- **Choosing the Right Location**:
  - Most herbs thrive in full sunlight, requiring about 6–8 hours of sun each day. Choose a south-facing window or an outdoor space that gets ample light.
  - For indoor growers, consider using a grow light to supplement natural light, especially in lower-light seasons.
- **Soil and pH Requirements**:
  - Alkaline herbs prefer well-draining soil with a slightly alkaline pH. You can create an ideal growing medium by mixing organic potting soil with compost and a bit of sand or perlite for drainage.
  - Test the pH of your soil with a simple soil pH test kit. For alkaline herbs, a pH of around 7.0 to 7.5 is ideal.
- **Containers and Garden Beds**:
  - Herbs grow well in containers as long as they have good drainage. Choose pots with drainage holes and place a layer of pebbles or stones at the bottom to prevent waterlogging.
  - If you're growing in a garden bed, ensure it's slightly elevated or well-drained to avoid soggy soil.
- **Mulching for Moisture Retention**:
  - Applying a thin layer of mulch around your herbs helps retain soil moisture and keeps roots cool, which is especially beneficial during hot seasons.

3. PLANTING ALKALINE HERBS: SEEDS VS. SEEDLINGS

Planting alkaline herbs can be done from seeds or seedlings, depending on the herb and your experience level. Starting from seeds can be more economical and rewarding, but seedlings offer a quicker, easier start.

- **Growing from Seeds**:
  - Many herbs, such as basil and dandelion, can be easily started from seeds. Sow the seeds according to the instructions on the packet, typically about 1/4 inch deep in moist soil.
  - Keep the soil consistently moist until seedlings emerge, then reduce watering slightly to prevent root rot.
- **Using Seedlings**:
  - Seedlings, or young plants, are available at nurseries and provide a head start, especially for herbs like nettle and burdock, which can take longer to mature.
  - When transplanting seedlings, dig a hole slightly

larger than the root ball, place the seedling in the hole, and fill in with soil. Water immediately to help the roots establish.
- **Spacing and Companion Planting**:
  » Herbs need space to grow, so avoid overcrowding. Place herbs like dandelion and burdock 12–18 inches apart to allow root expansion.
  » Consider companion planting by placing herbs that grow well together, such as chamomile and basil, in the same area. Companion planting can enhance growth and deter pests.

4. CARING FOR YOUR ALKALINE HERBS

Once your herbs are planted, regular care will help them thrive. Alkaline herbs are relatively low-maintenance, but they still require attention to watering, pruning, and pest control to stay healthy.

- **Watering Tips**:
  » Herbs generally prefer to dry out slightly between waterings. Water deeply once the top inch of soil feels dry.
  » Use a watering can with a fine spout to avoid splashing soil on the leaves, which can lead to fungal growth.
- **Pruning for Health and Growth**:
  » Pruning encourages new growth and prevents herbs from becoming too woody. Regularly trim leaves and stems, especially for herbs like basil and chamomile.
  » Pinch off the top leaves and flowers to promote bushier growth and prevent the plant from going to seed too soon.
- **Natural Pest Control**:
  » Herbs are usually resistant to pests, but aphids, spider mites, and caterpillars can sometimes be a problem. Spray plants with a natural solution of water and mild soap to deter pests.
  » You can also use companion plants like marigolds, which deter insects and promote a balanced garden environment.

5. HARVESTING ALKALINE HERBS

Harvesting is one of the most enjoyable parts of growing your own herbs. Knowing when and how to harvest ensures you get the highest potency and flavor from your plants.

- **When to Harvest**:
  » For leafy herbs like basil and lemon balm, harvest before the plant flowers, as this is when the leaves are most potent.
  » Root herbs, such as burdock and dandelion, are best harvested in the fall after the plant has stored nutrients in the roots.
- **How to Harvest**:
  » Use sharp scissors or garden shears to cut stems cleanly, which minimizes damage to the plant.
  » Harvest in the morning, after the dew has dried but before the sun is too intense. This preserves the essential oils in the herbs, enhancing flavor and potency.
- **Harvesting for Continuous Growth**:
  » For herbs like chamomile and basil, only harvest up to one-third of the plant at a time. This ensures the plant continues to grow and produce leaves for future harvests.

6. DRYING AND STORING YOUR HERBS

To extend the life of your harvest, drying and storing your herbs allows you to keep them on hand for teas, remedies, and cooking. Proper drying preserves the potency and flavor of the herbs, ensuring you have a consistent supply throughout the year.

- **Drying Herbs**:
  » Gather herbs in small bundles and hang them upside down in a warm, dry, and dark area. This process typically takes about 1–2 weeks, depending on the humidity.
  » Alternatively, you can use a dehydrator set on low or an oven on its lowest setting with the door slightly open.
- **Storing Dried Herbs**:
  » Store dried herbs in airtight glass jars, away from direct sunlight and heat. Label each jar with the herb's name and the date of drying.
  » Dried herbs maintain their potency for about 6–12 months, though some, like chamomile and peppermint, can retain flavor for longer.
- **Using Fresh vs. Dried Herbs**:
  » Fresh herbs are ideal for immediate use, but dried herbs work well for teas and remedies and tend to have a stronger, more concentrated flavor.

7. STARTING A SMALL INDOOR HERB GARDEN

If you lack outdoor space, you can still grow alkaline herbs indoors. An indoor herb garden is convenient and brings a touch of greenery and fresh scent to your home. Many herbs, such as basil, peppermint, and chamomile, adapt well to indoor growing conditions.

- **Choosing Containers**:
    - » Select small pots (6–8 inches in diameter) with drainage holes. Place a saucer beneath each pot to catch excess water.
    - » Consider using vertical planters or stacking shelves if space is limited.
- **Lighting Requirements**:
    - » Indoor herbs require bright, indirect sunlight for about 6–8 hours daily. Place them near a south-facing window or under a grow light for optimal growth.
    - » Rotate pots every week to ensure even light exposure.
- **Temperature and Humidity**:
    - » Herbs prefer temperatures between 60–75°F, so avoid placing them near drafty windows or heaters.
    - » To increase humidity, mist the leaves occasionally or place a small water tray nearby.

Growing alkaline herbs at home gives you direct access to fresh, healing plants, allowing you to experience the benefits of Dr. Sebi's teachings on a daily basis. By cultivating these herbs, you're not only building a sustainable source of natural remedies but also connecting with the cycles of nature and deepening your wellness journey. Each step, from planting and watering to harvesting and drying, is an opportunity to engage with the healing power of plants, making your herb garden a living, vibrant part of your self-care practice.

CHAPTER 2
SOIL, ENVIRONMENT, AND CARE

The quality of soil, the environment where your plants grow, and the care you give are fundamental to healthy, vibrant herbs. In this chapter, you'll find practical tips for each of these factors, ensuring your alkaline herbs grow strong and potent. By creating the right conditions, you not only ensure a bountiful harvest but also enhance the healing properties of each plant, making them more effective for your remedies.

1. PREPARING THE SOIL FOR ALKALINE HERBS

Soil is more than just dirt—it's a living ecosystem that provides essential nutrients to your plants. Alkaline herbs thrive best in slightly alkaline soil with a good mix of nutrients, proper drainage, and ample organic matter. A well-prepared soil base creates a strong foundation for healthy herbs.

- **Choosing the Right Soil Composition**:
  - **Loamy Soil**: A mix of sand, silt, and clay, loamy soil is ideal for alkaline herbs. It retains moisture well while allowing excess water to drain, providing roots with the oxygen and hydration they need.
  - **Organic Compost**: Adding organic compost to your soil enriches it with nutrients. Compost is rich in nitrogen, phosphorus, and potassium, which support root development, leaf growth, and flower production.
  - **Sand or Perlite**: To improve drainage, add sand or perlite to your soil mix, particularly if you're planting in pots or in a garden area that tends to hold water. Good drainage prevents root rot, a common issue in overly wet soil.
- **Adjusting Soil pH**:
  - Alkaline herbs prefer a soil pH of around 7.0 to 7.5. Test your soil's pH with a simple kit, which is available at garden stores or online.
  - **Raising Soil pH**: If your soil is too acidic, add garden lime, wood ash, or crushed eggshells to make it more alkaline. Use these amendments sparingly and retest the soil to avoid over-alkalinizing it.
- **Maintaining Nutrient-Rich Soil**:
  - Top-dress your soil with a thin layer of compost every few months to replenish nutrients, especially if you're growing your herbs in containers.
  - Consider using organic fertilizers like fish emulsion, seaweed extract, or worm castings. These provide a gentle nutrient boost without the risk of burning the plants, which can occur with chemical fertilizers.

2. SELECTING THE IDEAL ENVIRONMENT FOR ALKALINE HERBS

Herbs thrive best in environments that mimic their natural habitats. Whether you're growing indoors or outdoors, providing the right conditions for light, temperature, and air circulation is essential.

- **Light Requirements**:
  - **Outdoor Herbs**: Most alkaline herbs require 6–8 hours of sunlight daily. A south-facing garden spot is ideal, as it provides ample direct sunlight throughout the day.
  - **Indoor Herbs**: Place indoor herbs near a sunny window, ideally south or west-facing, for maximum light exposure. If natural light is insufficient, use a full-spectrum grow light positioned 12–18 inches above the plants.
- **Temperature and Humidity**:
  - Herbs typically prefer moderate temperatures between 60–75°F. If temperatures drop significantly at night, consider bringing potted herbs indoors or covering them to protect against cold snaps.
  - Use a humidity tray or mist your plants occasionally if you live in a dry climate. Herbs thrive in moderate humidity levels (around 40–60%), which you can achieve by placing plants near each other or using a room humidifier.
- **Air Circulation and Ventilation**:
  - Good air circulation helps prevent mold, mildew, and pests, which can affect herb quality. Space plants adequately in garden beds, allowing them to grow freely without crowding.
  - For indoor herbs, use a small fan to keep air circulating, which helps reduce stagnant air and discourages mold growth.

3. CARE TECHNIQUES FOR ALKALINE HERBS

Providing consistent care for your herbs ensures they remain healthy and productive. Watering, pruning, and natural pest control are essential aspects of herb care, helping you maintain vibrant plants that produce leaves, flowers, and roots rich in medicinal compounds.

- **Watering Tips**:
  - » Herbs prefer deep, infrequent watering rather than frequent light watering. Check the soil moisture by inserting your finger about an inch deep; if it feels dry, it's time to water.
  - » Water at the base of the plant to avoid wetting the leaves, which can lead to fungal infections. For potted herbs, ensure water drains freely from the pot's bottom to prevent waterlogging.
  - » Early morning is the best time to water, as it gives the plants a full day to absorb moisture and dries excess water off the leaves, reducing the risk of mold.
- **Pruning for Growth and Health**:
  - » Regular pruning encourages bushier growth, prevents herbs from becoming woody, and keeps them producing fresh leaves. Herbs like basil, chamomile, and lemon balm benefit from pruning every couple of weeks.
  - » Use clean, sharp scissors or pruning shears to snip off leaves and stems, focusing on cutting just above a pair of leaves to promote branching.
  - » Removing flowers, known as "deadheading," is essential for herbs that tend to bolt, such as basil and mint. This keeps the plants focused on leaf production rather than seed formation.
- **Natural Pest Control**:
  - » Herbs are generally resistant to pests, but occasional infestations can occur. Aphids, spider mites, and caterpillars are common pests that can damage herbs.
  - » Use a simple spray of water mixed with a few drops of mild soap to treat affected areas. Avoid harsh chemicals, as these can strip the plants of their natural oils and reduce their medicinal quality.
  - » Companion planting can also deter pests. For example, planting marigolds alongside your herbs repels insects, while planting mint nearby can discourage ants and aphids.

4. SEASONAL CARE FOR PERENNIAL AND ANNUAL HERBS

Different types of herbs require different care routines depending on the season. Perennial herbs (those that live for more than two years) and annuals (those that complete their lifecycle in one year) each have unique needs to keep them healthy and productive.

- **Perennial Herbs** (e.g., lemon balm, chamomile, rosemary):
  - » In spring, trim back old growth to make way for new shoots and apply a layer of compost to enrich the soil.
  - » In summer, prune regularly to maintain shape and encourage new growth, harvesting leaves as needed.
  - » In fall, reduce watering as temperatures cool, and prune plants lightly to prepare for winter dormancy. Cover herbs with mulch or bring pots indoors if you live in an area with harsh winters.
- **Annual Herbs** (e.g., basil, dill, cilantro):
  - » Plant annuals in spring after the last frost, providing ample sunlight and water as they grow.
  - » Harvest leaves frequently to encourage continued growth, but avoid cutting more than one-third of the plant at a time.
  - » Allow a few plants to flower and go to seed if you wish to save seeds for the next planting season.

5. CREATING A SUSTAINABLE CARE ROUTINE

A consistent care routine not only helps your herbs thrive but also keeps your garden manageable and enjoyable. Develop a weekly schedule for watering, pruning, and checking for pests, allowing you to tend to your herbs without overwhelming yourself.

- **Watering Routine**:
  - » Set a schedule based on your climate and the needs of your herbs. Generally, a deep watering once or twice a week is sufficient for outdoor herbs, while indoor herbs may require more frequent watering if the air is dry.
- **Pruning and Maintenance**:
  - » Schedule a pruning session every two weeks, using this time to also check for signs of stress, such as yellowing leaves or wilting. Early intervention can prevent minor issues from becoming major problems.
- **Seasonal Adjustments**:
  - » In summer, you may need to water more frequently, especially during dry spells. In winter, reduce water-

ing and keep an eye on temperature-sensitive herbs that may need extra protection from cold.

6. TROUBLESHOOTING COMMON CHALLENGES

Gardening is a learning process, and every gardener encounters challenges. Here are some common issues with growing herbs and natural solutions to keep your plants healthy.

- **Yellowing Leaves**:
    - » Yellow leaves can indicate overwatering, poor drainage, or nutrient deficiencies. Ensure pots have drainage holes, reduce watering, and consider adding organic fertilizer.
- **Wilting Plants**:
    - » Wilting may signal underwatering or extreme temperatures. Adjust your watering routine and consider moving the plant to a shadier or cooler spot if temperatures are too high.
- **Pest Infestations**:
    - » Regularly inspect plants for pests, particularly on the undersides of leaves. For minor infestations, remove pests by hand or use a mild soap spray. For larger infestations, consider using organic insecticidal soap or neem oil.
- **Leggy Growth**:
    - » Herbs growing tall with sparse leaves may indicate insufficient light. Move the plant to a sunnier spot or supplement with a grow light for indoor herbs.

Growing and caring for your own herbs is a process that connects you to the rhythms of nature. By nurturing your plants with the right soil, environment, and care, you're supporting their growth and ensuring they reach their full potential. Each step, from testing soil pH to pruning and watering, strengthens your connection to these healing plants. With time and attention, your alkaline herb garden will flourish, providing you with a sustainable, fresh source of natural remedies for daily health and well-being.

CHAPTER 3
HARVESTING AND STORAGE TIPS

Harvesting and storing your herbs correctly ensures they maintain their potency, flavor, and healing properties. By understanding when to harvest each type of herb and the best methods for drying and storing them, you can create a long-lasting supply of high-quality ingredients for teas, tinctures, and other natural remedies.

1. TIMING THE HARVEST FOR MAXIMUM POTENCY

Knowing when to harvest is crucial for obtaining the most medicinal value from your herbs. Each herb has an optimal harvest time, usually when its active compounds are at their highest concentration.

- **Leafy Herbs** (e.g., basil, lemon balm, nettle):
  » Harvest leafy herbs before they flower, as this is when their flavor and potency are strongest.
  » For perennial herbs like lemon balm, harvesting throughout the growing season encourages new growth and ensures a continuous supply.
  » Always harvest in the morning after the dew has dried but before the sun is too intense; this helps preserve essential oils and active compounds.
- **Flowering Herbs** (e.g., chamomile, lavender):
  » Harvest flowers as they begin to bloom, as they contain the highest levels of essential oils at this stage.
  » For herbs like chamomile, pick the flower heads individually, avoiding any that have started to wilt.
- **Root Herbs** (e.g., burdock, dandelion):
  » Roots are best harvested in the fall after the plant has stored nutrients in its roots to prepare for winter dormancy.
  » Use a garden fork or spade to loosen the soil around the root, taking care not to damage it as you dig it up.

2. HARVESTING TECHNIQUES FOR DIFFERENT HERBS

Using the right tools and techniques helps maintain the quality of the herbs and promotes healthy regrowth.

- **Leafy and Flowering Herbs**:
  » Use clean, sharp scissors or garden shears to avoid tearing the stems. Cut the leaves or flowers close to the base of the stem but leave at least one-third of the plant intact to allow for regrowth.
  » For herbs like mint and basil, prune just above a leaf pair to encourage bushier growth and prevent the plant from becoming too leggy.
- **Root Herbs**:
  » After loosening the soil, gently pull up the entire root system. Brush off excess dirt but avoid washing roots until you're ready to use or store them, as moisture can encourage mold during drying.
  » Trim off any fibrous root hairs or smaller side roots to focus on the main root, which contains the highest concentration of active compounds.

3. DRYING HERBS FOR LONG-TERM STORAGE

Proper drying techniques preserve the potency, flavor, and aroma of your herbs, allowing you to store them for months or even years.

- **Air Drying**:
  » Air drying is one of the best methods for preserving herbs, especially leafy and flowering varieties. Gather herbs into small bundles, tie them with string, and hang them upside down in a warm, dry, and dark area with good airflow.
  » This method takes about 1–2 weeks, depending on humidity levels. When fully dry, the leaves should crumble easily, and stems should snap rather than bend.
- **Using a Dehydrator**:
  » A dehydrator set at a low temperature (95–115°F) can dry herbs more quickly than air drying and is especially useful in humid climates.
  » Arrange the herbs in a single layer on the dehydrator trays and check them every few hours. Most herbs dry completely within 4–12 hours.
- **Oven Drying** (only as a last resort):
  » Use your oven on its lowest setting with the door slightly open to allow moisture to escape. Spread the herbs on a baking sheet lined with parchment paper.
  » Monitor them carefully to avoid overheating, as high temperatures can degrade essential oils and reduce the herbs' effectiveness.

4. STORING DRIED HERBS FOR POTENCY AND FRESHNESS

Once your herbs are fully dry, storing them correctly helps preserve their quality and medicinal properties. Protect dried herbs from light, air, and moisture to keep them fresh for as long as possible.

- **Airtight Containers**:
  » Use glass jars with airtight lids for the best results. Glass is non-porous and does not absorb the herbs' essential oils, ensuring the flavor and potency stay intact.
  » Avoid plastic containers, as they can leach chemicals and may allow air and moisture to seep in.
- **Storage Environment**:
  » Keep jars in a cool, dark place away from direct sunlight and heat, like a pantry or cabinet. Heat and light can degrade the herbs' active compounds over time.
  » Label each jar with the herb name and the date of drying, as potency can decrease over time, and it's best to use herbs within a year for maximum effect.
- **Checking for Freshness**:
  » Periodically check your stored herbs for signs of moisture or mold, especially if the storage area is humid. If you notice any dampness or unusual odors, dispose of the herbs to avoid contamination in other jars.

5. USING FRESH VS. DRIED HERBS IN REMEDIES

Fresh and dried herbs each have their benefits, and understanding when to use each form can help you get the most out of your herbal remedies.

- **Fresh Herbs**:
  » Fresh herbs are ideal for immediate use, especially in teas, poultices, and cooking. They contain higher moisture content, which gives them a mild flavor and aroma but also means they spoil faster.
  » For teas and infusions, you may need to use about twice as much fresh herb as you would dried, as fresh herbs are less concentrated.
- **Dried Herbs**:
  » Dried herbs are more concentrated, making them suitable for long-term storage and use in tinctures, capsules, and salves.
  » When using dried herbs, remember that their flavor and medicinal compounds are more potent, so adjust quantities accordingly. Typically, 1 tablespoon of dried herb is equivalent to 2 tablespoons of fresh herb.

6. EXTENDING THE SHELF LIFE OF DRIED HERBS

To get the most out of your stored herbs, there are a few simple practices that can help extend their shelf life and ensure they retain their potency.

- **Desiccant Packs**:
  » Placing a food-safe desiccant pack inside each jar can help absorb excess moisture, keeping your herbs dry and fresh for longer.
  » Replace the desiccant packs every few months or when you notice they're becoming saturated.
- **Freezing for Long-Term Storage**:
  » For delicate herbs that lose potency quickly, such as mint and basil, freezing can be a good alternative to drying. Chop the herbs, place them in an ice cube tray, cover with water or oil, and freeze.
  » Frozen herbs are best used within a few months and can be added directly to teas, soups, or infusions without thawing.
- **Using Dried Herbs Regularly**:
  » To avoid herbs sitting unused, incorporate them regularly into your teas, tinctures, or cooking. Regular use keeps your herbs rotated and ensures you're always working with fresh, potent ingredients.

Proper harvesting and storage techniques ensure that your herbs retain their potency, flavor, and healing properties long after they've left the garden. By timing your harvest correctly, drying and storing them with care, and knowing how to use both fresh and dried herbs, you can create a reliable, high-quality supply of natural remedies that support your wellness journey all year round. Each step in this process connects you to the healing power of plants, making your home-grown herbs a vital part of your holistic lifestyle.

BOOK 12
Heart Health and Dr. Sebi's Principles

Dr. Sebi's approach to heart health centers on maintaining an alkaline diet, reducing inflammation, and supporting the cardiovascular system with natural herbs and nutrients. By focusing on the body's electrical and cellular health, his philosophy emphasizes the role of herbs in promoting circulation, reducing blood pressure, and preventing plaque buildup in arteries. This book explores how to support heart health naturally using Dr. Sebi's methods, including specific herbs, lifestyle adjustments, and recipes for heart-boosting teas and tonics.

CHAPTER 1
HERBS FOR HEART HEALTH

A healthy heart is essential for longevity and quality of life. Herbs play a valuable role in supporting cardiovascular health by promoting blood flow, managing blood pressure, and reducing inflammation. Dr. Sebi advocated for natural remedies to nourish and protect the heart, aligning with his focus on alkalinity, detoxification, and a plant-based approach. This chapter provides an in-depth look at some of the best herbs for heart health and how to use them as part of a holistic lifestyle.

1. HAWTHORN BERRY: THE HEART'S ALLY

Hawthorn berry is one of the most well-regarded herbs for heart health and has been used traditionally to treat heart conditions. Known as "the heart's ally," hawthorn supports the heart by improving circulation, strengthening the heart muscle, and managing blood pressure.

- **Benefits of Hawthorn Berry:**
  - **Improves Circulation:** Hawthorn enhances blood flow by dilating blood vessels, allowing blood to flow more freely and reducing the heart's workload.
  - **Strengthens Heart Muscles:** It helps improve the heart's pumping ability, making it especially beneficial for those with weakened heart function.
  - **Reduces Blood Pressure:** The herb has mild hypotensive properties that help in lowering high blood pressure naturally.
- **How to Use Hawthorn Berry:**
  - **Hawthorn Berry Tea:** Steep 1 tablespoon of dried hawthorn berries in hot water for 10–15 minutes. Strain and enjoy daily to support heart function.
  - **Hawthorn Tincture:** A tincture made from hawthorn can be added to water or juice. Take 1–2 dropperfuls up to three times a day for an extra boost to cardiovascular health.

2. GARLIC: NATURE'S CHOLESTEROL REDUCER

Garlic is a potent herb with multiple cardiovascular benefits. It is known to help reduce cholesterol levels, lower blood pressure, and prevent plaque buildup in the arteries. Garlic also improves circulation, making it an essential herb in any heart health regimen.

- **Benefits of Garlic:**
  - **Reduces Cholesterol:** Garlic has been shown to lower LDL (bad cholesterol) levels while increasing HDL (good cholesterol).
  - **Prevents Plaque Build-Up:** The sulfur compounds in garlic help prevent plaque formation in arteries, reducing the risk of blockages.
  - **Lowers Blood Pressure:** Garlic's natural compounds help dilate blood vessels, reducing blood pressure and promoting better blood flow.
- **How to Use Garlic:**
  - **Garlic and Honey Heart Health Tonic:** Combine one clove of minced garlic with a tablespoon of raw honey. Take this mixture daily to support healthy cholesterol and blood pressure.
  - **Garlic Oil Capsules:** Garlic oil capsules are an easy way to consume garlic without the strong taste. Follow dosage recommendations on the packaging for best results.

3. CAYENNE PEPPER: THE CIRCULATORY STIMULANT

Cayenne pepper is an effective herb for stimulating blood flow and promoting cardiovascular health. The active compound in cayenne, capsaicin, supports heart health by improving circulation and helping to break up blood clots. Cayenne is often used in small doses to promote overall circulatory health.

- **Benefits of Cayenne Pepper:**
  - **Improves Circulation:** Cayenne stimulates blood flow and reduces plaque buildup in arteries.
  - **Normalizes Blood Pressure:** Cayenne helps regulate blood pressure by dilating blood vessels, which eases the pressure on artery walls.
  - **Reduces Blood Clots:** Cayenne helps break down fibrin, a substance that leads to blood clot formation.
- **How to Use Cayenne Pepper:**
  - **Cayenne Pepper Tea:** Add a pinch of cayenne to a cup of hot water with a squeeze of lemon and a bit of honey for a warming, heart-healthy drink.
  - **Cayenne Capsules:** For those who find cayenne too spicy, capsules are an effective alternative. Take with food to avoid stomach irritation.

4. HIBISCUS: A NATURAL BLOOD PRESSURE REGULATOR

Hibiscus is known for its beautiful flowers and rich red color, but it also has powerful health benefits for the cardiovascular system. Hibiscus tea has been shown to help lower blood pressure, making it a popular choice for those with hypertension. Additionally, hibiscus is rich in antioxidants, which help protect the heart from oxidative damage.

- **Benefits of Hibiscus**:
  - » **Lowers Blood Pressure**: Hibiscus acts as a natural diuretic, reducing blood volume and pressure on artery walls.
  - » **Reduces Cholesterol**: The antioxidants in hibiscus help lower LDL cholesterol and increase HDL cholesterol levels.
  - » **Protects Heart Cells**: Hibiscus is rich in anthocyanins and other antioxidants that protect heart cells from oxidative damage.
- **How to Use Hibiscus**:
  - » **Hibiscus Tea**: Steep 1–2 teaspoons of dried hibiscus flowers in hot water for 5–10 minutes. Drink up to two cups per day to manage blood pressure.
  - » **Hibiscus and Rose Tea Blend**: Blend hibiscus with dried rose petals for a refreshing, heart-supporting tea. This combination enhances the calming and anti-inflammatory effects of both herbs.

5. DANDELION: THE HEART DETOXIFIER

Dandelion, often considered a weed, is a powerful detoxifying herb that supports heart health by helping the body eliminate excess fluids and toxins. Dandelion's diuretic properties assist in reducing blood pressure and promoting a healthy balance of electrolytes.

- **Benefits of Dandelion**:
  - » **Acts as a Natural Diuretic**: Dandelion promotes the release of excess fluids without causing potassium depletion, as many pharmaceutical diuretics do.
  - » **Reduces Blood Pressure**: By helping the body get rid of extra fluid, dandelion reduces the volume of blood the heart has to pump, thereby lowering blood pressure.
  - » **Supports Liver Detoxification**: Dandelion supports liver function, which plays a key role in regulating cholesterol and filtering toxins from the blood.
- **How to Use Dandelion**:
  - » **Dandelion Leaf Tea**: Use 1 teaspoon of dried dandelion leaves or 1 tablespoon of fresh leaves per cup of hot water. Steep for 10 minutes and drink daily as a gentle diuretic.
  - » **Dandelion Root Coffee Substitute**: Roast dandelion root and brew as a coffee substitute. This acts as a heart-supporting detox drink, particularly beneficial for those trying to reduce caffeine intake.

6. MOTHERWORT: THE HEART CALMER

Motherwort is often used as a natural remedy for heart palpitations, anxiety, and mild hypertension. Known as a "cardiac tonic," motherwort helps relax the nervous system and reduces the frequency of irregular heartbeats. This herb is especially helpful for people with heart conditions related to stress and anxiety.

- **Benefits of Motherwort**:
  - » **Relieves Heart Palpitations**: Motherwort calms irregular heartbeats and reduces palpitations, especially those triggered by anxiety or stress.
  - » **Lowers Blood Pressure**: The herb's calming effects reduce overall blood pressure, easing the strain on the heart.
  - » **Reduces Anxiety**: Motherwort is mildly sedative, which helps reduce anxiety that can worsen cardiovascular issues.
- **How to Use Motherwort**:
  - » **Motherwort Tea**: Steep 1 teaspoon of dried motherwort in hot water for 10 minutes. Drink daily to promote heart calmness and reduce palpitations.
  - » **Motherwort Tincture**: Take 10–20 drops of motherwort tincture in water up to three times daily to support heart health and relaxation.

7. GINGER: THE HEART-HEALTHY ANTI-INFLAMMATORY

Ginger is a popular herb with anti-inflammatory properties that support cardiovascular health. It helps reduce inflammation in blood vessels, improves circulation, and lowers cholesterol, making it an excellent choice for those focusing on heart health.

- **Benefits of Ginger**:
  - » **Improves Circulation**: Ginger enhances blood flow and keeps blood vessels flexible, which can prevent hardening of the arteries.
  - » **Reduces Inflammation**: The anti-inflammatory compounds in ginger help protect blood vessels from inflammation and plaque buildup.

- » **Lowers Cholesterol**: Ginger may help reduce LDL cholesterol levels, supporting balanced cholesterol levels.
- **How to Use Ginger**:
  - » **Ginger Tea**: Add 1 teaspoon of freshly grated ginger to a cup of hot water, steep for 10 minutes, and drink daily to support circulation and lower cholesterol.
  - » **Ginger-Honey Paste**: Combine equal parts fresh ginger juice and honey, taking a teaspoon daily as a heart-healthy tonic.

PRACTICAL RECIPES FOR HEART HEALTH

These recipes incorporate heart-supporting herbs, making it easy to integrate them into your daily routine:

1. **Heart Health Tea Blend**:
   - » **Ingredients**: 1 tablespoon hawthorn berries, 1 teaspoon dandelion leaves, 1/2 teaspoon hibiscus flowers.
   - » **Instructions**: Combine all ingredients in a teapot with hot water, steep for 15 minutes, strain, and enjoy. Drink once daily.
2. **Cholesterol-Reducing Garlic and Lemon Tonic**:
   - » **Ingredients**: Juice of 1 lemon, 1 minced garlic clove, 1 tablespoon honey.
   - » **Instructions**: Mix lemon juice and garlic, then add honey. Take this tonic in the morning on an empty stomach for cholesterol support.
3. **Cooling Hibiscus and Mint Iced Tea**:
   - » **Ingredients**: 1 tablespoon dried hibiscus, 1 teaspoon dried mint, 4 cups water.
   - » **Instructions**: Steep hibiscus and mint in boiling water for 10 minutes. Strain, chill, and serve over ice. Perfect for warm days and heart health.

Incorporating these herbs into your daily routine provides a natural, effective way to support heart health according to Dr. Sebi's principles. Each herb offers specific benefits, from improving circulation to reducing cholesterol and blood pressure, allowing you to create a holistic approach to cardiovascular wellness. By blending these herbs in teas, tonics, and tinctures, you're harnessing nature's power to nurture and protect your heart for years to come.

CHAPTER 2
LOWERING BLOOD PRESSURE NATURALLY

High blood pressure, or hypertension, is a common health condition that can strain the heart, blood vessels, and other organs. Dr. Sebi's approach to managing blood pressure emphasizes natural remedies, an alkaline diet, and lifestyle modifications that reduce the need for pharmaceuticals. This chapter provides a practical guide to lowering blood pressure naturally, incorporating herbs, nutrition, and mindful habits.

1. HERBS FOR BLOOD PRESSURE MANAGEMENT

Certain herbs are particularly effective at helping regulate blood pressure by supporting the relaxation of blood vessels, improving circulation, and reducing stress. Here are a few herbs recommended in Dr. Sebi's approach for naturally lowering blood pressure:

- **Hibiscus**: Hibiscus tea is rich in antioxidants and acts as a natural diuretic, which helps reduce blood volume and pressure on artery walls. Studies have shown that drinking hibiscus tea daily can significantly lower blood pressure.
  - » **How to Use**: Steep 1–2 teaspoons of dried hibiscus flowers in hot water for 5–10 minutes, then strain. Drink up to two cups daily.
- **Garlic**: Garlic has been used for centuries to support cardiovascular health, as it helps relax blood vessels and improve circulation. It's particularly effective for lowering systolic (top number) blood pressure.
  - » **How to Use**: Crush or mince one garlic clove and consume it raw daily, or take it with a spoonful of honey. You can also use garlic in your meals as often as possible for ongoing benefits.
- **Olive Leaf**: Known for its vasodilating effects, olive leaf helps dilate blood vessels and reduce arterial stiffness, promoting better blood flow. Olive leaf also contains antioxidants that protect blood vessels from damage.
  - » **How to Use**: Take olive leaf extract in capsule or liquid form according to the product's dosage instructions, or drink olive leaf tea daily.
- **Basil**: Basil is rich in magnesium, which helps relax blood vessels and reduce blood pressure. It also contains eugenol, a compound known to lower blood pressure by blocking calcium channels in the blood vessels.
  - » **How to Use**: Add fresh basil to salads, smoothies, and cooking. Basil tea can also be made by steeping fresh or dried basil leaves in hot water for 5–10 minutes.

2. THE ROLE OF DIET IN BLOOD PRESSURE CONTROL

Diet plays a crucial role in blood pressure regulation, and Dr. Sebi's alkaline diet is well-suited for managing high blood pressure. An alkaline diet emphasizes whole, plant-based foods that reduce acidity and inflammation in the body, promoting overall heart health.

- **Increase Potassium-Rich Foods**: Potassium helps counteract the effects of sodium, a mineral that raises blood pressure. Foods rich in potassium include bananas, avocados, leafy greens, and sweet potatoes. Including these foods in your diet can help maintain balanced blood pressure levels.
- **Limit Sodium Intake**: Sodium causes the body to retain water, increasing blood volume and pressure. Dr. Sebi's diet naturally avoids high-sodium processed foods, focusing instead on fresh, whole foods that are lower in sodium.
- **Incorporate High-Fiber Foods**: Fiber-rich foods help reduce cholesterol levels and improve blood vessel elasticity, both of which support healthy blood pressure. Whole grains, fruits, vegetables, and legumes provide fiber that promotes cardiovascular health and prevents arterial stiffness.
- **Add Healthy Fats**: Healthy fats, such as those found in olive oil, avocados, and nuts, support heart health by reducing inflammation and maintaining flexible blood vessels. Avoid processed oils and trans fats, which can raise cholesterol and blood pressure.

3. DAILY HABITS FOR MANAGING BLOOD PRESSURE

Beyond diet and herbs, lifestyle habits play a major role in managing blood pressure. Here are some daily practices that align with Dr. Sebi's holistic approach:

- **Practice Mindful Breathing**: Deep breathing and mindfulness exercises help reduce stress, which is a significant contributor to high blood pressure. Incorporating a few minutes of mindful breathing each day can reduce stress hormones and promote relaxation.
  - » **How to Practice**: Take 5–10 minutes each morning

or before bed to sit comfortably and focus on slow, deep breaths. Inhale for a count of four, hold for four, and exhale for four.

- **Stay Active with Gentle Exercise**: Regular physical activity, such as walking, yoga, or cycling, improves cardiovascular fitness and supports blood pressure management. Exercise enhances blood flow and helps the heart pump more efficiently.
  » **Tip**: Aim for 30 minutes of moderate exercise daily, but choose activities that you enjoy, as consistency is key.
- **Limit Alcohol and Avoid Smoking**: Both alcohol and smoking increase blood pressure and damage blood vessels. Reducing alcohol consumption and avoiding tobacco products are essential steps in a heart-healthy lifestyle.
- **Get Adequate Sleep**: Lack of sleep increases stress hormones, which can lead to elevated blood pressure. Prioritize restful sleep by setting a regular sleep schedule and creating a calm bedtime routine to promote relaxation.

4. SIMPLE RECIPES FOR BLOOD PRESSURE SUPPORT

Here are a few easy-to-make recipes incorporating herbs and foods that support lower blood pressure:

- **Hibiscus and Basil Tea**:
  » **Ingredients**: 1 teaspoon dried hibiscus flowers, 1 teaspoon fresh or dried basil leaves, 2 cups hot water, honey (optional).
  » **Instructions**: Steep the hibiscus and basil in hot water for 10 minutes, strain, and add honey if desired. Drink daily to support balanced blood pressure.
- **Garlic and Avocado Spread**:
  » **Ingredients**: 1 ripe avocado, 1–2 cloves of minced garlic, juice of half a lemon, a pinch of sea salt.
  » **Instructions**: Mash the avocado and mix in the garlic, lemon juice, and sea salt. Use as a spread on wholegrain toast or as a dip with raw veggies. This spread provides potassium, healthy fats, and garlic for heart health.
- **Green Leafy Salad with Olive Oil Dressing**:
  » **Ingredients**: Mixed greens (spinach, arugula, kale), sliced cucumber, cherry tomatoes, 1 tablespoon extra-virgin olive oil, juice of half a lemon, black pepper to taste.
  » **Instructions**: Toss the greens, cucumber, and tomatoes together. Mix olive oil, lemon juice, and black pepper for a heart-healthy dressing, and drizzle over the salad. This salad offers fiber, potassium, and healthy fats to support blood pressure.

5. THE BENEFITS OF CONSISTENCY AND ROUTINE

Lowering blood pressure naturally is most effective when practiced consistently. Small, daily habits add up over time, leading to significant improvements in heart health. By regularly incorporating these herbs, foods, and lifestyle practices, you can support healthy blood pressure and protect your cardiovascular system.

- **Set a Routine**: Establish regular times to drink blood pressure-supporting teas, take herbal supplements, or engage in mindfulness practices. Having a routine helps integrate these habits into daily life, making it easier to maintain them long-term.
- **Track Your Progress**: Monitor your blood pressure regularly to see the positive effects of your natural approach. Tracking improvements can motivate you to stick with these heart-healthy practices.
- **Listen to Your Body**: Everyone's body responds differently to changes in diet and lifestyle. Pay attention to how you feel, and adjust as needed. Natural approaches to blood pressure management are adaptable and flexible, allowing you to find what works best for you.

By using herbs, making conscious dietary choices, and developing mindful habits, you can manage blood pressure in a way that aligns with Dr. Sebi's principles of holistic wellness. These practices not only support a healthy heart but also promote balance and well-being in all aspects of life. Embracing a natural approach to blood pressure can be empowering, allowing you to take an active role in your cardiovascular health for the long term.

CHAPTER 3
DIETARY TIPS FOR CARDIOVASCULAR HEALTH

A heart-healthy diet is foundational to maintaining cardiovascular wellness. Dr. Sebi's dietary approach focuses on plant-based, alkaline foods that provide essential nutrients, help reduce inflammation, and support optimal blood flow. In this chapter, you'll discover practical dietary tips that align with Dr. Sebi's philosophy, helping you make food choices that promote a healthy heart.

1. EMBRACE WHOLE, PLANT-BASED FOODS

A plant-based diet rich in whole, unprocessed foods is the cornerstone of Dr. Sebi's nutritional philosophy. Whole foods provide a variety of nutrients, antioxidants, and fiber, all of which play critical roles in cardiovascular health.

- **Focus on Fresh Vegetables and Fruits**:
  - » Vegetables like leafy greens, bell peppers, and cucumbers are packed with vitamins, minerals, and fiber that support the heart. Fruits such as berries, apples, and citrus fruits provide antioxidants that combat oxidative stress in the blood vessels.
  - » Aim for a colorful plate by including a variety of vegetables and fruits each day. The different colors signify a range of beneficial compounds, such as polyphenols, that support heart health.
- **Incorporate Fiber-Rich Foods**:
  - » Fiber is essential for maintaining healthy cholesterol levels and preventing plaque buildup in arteries. Whole grains like quinoa, amaranth, and spelt, as well as fiber-rich vegetables, help lower LDL cholesterol and support digestive health.
  - » Aiming for at least 25–30 grams of fiber daily can make a significant difference in cardiovascular health by reducing blood pressure and cholesterol levels.

2. PRIORITIZE ALKALINE FOODS

Dr. Sebi advocated for an alkaline diet to promote balance in the body. An alkaline diet reduces inflammation, improves cellular health, and minimizes stress on the cardiovascular system. Acidic foods, like processed foods and red meat, can contribute to inflammation and heart disease.

- **Leafy Greens and Sea Vegetables**:
  - » Leafy greens such as kale, arugula, and dandelion greens are highly alkaline and rich in antioxidants, fiber, and minerals. Sea vegetables like sea moss and bladderwrack contain iodine and other trace minerals that support cellular health.
  - » Incorporate a daily serving of leafy greens in salads, smoothies, or steamed as a side to help maintain an alkaline environment in the body.
- **Avoid Processed and Acidic Foods**:
  - » Foods high in sugar, refined grains, and trans fats are inflammatory and can increase blood pressure and cholesterol. Reducing or eliminating processed foods can significantly improve heart health.
  - » Replace acidic foods with natural, whole foods that are minimally processed, focusing on plant-based sources for optimal nutrient density.

3. INCORPORATE HEART-HEALTHY FATS

While Dr. Sebi's approach discourages high-fat animal products, it does encourage healthy plant-based fats that are beneficial for the heart. Healthy fats from sources like avocados, nuts, and olive oil provide essential fatty acids that support cardiovascular health without raising cholesterol.

- **Avocados and Olives**:
  - » Both avocados and olives are rich in monounsaturated fats, which can help lower LDL cholesterol while raising HDL (good) cholesterol. These foods are also high in fiber and potassium, both of which are beneficial for heart health.
  - » Add sliced avocado to salads or use olive oil as a dressing to gain the benefits of heart-healthy fats.
- **Nuts and Seeds**:
  - » Nuts like walnuts, almonds, and pumpkin seeds are excellent sources of heart-healthy omega-3 and omega-6 fatty acids, as well as magnesium, which helps relax blood vessels and regulate blood pressure.
  - » Include a handful of unsalted nuts as a snack, or sprinkle seeds onto salads and smoothie bowls for added heart benefits.

4. OPT FOR NATURAL SOURCES OF POTASSIUM

Potassium helps balance sodium levels in the body, which is essential for blood pressure control. Dr. Sebi's diet includes potassium-rich foods, particularly fruits and vegetables, that help relax blood vessels and prevent fluid retention.

- **Potassium-Rich Foods:**
  - » Foods like bananas, sweet potatoes, spinach, and coconut water are high in potassium, which helps to counteract the effects of sodium on blood pressure. Including these foods daily can support cardiovascular health by reducing strain on the heart.
  - » Coconut water is a great hydrating option that supplies both potassium and magnesium, making it an ideal choice for supporting electrolyte balance.

5. CHOOSE WHOLE GRAINS OVER REFINED GRAINS

Whole grains provide essential fiber, vitamins, and minerals that contribute to heart health, unlike refined grains, which can raise blood sugar and inflammation levels.

- **Whole Grains**:
  - » Grains like quinoa, amaranth, and wild rice are unprocessed and rich in fiber, supporting cholesterol regulation and blood vessel health.
  - » Replace refined grains, such as white bread and white rice, with whole grains to maintain balanced blood sugar levels and provide long-lasting energy, reducing stress on the heart.

6. USE HERBS AND SPICES FOR FLAVOR AND HEART BENEFITS

Certain herbs and spices not only add flavor to meals but also offer cardiovascular benefits. Many of these, such as garlic, cayenne pepper, and turmeric, have anti-inflammatory and blood pressure-lowering effects.

- **Garlic and Ginger**:
  - » Garlic and ginger both promote blood circulation, reduce inflammation, and have mild blood-thinning properties, which can lower the risk of blood clots and high blood pressure.
  - » Use fresh garlic in salads, sauces, and dressings, and add ginger to teas and smoothies to support heart health.
- **Cayenne Pepper and Turmeric**:
  - » Cayenne pepper contains capsaicin, a compound that helps reduce blood pressure by improving blood flow. Turmeric contains curcumin, an anti-inflammatory agent that protects blood vessels from damage.
  - » Add a pinch of cayenne to soups and stews or incorporate turmeric into smoothies and curries for anti-inflammatory benefits.

7. HYDRATE WITH HEART-HEALTHY BEVERAGES

Proper hydration is key to maintaining blood volume and pressure. Choosing heart-supporting beverages can provide additional nutrients while helping the body stay hydrated.

- **Herbal Teas**:
  - » Teas like hibiscus, green tea, and nettle are rich in antioxidants and help reduce blood pressure. Hibiscus tea, in particular, acts as a natural diuretic, which helps regulate blood volume and pressure.
  - » Drink 1–2 cups of herbal tea daily to support blood pressure and hydration. Hibiscus tea, with its high antioxidant content, can be particularly beneficial for cardiovascular health.
- **Coconut Water**:
  - » Coconut water is a natural source of potassium and magnesium, which support blood pressure regulation and prevent muscle cramping. It's an excellent hydrating option, especially for those who need to manage blood pressure.
  - » Enjoy coconut water as a refreshing beverage or mix it into smoothies to replace sugary drinks and sodas.

8. SIMPLE RECIPES TO SUPPORT CARDIOVASCULAR HEALTH

Incorporating these foods into your daily diet doesn't have to be complicated. Here are a couple of easy recipes to support heart health:

- **Heart-Healthy Green Smoothie:**
  - » **Ingredients**: 1 cup coconut water, 1 banana, 1 handful of spinach, 1/2 avocado, 1 tablespoon chia seeds.
  - » **Instructions**: Blend all ingredients until smooth. This smoothie provides potassium, fiber, and healthy fats that support heart health.
- **Garlic and Olive Oil Salad Dressing**:
  - » **Ingredients**: 2 cloves minced garlic, 1/4 cup extra-virgin olive oil, juice of 1 lemon, salt and pepper to taste.
  - » **Instructions**: Combine all ingredients and whisk well. Use this dressing over mixed greens or roasted vegetables for a flavorful, heart-healthy addition.

By following these dietary tips, you're nourishing your heart and supporting your cardiovascular system in alignment with Dr. Sebi's principles. The focus on whole, alkaline foods, plant-based fats, and nutrient-dense choices not only promotes heart health but also contributes to overall wellness and vitality. Through mindful food choices and simple recipes, you can take proactive steps to protect your heart for years to come.

BOOK 13
Managing Diabetes Naturally

Dr. Sebi's philosophy promotes natural methods for managing chronic health conditions like diabetes. By emphasizing an alkaline, plant-based diet, he focused on helping the body restore balance and improve metabolic function. This book explores how to manage diabetes using natural methods, particularly through an alkaline diet, lifestyle changes, and the strategic use of herbs to support healthy blood sugar levels.

CHAPTER 1
ALKALINE DIET'S IMPACT ON BLOOD SUGAR

Diabetes is a chronic condition characterized by high blood sugar levels resulting from insulin resistance or the body's inability to produce insulin effectively. Traditional treatments often include medication and lifestyle changes, but Dr. Sebi's approach emphasizes the healing potential of an alkaline diet to help restore the body's natural balance and improve blood sugar regulation. This chapter delves into how an alkaline diet can positively impact blood sugar levels, reduce insulin resistance, and enhance overall health.

1. UNDERSTANDING DIABETES AND BLOOD SUGAR BALANCE

To understand the impact of an alkaline diet on blood sugar, it's helpful to first understand diabetes and how blood sugar is regulated in the body.

- **Blood Sugar Regulation**:
  » Blood sugar levels are primarily regulated by insulin, a hormone produced by the pancreas. Insulin helps glucose (sugar) enter cells, where it is used for energy. When insulin doesn't function properly, blood sugar levels remain elevated, leading to health complications.
  » In Type 2 diabetes, the body becomes resistant to insulin, causing higher blood glucose levels. In Type 1 diabetes, the body does not produce insulin, requiring external insulin management.
- **Factors Affecting Blood Sugar**:
  » Several factors impact blood sugar, including diet, physical activity, stress, and overall metabolic health. Foods high in refined sugars and carbohydrates can cause rapid spikes in blood sugar, while fiber, protein, and healthy fats can help stabilize it.

2. THE ALKALINE DIET AND BLOOD SUGAR MANAGEMENT

An alkaline diet focuses on consuming foods that reduce acidity in the body, emphasizing plant-based, whole foods over processed and refined options. Dr. Sebi's alkaline diet specifically aims to reduce inflammation, balance pH levels, and support cellular health—all of which play a role in managing blood sugar levels.

- **Reducing Acidity and Inflammation**:
  » Inflammation is often linked to insulin resistance, as chronic inflammation can impair cellular response to insulin. An alkaline diet reduces inflammation by avoiding acidic, processed foods and focusing on whole, nutrient-rich plant foods.
  » High-acid foods, such as red meat, dairy, refined sugars, and processed grains, contribute to metabolic acidosis, a condition that can disrupt cellular function and worsen insulin resistance.
- **Maintaining Balanced Blood pH Levels**:
  » Although the body regulates its pH within a narrow range, an alkaline diet may reduce stress on organs involved in maintaining this balance, such as the kidneys and liver. By easing the body's acid load, the alkaline diet helps reduce metabolic stress, which can improve blood sugar regulation.
- **Supporting Cellular Health**:
  » Foods rich in antioxidants, vitamins, and minerals support cellular health and improve the body's response to insulin. Alkaline foods, like leafy greens, cucumbers, and avocados, provide essential nutrients that support metabolic health.

3. KEY ALKALINE FOODS FOR BLOOD SUGAR MANAGEMENT

Certain alkaline foods are particularly effective at helping regulate blood sugar levels, manage insulin resistance, and reduce the risk of complications associated with diabetes.

- **Leafy Greens (Kale, Spinach, Swiss Chard)**:
  » Leafy greens are low in calories and carbohydrates but rich in fiber, magnesium, and other essential nutrients that help control blood sugar levels. Magnesium has been shown to improve insulin sensitivity, making these greens ideal for diabetes management.
  » **How to Use**: Add greens to salads, smoothies, or steamed dishes to increase fiber intake and provide steady energy.
- **Cucumbers**:
  » Cucumbers are hydrating, low in carbohydrates, and help stabilize blood sugar levels. They have a cooling, alkaline effect on the body and are an excellent source of antioxidants.

- **How to Use**: Enjoy cucumbers in salads, smoothies, or even as a hydrating snack.
- **Avocados**:
  - Avocados provide healthy fats and fiber, both of which help stabilize blood sugar levels by slowing digestion and preventing rapid spikes.
  - **How to Use**: Add avocado to salads, spreads, or enjoy it with a dash of lime and sea salt as a snack.
- **Sea Vegetables (Sea Moss, Bladderwrack)**:
  - Sea vegetables are packed with trace minerals and iodine, supporting thyroid health and metabolic balance. They also contain alginates, which help regulate blood sugar by slowing glucose absorption.
  - **How to Use**: Add powdered sea moss or bladderwrack to smoothies, soups, or other recipes for a mineral boost.
- **Berries (Blueberries, Strawberries, Blackberries)**:
  - Berries are low-glycemic fruits that provide fiber and antioxidants, supporting cellular health and reducing oxidative stress, which is beneficial for insulin sensitivity.
  - **How to Use**: Add a handful of berries to smoothies, salads, or as a topping on oatmeal.

4. DIETARY TIPS TO SUPPORT BLOOD SUGAR CONTROL

Dr. Sebi's alkaline diet can be enhanced with dietary strategies that focus on blood sugar stability. Here are a few key tips:

- **Prioritize Fiber-Rich Foods**:
  - Fiber slows down the absorption of sugars into the bloodstream, helping to prevent blood sugar spikes. Foods like vegetables, whole grains, and legumes are excellent sources of fiber.
  - **Tip**: Incorporate fiber-rich foods into every meal, such as adding leafy greens to breakfast smoothies or including a side salad with lunch and dinner.
- **Balance Meals with Healthy Fats and Protein**:
  - Healthy fats and plant-based protein stabilize blood sugar and provide longer-lasting energy. Foods like nuts, seeds, and avocados can be easily included in meals to add a balance of macronutrients.
  - **Tip**: Include a source of healthy fat with each meal, such as a handful of nuts with breakfast or olive oil on salads.
- **Avoid Processed Carbohydrates**:
  - Processed carbs, like white bread, pasta, and sugary snacks, cause rapid blood sugar spikes and crashes, increasing insulin resistance over time.
  - **Tip**: Opt for whole, unprocessed foods whenever possible, choosing whole grains like quinoa or amaranth over refined options.
- **Stay Hydrated**:
  - Proper hydration is essential for blood sugar control, as dehydration can lead to higher blood sugar levels. Drinking plenty of water helps the kidneys filter excess sugar out of the blood.
  - **Tip**: Aim to drink at least eight cups of water daily and incorporate hydrating foods like cucumbers and melons.

5. HERBAL SUPPORT FOR BLOOD SUGAR REGULATION

In addition to an alkaline diet, certain herbs can further support blood sugar control and improve insulin sensitivity. Here are some effective herbs to consider:

- **Bitter Melon**:
  - Bitter melon contains compounds that mimic insulin, helping cells absorb glucose more effectively. Studies show it can reduce blood sugar levels and improve insulin sensitivity.
  - **How to Use**: Brew bitter melon tea or take it as a supplement. Consuming bitter melon with meals can enhance blood sugar regulation.
- **Fenugreek**:
  - Fenugreek seeds are high in soluble fiber, which can improve glucose control by slowing sugar absorption. It also contains compounds that enhance insulin production.
  - **How to Use**: Soak fenugreek seeds in water overnight and drink the water in the morning. Fenugreek can also be added to soups and salads.
- **Cinnamon**:
  - Cinnamon has been shown to lower fasting blood glucose levels and improve insulin sensitivity. It also contains antioxidants that support overall metabolic health.
  - **How to Use**: Add a pinch of cinnamon to smoothies, oatmeal, or herbal teas for natural blood sugar support.

6. MEAL TIMING AND PORTION CONTROL

Meal timing and portion sizes play a critical role in managing blood sugar. Smaller, well-balanced meals consumed throughout the day can help prevent large spikes and dips in blood sugar.

- **Eat Smaller, More Frequent Meals**:
  - » Consuming smaller, balanced meals every 3–4 hours can help regulate blood sugar levels and prevent large fluctuations. This approach can reduce hunger and improve energy levels.
  - » **Tip**: Plan meals and snacks that combine fiber, healthy fats, and protein to maintain steady blood sugar.
- **Practice Portion Control**:
  - » Overeating, even healthy foods, can lead to high blood sugar levels. Eating controlled portions helps manage caloric intake and improves blood sugar regulation.
  - » **Tip**: Use smaller plates, eat slowly, and pay attention to hunger cues to avoid overeating.

7. ALKALINE RECIPE IDEAS FOR BLOOD SUGAR SUPPORT

Here are a few simple recipes incorporating blood sugar-friendly, alkaline foods:

- **Green Alkaline Smoothie**:
  - » **Ingredients**: 1 handful spinach, 1/2 avocado, 1/2 cucumber, 1/2 cup unsweetened almond milk, 1 teaspoon chia seeds.
  - » **Instructions**: Blend all ingredients until smooth. This smoothie provides fiber, healthy fats, and essential minerals for blood sugar stability.
- **Berry and Sea Moss Chia Pudding**:
  - » **Ingredients**: 1 cup almond milk, 2 tablespoons chia seeds, 1/4 cup berries, 1 teaspoon sea moss gel, 1/2 teaspoon cinnamon.
  - » **Instructions**: Mix almond milk, chia seeds, sea moss gel, and cinnamon. Refrigerate overnight, then top with berries before serving. This recipe combines fiber, antioxidants, and healthy fats.

By following an alkaline diet rich in whole, plant-based foods and integrating these strategies, you can support healthy blood sugar levels naturally. The focus on alkaline foods, fiber, healthy fats, and herbal supplements aligns with Dr. Sebi's approach to managing diabetes, empowering you to take charge of your health and reduce reliance on pharmaceuticals. Embracing these dietary changes promotes balanced blood sugar, improves insulin sensitivity, and supports long-term metabolic health.

CHAPTER 2
KEY HERBS FOR DIABETES SUPPORT

Herbal remedies have long been used to manage diabetes by helping regulate blood sugar, improve insulin sensitivity, and reduce the risk of complications. Dr. Sebi's approach includes specific herbs that support metabolic function, address underlying imbalances, and contribute to cellular health. This chapter provides an overview of some of the most effective herbs for diabetes support, offering practical usage tips and explanations of each herb's role in managing blood sugar.

1. BITTER MELON: NATURE'S INSULIN MIMICKER

Bitter melon is a powerful herb for managing diabetes. Known for its unique bitter taste, it contains compounds that mimic insulin, helping lower blood sugar levels naturally. Bitter melon has been used in traditional medicine for centuries and is especially beneficial for individuals with Type 2 diabetes.

- **Key Benefits of Bitter Melon**:
  - » **Lowers Blood Sugar**: Bitter melon contains charantin, an insulin-like compound that promotes glucose uptake by cells, helping to lower blood sugar levels.
  - » **Improves Insulin Sensitivity**: By improving how cells respond to insulin, bitter melon supports better blood sugar regulation.
  - » **Reduces Inflammation**: Bitter melon's antioxidant properties help reduce inflammation, a common issue in those with diabetes.
- **How to Use Bitter Melon**:
  - » **Bitter Melon Tea**: Slice fresh or dried bitter melon, add to hot water, and steep for 10–15 minutes. Drink this tea once or twice daily for blood sugar support.
  - » **Bitter Melon Capsules**: Bitter melon supplements are available in capsule form, making it easy to add to your routine. Follow the dosage recommendations on the packaging.

2. FENUGREEK: THE FIBER-PACKED SEED FOR BLOOD SUGAR BALANCE

Fenugreek seeds are rich in soluble fiber, which slows the digestion and absorption of carbohydrates, helping prevent spikes in blood sugar. Fenugreek also contains compounds that enhance insulin sensitivity, making it an effective herb for diabetes management.

- **Key Benefits of Fenugreek**:
  - » **Regulates Blood Sugar**: The fiber in fenugreek helps manage blood sugar by slowing carbohydrate absorption, preventing sudden spikes.
  - » **Boosts Insulin Production**: Fenugreek contains compounds that encourage the pancreas to produce insulin, which can be particularly helpful for individuals with Type 2 diabetes.
  - » **Reduces Cholesterol**: Fenugreek seeds also help lower LDL (bad cholesterol), supporting overall heart health in people with diabetes.
- **How to Use Fenugreek**:
  - » **Fenugreek Water**: Soak 1–2 tablespoons of fenugreek seeds in water overnight. Strain and drink the water in the morning on an empty stomach to help regulate blood sugar.
  - » **Fenugreek Powder**: Add ground fenugreek seeds to smoothies, soups, or salads for a fiber boost. Start with small amounts, as fenugreek has a strong flavor.

3. GYMNEMA SYLVESTRE: THE SUGAR DESTROYER

Gymnema Sylvestre, known as the "sugar destroyer" in Ayurvedic medicine, is renowned for its ability to reduce sugar cravings and block sugar absorption. It is especially useful for individuals working to reduce sugar intake and manage blood sugar levels.

- **Key Benefits of Gymnema Sylvestre**:
  - » **Reduces Sugar Cravings**: Gymnema reduces the taste of sweetness, which can help reduce sugar cravings and support healthy eating habits.
  - » **Blocks Sugar Absorption**: The herb prevents the intestines from absorbing excess sugar, helping to maintain stable blood sugar levels after meals.
  - » **Improves Insulin Function**: Gymnema has been shown to support the function of insulin-producing cells in the pancreas, which can benefit those with Type 2 diabetes.
- **How to Use Gymnema Sylvestre**:
  - » **Gymnema Tea**: Steep 1 teaspoon of dried Gymnema

leaves in hot water for 5–10 minutes. Drink before meals to help block sugar absorption.
- » **Gymnema Capsules**: Capsules offer a convenient option for those who may not enjoy the taste of Gymnema tea. Take as directed on the packaging.

4. CINNAMON: THE BLOOD SUGAR STABILIZER

Cinnamon is a widely available herb with potent blood sugar-regulating properties. This warming spice has been shown to improve insulin sensitivity and reduce fasting blood sugar levels, making it a simple yet effective tool for managing diabetes.

- **Key Benefits of Cinnamon**:
  - » **Improves Insulin Sensitivity**: Cinnamon helps improve insulin sensitivity, allowing glucose to enter cells more effectively and reduce blood sugar.
  - » **Lowers Fasting Blood Sugar**: Research has shown that cinnamon can lower fasting blood glucose levels, making it beneficial for those with Type 2 diabetes.
  - » **Reduces Oxidative Stress**: Cinnamon contains powerful antioxidants that protect cells from damage, which is crucial for preventing complications of diabetes.
- **How to Use Cinnamon**:
  - » **Cinnamon Tea**: Add 1/2 teaspoon of ground cinnamon to hot water and let steep for 5–10 minutes. Drink daily to support blood sugar levels.
  - » **Add to Meals**: Sprinkle cinnamon on oatmeal, smoothies, or fruit for a blood sugar-friendly flavor boost.

5. HOLY BASIL: THE ANTI-STRESS BLOOD SUGAR HERB

Holy basil, also known as tulsi, is an adaptogenic herb that helps the body adapt to stress. It is particularly beneficial for diabetes management because stress can significantly impact blood sugar levels. Holy basil also contains compounds that directly help regulate blood sugar.

- **Key Benefits of Holy Basil**:
  - » **Reduces Blood Sugar**: Holy basil has hypoglycemic effects that help lower blood sugar levels naturally.
  - » **Manages Stress**: As an adaptogen, holy basil reduces stress hormones, which helps prevent stress-induced blood sugar spikes.
  - » **Anti-Inflammatory Properties**: Holy basil is rich in antioxidants, which reduce inflammation and support immune health in people with diabetes.
- **How to Use Holy Basil**:
  - » **Holy Basil Tea**: Steep fresh or dried holy basil leaves in hot water for 5–10 minutes. Drink 1–2 cups daily to support stress management and blood sugar levels.
  - » **Holy Basil Supplements**: Holy basil is available in capsule form, offering a convenient way to incorporate it into your routine. Follow dosage instructions on the packaging.

6. NOPAL CACTUS: THE BLOOD SUGAR BALANCER

Nopal cactus, also known as prickly pear cactus, is rich in fiber and antioxidants, which support blood sugar balance and help reduce post-meal glucose spikes. Nopal is commonly used in traditional Mexican medicine for managing diabetes and supporting metabolic health.

- **Key Benefits of Nopal Cactus**:
  - » **Slows Glucose Absorption**: The high fiber content of nopal cactus helps prevent sudden increases in blood sugar after meals.
  - » **Reduces Insulin Resistance**: Compounds in nopal cactus improve insulin sensitivity, allowing cells to absorb glucose more effectively.
  - » **Supports Digestive Health**: The fiber in nopal also supports healthy digestion, which can help regulate blood sugar levels over time.
- **How to Use Nopal Cactus**:
  - » **Nopal Juice**: Blend fresh nopal cactus with water and a squeeze of lime. Drink this juice daily to support blood sugar levels and improve digestion.
  - » **Nopal Powder**: Nopal powder can be added to smoothies or soups for a convenient way to incorporate this blood sugar-balancing herb.

7. ALOE VERA: THE HEALING PLANT

Aloe vera is known for its healing properties, and studies suggest that it may also benefit blood sugar regulation. Aloe vera gel contains compounds that improve glucose metabolism and enhance insulin sensitivity.

- **Key Benefits of Aloe Vera**:
  - » **Improves Insulin Sensitivity**: Aloe vera has compounds that help cells respond better to insulin, supporting stable blood sugar levels.
  - » **Supports Gut Health**: Aloe vera promotes healthy digestion, which is beneficial for blood sugar control as digestive health directly impacts metabolism.
  - » **Reduces Inflammation**: Aloe vera's anti-inflamma-

tory properties help manage oxidative stress, which can worsen insulin resistance.

- **How to Use Aloe Vera**:
  - » **Aloe Vera Juice**: Consume 1 tablespoon of aloe vera gel mixed with water or juice daily. Avoid excess consumption, as aloe can have a laxative effect.
  - » **Add to Smoothies**: Fresh aloe gel can be blended into smoothies for added health benefits.

8. PRACTICAL TIPS FOR USING HERBS FOR BLOOD SUGAR SUPPORT

Incorporating herbs into your daily routine can make a significant difference in blood sugar management. Here are some tips for getting the most out of these herbs:

- **Create a Routine**: Take herbal teas or supplements at the same time each day to establish a consistent routine that supports blood sugar stability.
- **Start Slowly**: Introduce one herb at a time and observe how your body responds. This can help you identify which herbs are most effective for your individual needs.
- **Combine with Lifestyle Changes**: Herbal support is most effective when combined with a balanced diet, regular exercise, and stress management. Aim to make holistic lifestyle adjustments alongside herbal usage.
- **Consult with a Healthcare Professional**: Always consult with a healthcare provider, especially if you're on medication, as some herbs can interact with pharmaceuticals.

These herbs, when used alongside an alkaline diet and lifestyle changes, can offer natural support for managing diabetes. By regulating blood sugar, improving insulin sensitivity, and reducing inflammation, these herbs align with Dr. Sebi's approach to holistic health. With consistent use, they contribute to metabolic balance and help reduce the risk of complications, empowering you to take control of your health naturally.

CHAPTER 3
DETOX AND PANCREATIC HEALTH

The pancreas is a critical organ for blood sugar regulation and overall metabolic health. It produces insulin, which helps regulate blood glucose levels, and secretes digestive enzymes essential for breaking down food. When the pancreas is compromised, it can lead to insulin resistance, Type 2 diabetes, and other metabolic disorders. Detoxifying the body, especially the pancreas, liver, and digestive tract, can support pancreatic health, allowing for improved insulin production and sensitivity. This chapter explores how detox practices and an alkaline lifestyle can enhance pancreatic function and aid in managing diabetes naturally.

1. WHY DETOXIFICATION IS ESSENTIAL FOR PANCREATIC HEALTH

Detoxification is the process of eliminating toxins from the body, which helps restore balance and prevent organ stress. A buildup of toxins—due to processed foods, environmental pollution, and stress—can strain the pancreas and other organs, compromising their function and contributing to blood sugar imbalances.

- **Toxins and Insulin Resistance**:
  » Toxins, especially those stored in fatty tissue, can interfere with insulin function, causing the cells to become less responsive, a condition known as insulin resistance. Detoxification helps reduce this toxin load, allowing cells to respond to insulin more effectively.
- **Liver and Pancreas Connection**:
  » The liver and pancreas work closely together in blood sugar regulation. A healthy liver helps maintain steady glucose levels by storing and releasing sugar when needed. Detoxifying the liver reduces its toxic burden, indirectly supporting pancreatic health and improving insulin production.
- **Reducing Inflammation**:
  » Inflammation is a key contributor to insulin resistance. A detox program reduces inflammation by removing inflammatory foods and supporting cellular repair, making it easier for the pancreas to function properly and produce insulin effectively.

2. KEY STEPS IN DETOXIFYING FOR PANCREATIC HEALTH

Detoxification is most effective when done gradually and consistently. Here are key steps to support detoxification and improve pancreatic health, aligned with Dr. Sebi's holistic approach.

- **Follow an Alkaline Diet**:
  » An alkaline diet rich in fruits, vegetables, nuts, and seeds reduces acidity and inflammation, creating a supportive environment for the pancreas and other organs.
  » **Tip**: Incorporate alkaline foods daily, such as leafy greens, cucumbers, sea vegetables, and avocados. Avoid acidic foods like red meat, refined sugars, and processed grains, which can increase inflammation.
- **Increase Hydration with Herbal Infusions**:
  » Staying hydrated is essential for flushing out toxins. Herbal infusions and teas provide hydration while delivering additional detoxifying benefits.
  » **Detox Herbs**: Dandelion root, burdock root, and nettle leaf are excellent for liver and kidney detoxification, helping to reduce the toxic burden on the pancreas.
  » **Tip**: Drink 1–2 cups of detox tea daily to support liver and pancreatic health.
- **Incorporate Fiber-Rich Foods**:
  » Fiber binds to toxins and helps them move through the digestive system, promoting their removal from the body. This reduces the strain on the pancreas and improves blood sugar regulation.
  » **Fiber Sources**: Leafy greens, chia seeds, flaxseeds, and whole grains like quinoa are rich in fiber. Include them in each meal to enhance detoxification.
- **Prioritize Antioxidant-Rich Foods**:
  » Antioxidants protect the pancreas from oxidative stress and support cellular repair. Berries, leafy greens, and cruciferous vegetables are high in antioxidants, aiding in the detox process and reducing pancreatic stress.
  » **Tip**: Aim to include a variety of colorful vegetables and fruits in your daily meals for a wide spectrum of antioxidants.

3. HERBS FOR DETOXIFICATION AND PANCREATIC SUPPORT

Herbs play an important role in detoxification, especially in supporting the pancreas and liver. Certain herbs help cleanse the blood, reduce inflammation, and promote pancreatic health, making them invaluable for managing diabetes naturally.

- **Dandelion Root**:
  » Dandelion root is a powerful liver cleanser that helps reduce toxin buildup, indirectly benefiting the pancreas. It stimulates bile production, which aids in the digestion of fats and helps remove toxins from the liver.
  » **How to Use**: Brew dandelion root tea by simmering 1 tablespoon of dried root in water for 10–15 minutes. Drink daily to support liver and pancreatic detoxification.

- **Milk Thistle**:
  » Milk thistle contains silymarin, a compound that supports liver regeneration and detoxification. By improving liver health, milk thistle reduces strain on the pancreas and promotes better blood sugar regulation.
  » **How to Use**: Take milk thistle as a supplement or in tea form. For tea, steep 1 teaspoon of milk thistle seeds in hot water for 10 minutes.

- **Burdock Root**:
  » Burdock root is a blood purifier that helps remove toxins from the bloodstream. This reduces stress on the pancreas and promotes better metabolic function, making it beneficial for those managing diabetes.
  » **How to Use**: Use burdock root in a tea or tincture form. For tea, simmer 1 teaspoon of dried burdock root in hot water for 10 minutes.

- **Licorice Root**:
  » Licorice root has anti-inflammatory and adrenal-supporting properties, helping to reduce stress on the pancreas. It also helps regulate blood sugar levels and can improve insulin sensitivity.
  » **How to Use**: Steep 1/2 teaspoon of licorice root in hot water for 5–10 minutes. Drink as needed to support blood sugar levels and pancreatic health. Avoid overuse, as licorice can raise blood pressure in some individuals.

4. FASTING AND INTERMITTENT FASTING FOR PANCREATIC HEALTH

Fasting has been shown to improve insulin sensitivity, reduce inflammation, and allow the pancreas time to rest and repair. Intermittent fasting or periodic fasting, done carefully, can be a powerful tool for supporting pancreatic health.

- **Intermittent Fasting**:
  » This practice involves fasting for a portion of the day and eating during a specified window (e.g., fasting for 16 hours and eating within an 8-hour window). Intermittent fasting has been shown to reduce insulin resistance and improve blood sugar control.
  » **How to Practice**: Start by gradually extending the fasting period, beginning with 12 hours and increasing to 16 hours if it feels comfortable.

- **Juice Fasting**:
  » Fresh, low-sugar vegetable juices support detoxification and provide essential nutrients without placing a heavy digestive load on the pancreas. Juicing can be done as a one-day fast or as part of a larger detox plan.
  » **Suggested Juices**: Green juices made from cucumber, celery, lemon, and leafy greens are nutrient-rich and detoxifying. Avoid high-sugar fruits to prevent blood sugar spikes.

5. STRESS MANAGEMENT FOR DETOX AND PANCREATIC HEALTH

Chronic stress affects blood sugar regulation and can exacerbate pancreatic stress. Managing stress is crucial for supporting detoxification and reducing the body's demand for insulin.

- **Mindfulness and Deep Breathing**:
  » Mindful practices, such as meditation and deep breathing, help reduce stress hormones, which in turn support stable blood sugar levels. These practices promote relaxation, reducing the toxic burden that stress places on the pancreas.
  » **Tip**: Dedicate 10–15 minutes each day to mindfulness or breathing exercises, especially before meals, to support digestion and blood sugar regulation.

- **Gentle Exercise**:
  » Regular, low-impact exercise like walking, yoga, or swimming supports detoxification by promoting lymphatic drainage and increasing blood circulation. Exercise also improves insulin sensitivity, reducing strain on the pancreas.
  » **Tip**: Aim for at least 30 minutes of gentle exercise

daily, which can be broken up into shorter sessions if needed.

6. SAMPLE DETOX ROUTINE FOR PANCREATIC HEALTH

A gentle detox routine, aligned with Dr. Sebi's principles, can help rejuvenate the pancreas, reduce insulin resistance, and improve overall metabolic health. Here's a sample three-day detox plan to support pancreatic health.

- **Day 1: Pre-Cleanse with Hydration and Alkaline Foods**:
  » Start the day with a glass of warm water and lemon to stimulate digestion.
  » Focus on eating raw, alkaline foods throughout the day, such as salads with leafy greens, cucumbers, and avocados.
  » Drink 1–2 cups of dandelion tea to support liver and pancreatic function.
- **Day 2: Juice Fast and Herbal Support**:
  » Drink green vegetable juices (cucumber, celery, kale, lemon) throughout the day, avoiding high-sugar fruits.
  » Incorporate herbal teas such as milk thistle and burdock root to support liver detoxification.
  » Stay hydrated with water and coconut water to maintain electrolyte balance.
- **Day 3: Reintroducing Alkaline Foods**:
  » Begin reintroducing solid foods with a light smoothie made from leafy greens, cucumber, and avocado.
  » Enjoy a fiber-rich salad with a variety of raw vegetables for lunch, and a light, steamed vegetable dish for dinner.
  » Continue drinking detox teas to support ongoing liver and pancreatic health.

Through a focused detox routine and the incorporation of key herbs, you can create an environment that allows the pancreas to rest and regenerate. Dr. Sebi's approach to detox and pancreatic health provides a foundation for naturally managing blood sugar, improving insulin sensitivity, and promoting holistic wellness. By practicing these steps consistently, you support the body's natural healing processes, making it easier to manage diabetes without relying heavily on pharmaceuticals.

BOOK 14
Supporting Autoimmune Health

Autoimmune conditions occur when the immune system mistakenly attacks the body's own cells, causing inflammation and damage to healthy tissues. Dr. Sebi's approach to managing autoimmune conditions centers on maintaining an alkaline diet, reducing inflammation, and using specific herbs to bring the immune system back into balance. This book provides insights into managing autoimmune health naturally, with dietary and herbal strategies that support a balanced immune response and reduce symptom flare-ups.

CHAPTER 1
FOODS AND HERBS FOR IMMUNE BALANCE

Managing autoimmune conditions naturally requires a holistic approach that focuses on reducing inflammation, supporting gut health, and balancing the immune system. The foods and herbs recommended in this chapter are known for their immune-modulating properties, helping the body maintain a balanced immune response without overstimulation. By following an alkaline, plant-based diet and incorporating these powerful herbs, you can create a supportive foundation for autoimmune health.

1. UNDERSTANDING AUTOIMMUNE IMBALANCE AND INFLAMMATION

Autoimmune conditions such as lupus, rheumatoid arthritis, Hashimoto's thyroiditis, and multiple sclerosis are characterized by an overactive immune response that leads to chronic inflammation. This imbalance can be triggered by various factors, including genetics, environmental toxins, poor diet, and chronic stress.

- **The Role of Inflammation**:
    - » In autoimmune conditions, the immune system attacks healthy tissues, mistaking them for harmful invaders. This response results in chronic inflammation, which can worsen symptoms and damage tissues over time.
    - » Reducing inflammation through diet and herbal support is key to managing autoimmune conditions, as it helps ease symptoms and protects healthy cells from immune attacks.
- **Diet and Immune Balance**:
    - » Dr. Sebi's alkaline diet emphasizes whole, plant-based foods that reduce acidity and inflammation. Consuming foods that are low in toxins and high in antioxidants helps reduce the immune system's burden, creating a more balanced internal environment.
    - » By focusing on nutrient-dense, alkaline foods, you can support immune function without overstimulating it, which is essential for those managing autoimmune diseases.

2. ALKALINE FOODS FOR REDUCING INFLAMMATION AND SUPPORTING IMMUNE HEALTH

Dr. Sebi's alkaline food principles focus on foods that help maintain a balanced pH, are rich in antioxidants, and provide essential nutrients to reduce inflammation. Here are some of the best foods to include in your diet for immune balance:

- **Leafy Greens (Kale, Spinach, Dandelion Greens)**:
    - » Leafy greens are highly alkaline, rich in vitamins A, C, and K, and provide antioxidants that protect against cellular damage. These greens also contain chlorophyll, which supports detoxification and reduces inflammation.
    - » **How to Use**: Add leafy greens to salads, smoothies, or lightly sauté them to preserve nutrients. Aim for at least one serving per meal.
- **Cruciferous Vegetables (Broccoli, Cauliflower, Brussels Sprouts)**:
    - » Cruciferous vegetables contain compounds like sulforaphane, which reduce inflammation and support liver detoxification, an essential process for immune health.
    - » **How to Use**: Steam or roast cruciferous vegetables and include them in meals throughout the week. These vegetables provide fiber and antioxidants that support both gut and immune health.
- **Berries (Blueberries, Strawberries, Blackberries)**:
    - » Berries are low in sugar and high in antioxidants, particularly anthocyanins, which protect cells from oxidative stress. These antioxidants help reduce inflammation and support immune balance.
    - » **How to Use**: Enjoy a handful of berries as a snack, add them to smoothies, or sprinkle them on salads for a burst of flavor and nutrients.
- **Avocado**:
    - » Avocado provides healthy monounsaturated fats that help reduce inflammation and support cellular health. Rich in potassium, magnesium, and fiber, avocados also contribute to electrolyte balance and digestive health, which are important for immune function.
    - » **How to Use**: Add avocado to salads, smoothies, or make a simple guacamole for a nutrient-dense, anti-inflammatory snack.

- **Quinoa and Amaranth**:
  - » Quinoa and amaranth are both alkaline pseudo-grains rich in protein, fiber, and essential minerals like magnesium, which supports nerve and muscle function. They help maintain steady blood sugar levels, reducing stress on the immune system.
  - » **How to Use**: Use quinoa or amaranth as a base for salads, stews, or side dishes to add nutrient-dense, alkaline grains to your diet.

3. KEY HERBS FOR IMMUNE BALANCE AND ANTI-INFLAMMATORY SUPPORT

Certain herbs are particularly beneficial for managing autoimmune conditions because they help regulate immune activity, reduce inflammation, and support overall wellness. These herbs align with Dr. Sebi's emphasis on plant-based healing and natural immune support.

- **Turmeric**:
  - » Turmeric contains curcumin, a powerful anti-inflammatory compound that has been shown to reduce symptoms in autoimmune conditions by inhibiting inflammatory pathways. It also acts as an antioxidant, protecting cells from damage.
  - » **How to Use**: Use 1/2 teaspoon of turmeric powder daily in smoothies, soups, or teas. To enhance absorption, combine turmeric with black pepper or a source of healthy fat like olive oil or avocado.
- **Ashwagandha**:
  - » An adaptogen, ashwagandha helps the body respond to stress, which is crucial for autoimmune health, as chronic stress can exacerbate immune responses. Ashwagandha also has anti-inflammatory properties, supporting balanced immune function.
  - » **How to Use**: Take ashwagandha in capsule form or as a powder added to smoothies. A typical daily dose ranges from 300 to 500 mg. It's best taken in the evening, as it has calming effects.
- **Ginger**:
  - » Ginger is another potent anti-inflammatory herb that helps reduce pain and swelling, particularly for individuals with rheumatoid arthritis and similar autoimmune conditions. It also supports digestion, which is vital for immune health.
  - » **How to Use**: Fresh ginger can be added to teas, smoothies, or grated into salad dressings. For concentrated benefits, consume 1–2 teaspoons of grated ginger daily or take ginger capsules.
- **Holy Basil**:
  - » Known as tulsi, holy basil is a powerful adaptogen with immune-modulating properties. It reduces inflammation, protects against oxidative stress, and helps the body cope with stress, which is essential for managing autoimmune symptoms.
  - » **How to Use**: Brew holy basil tea by steeping 1–2 teaspoons of dried leaves in hot water for 5–10 minutes. Drink daily to support immune balance and reduce inflammation.
- **Reishi Mushroom**:
  - » Reishi mushrooms have immunomodulatory properties, meaning they help balance immune system activity. They are also rich in antioxidants, which protect cells from damage. Reishi is particularly beneficial for autoimmune conditions as it reduces immune overactivity.
  - » **How to Use**: Reishi is available in powder or capsule form. Add 1/2 teaspoon of reishi powder to teas, smoothies, or soups. Follow recommended dosages for capsules based on the product instructions.

4. SUPPORTING GUT HEALTH FOR IMMUNE BALANCE

A significant portion of the immune system is located in the gut, making gut health essential for immune balance. Foods and herbs that support digestive health can help modulate the immune response, reducing the likelihood of autoimmune flare-ups.

- **Probiotic-Rich Foods**:
  - » Probiotics support a balanced gut microbiome, which in turn helps regulate immune activity. Fermented foods such as sauerkraut, kimchi, and coconut yogurt introduce beneficial bacteria that promote gut health.
  - » **How to Use**: Include a small serving of probiotic-rich foods daily. If fermented foods are too strong for you, consider a high-quality probiotic supplement with a variety of strains.
- **Fiber-Rich Foods**:
  - » Fiber feeds beneficial bacteria in the gut, promoting a healthy microbiome. Vegetables, fruits, and whole grains provide soluble and insoluble fiber that supports digestion and immune health.
  - » **How to Use**: Aim for at least 25–30 grams of fiber daily from various plant-based sources like leafy greens, berries, and quinoa.
- **Slippery Elm and Marshmallow Root**:
  - » These mucilaginous herbs coat the digestive tract and reduce inflammation, creating a soothing effect that

DR. SEBI HERBAL BIBLE [30 BOOKS IN 1] 123

can be helpful for those with autoimmune conditions involving digestive symptoms.
- » **How to Use**: Take slippery elm or marshmallow root in tea form, especially during flare-ups. Steep 1–2 teaspoons of the herb in hot water for 5–10 minutes.

5. LIFESTYLE PRACTICES FOR IMMUNE BALANCE

Supporting immune health isn't just about diet and herbs; lifestyle practices play a significant role in managing autoimmune conditions. Regular habits that reduce stress, promote restful sleep, and encourage movement help maintain immune balance.

- **Mindfulness and Stress Management**:
  - » Chronic stress can worsen autoimmune symptoms by triggering inflammatory responses. Practicing mindfulness techniques, such as meditation, deep breathing, or yoga, helps reduce stress hormones and promote relaxation.
  - » **Tip**: Dedicate 10–15 minutes each day to a calming activity, especially during times of high stress or flare-ups.
- **Regular Movement**:
  - » Gentle exercise, such as walking, stretching, or tai chi, supports circulation and reduces inflammation. Physical activity also helps detoxify the body and relieve stress, which can benefit immune health.
  - » **Tip**: Aim for at least 30 minutes of movement daily. Choose activities that feel supportive rather than strenuous, as intense exercise can sometimes trigger flare-ups.
- **Quality Sleep**:
  - » Quality sleep is essential for immune regulation, as the body repairs and regenerates cells during rest. Poor sleep can contribute to increased inflammation, making it harder to manage autoimmune symptoms.
  - » **Tip**: Create a calming bedtime routine, avoid screen time an hour before bed, and aim for 7–8 hours of sleep each night.

6. SAMPLE DAILY ROUTINE FOR IMMUNE BALANCE

A consistent routine incorporating these dietary and lifestyle practices can help support immune balance and reduce autoimmune symptoms. Here's a sample day:

- **Morning**:
  - » Start with a glass of water and a squeeze of lemon to stimulate digestion.
  - » Breakfast: Smoothie with spinach, berries, chia seeds, and a teaspoon of turmeric.
  - » Gentle stretching or a 15-minute meditation session.
- **Mid-Morning**:
  - » Holy basil tea with a small handful of almonds.
- **Lunch**:
  - » Quinoa salad with mixed greens, avocado, cruciferous vegetables, and a drizzle of olive oil.
- **Afternoon**:
  - » Reishi mushroom tea or a cup of ginger tea.
- **Dinner**:
  - » Steamed vegetables with a serving of amaranth or quinoa and a side of probiotic-rich sauerkraut.
- **Evening**:
  - » Wind down with a relaxing activity like reading or gentle yoga. Avoid heavy meals close to bedtime.

Following a daily routine with immune-supporting foods, herbs, and lifestyle practices can create a balanced environment for autoimmune health. By aligning with Dr. Sebi's approach, focusing on anti-inflammatory, alkaline foods, and adding herbs that regulate immune function, you support your body in managing autoimmune symptoms naturally. These practices promote overall wellness and help maintain a balanced immune response, improving quality of life and reducing the frequency of flare-ups.

CHAPTER 2

DETOX PROTOCOLS FOR AUTOIMMUNE WELLNESS

Detoxifying the body is an effective way to support immune balance, especially for those with autoimmune conditions. By removing toxins, reducing inflammation, and nourishing the body with plant-based nutrients, detoxification can help reduce symptom flare-ups and promote overall wellness. This chapter introduces gentle, effective detox protocols tailored for autoimmune health, focusing on foods, herbs, and practices that support a balanced immune response.

1. WHY DETOXIFICATION IS ESSENTIAL FOR AUTOIMMUNE HEALTH

Detoxification helps clear the body of harmful substances that can trigger or worsen autoimmune reactions. Environmental pollutants, processed foods, and toxins from everyday products all place an extra burden on the immune system, which can exacerbate autoimmune symptoms. By implementing a detox protocol, you can help alleviate these stressors, allowing the body to focus on healing and balancing the immune response.

- **Reducing Toxic Load**:
  » Toxins from food, air, and personal care products accumulate in the body over time, potentially disrupting immune function. Detoxification reduces the toxic load, giving the immune system a chance to recalibrate and reduce hyperactivity associated with autoimmune conditions.
- **Supporting Inflammation Reduction**:
  » Chronic inflammation is a hallmark of autoimmune disorders. By focusing on anti-inflammatory, detoxifying foods and practices, you can help reduce inflammation and support immune health.
- **Promoting Alkaline Balance**:
  » Dr. Sebi's principles emphasize an alkaline diet, which helps reduce acidity in the body. A more alkaline environment supports cellular health and makes it easier for the immune system to function optimally without overreacting.

2. KEY FOODS FOR AUTOIMMUNE DETOXIFICATION

Following an alkaline diet rich in detoxifying foods helps reduce inflammation, support liver function, and improve gut health—all of which are essential for autoimmune wellness. Here are some of the best foods to include during a detox:

- **Leafy Greens (Spinach, Kale, Dandelion Greens)**:
  » These greens are highly alkaline, fiber-rich, and packed with antioxidants that support liver detoxification and reduce inflammation. Dandelion greens also have mild diuretic effects, helping the body flush out toxins.
  » **How to Use**: Add leafy greens to salads, smoothies, or lightly steam them as a side dish. Aim for at least two servings of greens daily during the detox.
- **Cucumbers and Celery**:
  » Both cucumbers and celery are hydrating and rich in antioxidants, making them excellent for detox. They also support kidney health, helping the body eliminate waste products.
  » **How to Use**: Include cucumbers and celery in salads, green juices, or as snacks. They are particularly beneficial when consumed raw.
- **Cruciferous Vegetables (Broccoli, Brussels Sprouts, Cauliflower)**:
  » Cruciferous vegetables contain compounds like sulforaphane, which support liver detoxification and have anti-inflammatory effects. They are beneficial for managing immune system balance.
  » **How to Use**: Steam or lightly cook cruciferous vegetables to preserve their detoxifying properties, and include them in meals at least once daily.
- **Berries (Blueberries, Blackberries, Strawberries)**:
  » Berries are high in antioxidants and low in sugar, making them ideal for reducing inflammation and supporting immune health. Their antioxidants help combat oxidative stress, which is common in autoimmune conditions.
  » **How to Use**: Add a handful of berries to your morning smoothie or eat them as a snack.
- **Lemon and Lime**:

- » These citrus fruits are high in vitamin C, which supports immune function and helps detoxify the liver. Lemon and lime also help alkalize the body and promote better digestion.
- » **How to Use**: Start each day with a glass of warm water and a squeeze of fresh lemon or lime to stimulate digestion and support liver function.

3. HERBS TO SUPPORT AUTOIMMUNE DETOXIFICATION

Certain herbs are especially helpful for detoxification in individuals with autoimmune conditions. These herbs aid the liver, support gut health, and reduce inflammation, making them ideal for a balanced immune system.

- **Dandelion Root**:
  - » Dandelion root is a potent liver cleanser that helps eliminate toxins. Its mild diuretic effects also aid the kidneys in flushing out waste.
  - » **How to Use**: Brew dandelion root tea by steeping 1 tablespoon of dried root in hot water for 10–15 minutes. Drink 1–2 cups daily during the detox.
- **Milk Thistle**:
  - » Milk thistle contains silymarin, a compound that promotes liver health and protects cells from damage. It supports liver regeneration, making it especially useful during a detox.
  - » **How to Use**: Take milk thistle in capsule or tincture form, following the dosage recommendations on the product label.
- **Burdock Root**:
  - » Burdock root is known for its blood-purifying properties, helping to cleanse the bloodstream and reduce inflammation. It is beneficial for those with skin-related autoimmune symptoms.
  - » **How to Use**: Brew burdock root tea or add burdock root powder to smoothies. For tea, simmer 1 teaspoon of dried root in water for 10–15 minutes.
- **Ginger**:
  - » Ginger has powerful anti-inflammatory and digestive properties. It helps soothe the digestive system, reducing inflammation and promoting better detoxification.
  - » **How to Use**: Add fresh ginger to teas, smoothies, or juices. Drink ginger tea once or twice daily to support digestion and reduce inflammation.

4. SIMPLE DETOX PRACTICES FOR AUTOIMMUNE HEALTH

In addition to diet, certain daily practices enhance the detox process and support immune balance. These practices are gentle and effective for those managing autoimmune symptoms, promoting a balanced and relaxed state for the body.

- **Hydration and Herbal Infusions**:
  - » Staying hydrated helps flush out toxins through the kidneys and supports immune function. Herbal infusions, such as nettle and chamomile, provide hydration and have calming, anti-inflammatory effects.
  - » **Tip**: Drink at least 8–10 cups of water daily, and include 1–2 cups of herbal tea to support detoxification.
- **Dry Brushing**:
  - » Dry brushing stimulates lymphatic circulation, which helps remove toxins and reduce inflammation. It also supports skin health, making it beneficial for autoimmune conditions affecting the skin.
  - » **How to Use**: Before showering, use a dry brush with gentle, upward strokes toward the heart. Focus on areas where lymph nodes are concentrated, like the underarms and groin.
- **Gentle Exercise**:
  - » Light physical activity promotes circulation and supports detoxification through sweat. Gentle practices like yoga, walking, or tai chi are particularly helpful for autoimmune health as they reduce stress without overstressing the body.
  - » **Tip**: Aim for 20–30 minutes of gentle exercise daily, focusing on movements that support relaxation and deep breathing.

5. SAMPLE 3-DAY AUTOIMMUNE DETOX ROUTINE

Here's a simple 3-day detox routine designed to reduce inflammation, support immune balance, and promote detoxification. Each day focuses on whole, alkaline foods and incorporates herbs and practices that are gentle on the body.

- **Day 1**:
  - » **Morning**: Start with a glass of warm water with lemon. Have a smoothie with spinach, cucumber, blueberries, and ginger.
  - » **Mid-Morning**: Drink a cup of dandelion tea.
  - » **Lunch**: Large salad with leafy greens, avocado, cucumber, and lemon-tahini dressing.
  - » **Afternoon**: Snack on a handful of berries and drink a cup of burdock root tea.

- » **Dinner**: Steamed cruciferous vegetables (broccoli, Brussels sprouts) with quinoa and fresh herbs.
- **Day 2**:
  - » **Morning**: Begin with warm water and lemon. Have a smoothie with kale, celery, lemon, and a teaspoon of ground flaxseed.
  - » **Mid-Morning**: Drink a cup of milk thistle tea.
  - » **Lunch**: Quinoa bowl with mixed greens, avocado, cucumbers, and a sprinkle of chia seeds.
  - » **Afternoon**: Drink ginger tea and snack on sliced cucumber and celery.
  - » **Dinner**: Light vegetable soup with leafy greens, garlic, and turmeric.
- **Day 3**:
  - » **Morning**: Start with lemon water. Smoothie with dandelion greens, a handful of berries, and fresh ginger.
  - » **Mid-Morning**: Nettle tea with a slice of lemon.
  - » **Lunch**: Salad with mixed greens, radishes, avocado, and a drizzle of olive oil and apple cider vinegar.
  - » **Afternoon**: Snack on berries and drink a cup of chamomile tea.
  - » **Dinner**: Steamed vegetables and a small serving of quinoa with turmeric and black pepper.

Following a gentle detox protocol helps reduce inflammation and supports immune balance, giving the body the resources it needs to manage autoimmune conditions naturally. By choosing anti-inflammatory, detoxifying foods, herbs, and lifestyle practices, you create a supportive environment for immune health, helping alleviate symptoms and promote long-term wellness. This approach aligns with Dr. Sebi's philosophy, providing a foundation for balanced and sustainable health.

CHAPTER 3
GUT HEALTH AND INFLAMMATION REDUCTION

Gut health is foundational to managing autoimmune health, as a significant portion of the immune system resides in the gut. When the gut is out of balance—due to poor diet, stress, or environmental toxins—it can lead to systemic inflammation, worsening autoimmune symptoms. Strengthening gut health can reduce inflammation, support immune balance, and help alleviate the severity and frequency of flare-ups. This chapter explores how gut health influences inflammation and offers practical strategies for nurturing a healthy gut environment.

1. THE GUT-INFLAMMATION CONNECTION IN AUTOIMMUNE HEALTH

The gut plays a central role in regulating immune responses and managing inflammation. When gut health is compromised, the body becomes more susceptible to inflammation and autoimmune reactions.

- **Leaky Gut and Autoimmune Flare-Ups:**
  - » "Leaky gut" refers to a condition where the intestinal lining becomes permeable, allowing undigested food particles, toxins, and bacteria to enter the bloodstream. This process triggers immune responses and inflammation, which can worsen autoimmune symptoms.
  - » Maintaining a healthy gut barrier through diet and lifestyle helps prevent leaky gut, thereby reducing immune hyperactivity and inflammation.
- **The Role of Gut Microbiome in Immune Balance:**
  - » The gut is home to trillions of beneficial bacteria that play a key role in immune regulation. An imbalance in gut bacteria (dysbiosis) is associated with increased inflammation and may contribute to autoimmune disorders.
  - » Supporting a balanced gut microbiome with probiotic-rich foods and prebiotics helps reduce inflammation and supports a balanced immune response.

2. FOODS FOR GUT HEALTH AND INFLAMMATION REDUCTION

Dr. Sebi's approach emphasizes alkaline, plant-based foods that support gut health, reduce inflammation, and create an environment conducive to healing. Here are some of the best foods for nurturing a healthy gut and reducing inflammation.

- **Leafy Greens (Spinach, Kale, Swiss Chard):**
  - » Leafy greens are rich in fiber, antioxidants, and nutrients that support a healthy gut microbiome. They contain prebiotic fibers that feed beneficial bacteria, promoting a balanced microbiome.
  - » **How to Use:** Include leafy greens in salads, smoothies, or steam them as a side dish. Aim to consume at least one serving of leafy greens daily.
- **Fermented Foods (Sauerkraut, Kimchi, Coconut Yogurt):**
  - » Fermented foods are natural sources of probiotics, which support gut health by introducing beneficial bacteria. These foods improve digestion and help reduce inflammation, making them ideal for autoimmune wellness.
  - » **How to Use:** Start with small amounts of fermented foods to avoid overstimulation. Aim for 1–2 tablespoons daily, adding them to salads or enjoying as a condiment.
- **Bone Broth (Vegetable-Based for Plant-Based Diet):**
  - » While traditional bone broth is a known gut-healer, plant-based alternatives using nutrient-dense vegetables (like seaweed, mushrooms, and root vegetables) can provide similar benefits. Broths help soothe the digestive lining and reduce inflammation in the gut.
  - » **How to Use:** Simmer vegetables, herbs, and seaweed in water to create a nourishing, anti-inflammatory broth. Enjoy as a warming drink or use it as a base for soups.
- **Berries (Blueberries, Raspberries, Blackberries):**
  - » Berries are high in antioxidants and low in sugar, making them excellent for reducing inflammation. Their fiber content supports healthy digestion, providing nourishment for beneficial gut bacteria.
  - » **How to Use:** Add a handful of berries to smoothies, salads, or eat them as a snack. Berries are an excellent choice for reducing oxidative stress and inflammation.
- **Garlic and Onions:**
  - » Garlic and onions contain prebiotic fibers that feed beneficial bacteria, supporting a balanced gut microbiome. They also have anti-inflammatory and

antimicrobial properties, helping to keep the gut free of harmful pathogens.
- **How to Use**: Incorporate garlic and onions into meals whenever possible. For maximum benefits, let crushed garlic sit for 10 minutes before cooking to enhance its beneficial compounds.

3. HERBS TO SUPPORT GUT HEALTH AND REDUCE INFLAMMATION

Certain herbs have powerful anti-inflammatory and gut-soothing properties, making them ideal for managing autoimmune symptoms. These herbs help reduce inflammation, support digestion, and promote a healthy gut lining, which are essential for reducing autoimmune flare-ups.

- **Slippery Elm**:
  - Slippery elm is a mucilaginous herb that coats and soothes the digestive tract, helping to repair leaky gut and reduce inflammation. It also supports the growth of beneficial bacteria in the gut.
  - **How to Use**: Mix 1/2 teaspoon of slippery elm powder with water and drink before meals. Start with small doses to assess tolerance and gradually increase as needed.
- **Licorice Root**:
  - Licorice root, particularly in its deglycyrrhizinated (DGL) form, helps soothe the digestive tract and reduce inflammation. It promotes healing of the gut lining and is beneficial for those with leaky gut.
  - **How to Use**: Take DGL licorice in chewable tablet form before meals or as a tea. Avoid using regular licorice root if you have high blood pressure, as it can raise blood pressure in some individuals.
- **Ginger**:
  - Ginger is a warming, anti-inflammatory herb that supports digestion and helps reduce gut inflammation. It can alleviate nausea and bloating, which are common symptoms for those with digestive imbalances.
  - **How to Use**: Add fresh ginger to teas, smoothies, or grated into salad dressings. Drink ginger tea before meals to support digestion and reduce inflammation.
- **Marshmallow Root**:
  - Marshmallow root is another mucilaginous herb that coats and protects the gut lining, helping to repair damage from leaky gut and reduce inflammation.
  - **How to Use**: Make a cold infusion by soaking 1–2 tablespoons of marshmallow root in cold water overnight, then strain and drink. Marshmallow root is gentle and can be taken daily to soothe the digestive tract.

4. LIFESTYLE PRACTICES TO SUPPORT GUT HEALTH AND INFLAMMATION REDUCTION

Supporting gut health goes beyond diet and herbs; lifestyle practices can also make a significant difference. Consistent daily habits that reduce stress, promote relaxation, and support digestion are essential for those with autoimmune conditions.

- **Mindful Eating**:
  - Eating mindfully helps improve digestion by allowing the body to properly break down food, reducing bloating and discomfort. Eating in a relaxed state also supports better absorption of nutrients, which is essential for gut health.
  - **Tip**: Take time to chew your food thoroughly, avoid distractions while eating, and practice gratitude before meals to create a calming eating environment.
- **Stress Management**:
  - Chronic stress affects gut health and can worsen inflammation, as stress hormones impact the gut lining and microbiome. Reducing stress helps support a balanced immune response.
  - **Tip**: Incorporate stress-reducing activities into your daily routine, such as meditation, deep breathing, or gentle stretching.
- **Gentle Movement**:
  - Exercise stimulates digestion, promotes circulation, and reduces stress—all of which support gut health and reduce inflammation. Gentle activities, such as walking, yoga, or tai chi, are particularly beneficial.
  - **Tip**: Aim for 20–30 minutes of gentle exercise daily, focusing on movements that support relaxation rather than high intensity.
- **Hydration**:
  - Staying well-hydrated is essential for digestion and detoxification. Proper hydration supports bowel regularity, reduces bloating, and helps flush toxins from the body.
  - **Tip**: Drink at least eight cups of water daily, and consider including herbal teas like chamomile or peppermint to support digestion.

5. SAMPLE DAY FOR GUT HEALTH AND INFLAMMATION REDUCTION

Here's a sample day that incorporates foods, herbs, and lifestyle practices for gut health and inflammation reduction. Following a routine like this can support gut health, balance inflammation, and reduce the risk of autoimmune flare-ups.

- **Morning**:
  » Start with a glass of warm water and lemon to stimulate digestion.
  » **Breakfast**: Smoothie with spinach, blueberries, avocado, and a teaspoon of ground flaxseed for fiber and anti-inflammatory benefits.
- **Mid-Morning**:
  » Drink a cup of ginger tea to support digestion and reduce inflammation.
- **Lunch**:
  » Large salad with leafy greens, cucumber, carrots, and sauerkraut for probiotics. Top with avocado and a dressing made from olive oil, lemon, and garlic.
- **Afternoon Snack**:
  » Enjoy a handful of berries and a small serving of coconut yogurt for probiotics and antioxidants.
- **Dinner**:
  » Steamed cruciferous vegetables (broccoli, cauliflower) with quinoa and fresh herbs. Add a serving of plant-based broth with anti-inflammatory ingredients like turmeric and ginger.
- **Evening**:
  » Wind down with a cup of chamomile or slippery elm tea, both of which support gut health and promote relaxation.

By focusing on gut health and inflammation reduction, you can help manage autoimmune symptoms naturally. Dr. Sebi's approach emphasizes plant-based, alkaline foods, beneficial herbs, and mindful lifestyle practices that support the gut, reduce inflammation, and promote a balanced immune system. With these practices, you create a foundation for improved well-being, reduced autoimmune flare-ups, and long-term health stability.

BOOK 15
Herbal Support for Viral Infections

Viruses present unique challenges to the immune system, often requiring targeted support for both prevention and recovery. Dr. Sebi's approach to viral management emphasizes maintaining an alkaline environment in the body, as viruses thrive in acidic conditions. By focusing on an alkaline, plant-based diet and incorporating supportive herbs, you can strengthen the immune system, support the body's natural defenses, and reduce the frequency and severity of viral infections.

CHAPTER 1
ALKALINE DIET FOR VIRAL MANAGEMENT

The foundation of Dr. Sebi's approach to viral management is an alkaline diet. By focusing on alkaline foods, the body can maintain a balanced pH level that reduces the environment in which viruses thrive. An alkaline diet also supports the immune system by reducing inflammation, enhancing detoxification, and providing essential nutrients that fortify the body's defenses. This chapter covers the basics of an alkaline diet for managing viral infections and how to implement this approach in daily life to boost immunity and resilience against viruses.

1. THE ROLE OF PH BALANCE IN VIRAL INFECTIONS

The body's internal pH balance plays a crucial role in immune function. Viruses and other pathogens are more likely to thrive in acidic environments, which can be exacerbated by processed foods, refined sugars, and high-stress levels.

- **Acidity and Viral Growth**:
  » Acidic conditions in the body, often due to a diet high in processed foods and low in nutrients, provide an environment in which viruses can thrive. These acidic conditions place additional stress on the immune system, making it more difficult to fend off infections.
- **Alkalinity and Immune Function**:
  » An alkaline diet, rich in plant-based foods, helps to neutralize excess acidity in the body, creating an internal environment less favorable for viral activity. By supporting detoxification and reducing inflammation, an alkaline diet allows the immune system to function more effectively.

2. KEY ALKALINE FOODS FOR VIRAL MANAGEMENT

Certain alkaline foods are especially supportive of immune function and viral management, thanks to their nutrient density, antioxidants, and anti-inflammatory properties. These foods work together to strengthen the body's natural defenses, making it harder for viruses to take hold.

- **Leafy Greens (Spinach, Kale, Dandelion Greens)**:
  » Leafy greens are rich in chlorophyll, which helps alkalize the body and supports detoxification. These greens also provide essential vitamins A and C, both of which support immune function and help the body fight off infections.
  » **How to Use**: Include leafy greens in smoothies, salads, or lightly sautéed. Aim to consume at least one serving of leafy greens each day.
- **Berries (Blueberries, Blackberries, Strawberries)**:
  » Berries are high in antioxidants, particularly vitamin C, which helps boost immune defenses and combat oxidative stress. Their low glycemic index and fiber content make them ideal for a balanced immune response.
  » **How to Use**: Add a handful of berries to smoothies, oatmeal, or eat them as a snack. Berries can be enjoyed daily for ongoing immune support.
- **Citrus Fruits (Lemons, Limes, Oranges)**:
  » Citrus fruits are rich in vitamin C, an essential nutrient for immune health. They also have a slightly alkalizing effect on the body once digested, helping maintain pH balance.
  » **How to Use**: Start each morning with a glass of warm lemon water to support detoxification. Citrus fruits can be added to salads, smoothies, or enjoyed as a snack.
- **Garlic**:
  » Garlic is a powerful antiviral and immune-supportive food. Its active compound, allicin, has been shown to boost immune cell activity and support the body's ability to combat viral infections.
  » **How to Use**: Incorporate raw or lightly cooked garlic into meals for maximum benefit. Crushing or chopping garlic before use and letting it sit for a few minutes enhances its antiviral properties.
- **Ginger**:
  » Ginger is a warming, anti-inflammatory root that supports immune health by enhancing circulation and reducing inflammation. It has antiviral properties that make it a valuable addition to a diet for viral management.
  » **How to Use**: Add fresh ginger to teas, soups, or smoothies. Ginger tea is especially effective for boosting immunity during colder months or during viral outbreaks.
- **Avocado**:
  » Avocados are rich in healthy fats, particularly mono-

unsaturated fats, which help reduce inflammation. They also provide essential nutrients like vitamin E, which is important for immune function.
- » **How to Use**: Add avocado to salads, smoothies, or enjoy it as a topping on toast. Its versatility makes it easy to include in daily meals for consistent immune support.
- **Sea Vegetables (Sea Moss, Bladderwrack)**:
  - » Sea vegetables are highly alkaline and rich in iodine, a mineral essential for immune health. Sea moss, in particular, contains compounds that help the body fight off viruses and reduce mucus, making it ideal for respiratory health.
  - » **How to Use**: Add sea moss gel to smoothies or soups. Bladderwrack can be taken in powdered form or as a supplement to support thyroid and immune health.

3. FOODS TO AVOID FOR VIRAL HEALTH

While adding alkaline foods to the diet is essential, it's equally important to avoid foods that increase acidity and place additional stress on the immune system. The following foods can worsen inflammation and create an environment conducive to viral activity:

- **Refined Sugars**:
  - » Sugar suppresses immune function, feeds harmful bacteria, and contributes to an acidic environment in the body. High sugar intake has been linked to increased susceptibility to infections and slower recovery times.
  - » **Tip**: Replace refined sugars with natural options like raw honey or maple syrup, but use these sparingly as well.
- **Processed Foods**:
  - » Processed foods are high in additives, preservatives, and unhealthy fats that increase inflammation. These foods often lack the nutrients needed to support a strong immune response.
  - » **Tip**: Focus on whole, plant-based foods and avoid packaged snacks and meals. Preparing meals at home ensures better control over ingredients and nutrient quality.
- **Dairy Products**:
  - » Dairy can increase mucus production and inflammation, particularly in the respiratory system. This can exacerbate symptoms of viral infections, especially those affecting the lungs.
  - » **Tip**: Replace dairy with plant-based alternatives like almond or coconut milk, which are less likely to contribute to inflammation.
- **Red Meat**:
  - » Red meat is acidic and can contribute to inflammation, making it harder for the immune system to function optimally. Its high fat content also increases the risk of oxidative stress.
  - » **Tip**: Opt for plant-based sources of protein, such as legumes, nuts, seeds, and leafy greens.

4. PRACTICAL TIPS FOR IMPLEMENTING AN ALKALINE DIET FOR VIRAL MANAGEMENT

Transitioning to an alkaline diet for viral management doesn't have to be complicated. By following these tips, you can gradually incorporate more alkaline foods and reduce acidic, inflammatory foods in your daily diet.

- **Start with an Alkaline Breakfast**:
  - » Begin the day with a smoothie made from leafy greens, berries, ginger, and a tablespoon of sea moss. This helps alkalize the body, provides essential vitamins, and gives an immune boost first thing in the morning.
- **Hydrate with Alkaline Water and Herbal Teas**:
  - » Proper hydration is essential for immune health, and alkaline water or herbal teas can help maintain pH balance. Herbal teas like ginger, dandelion, and nettle support detoxification and immune function.
  - » **Tip**: Aim for 8–10 cups of water and herbal teas daily to stay hydrated and support immunity.
- **Add Garlic and Ginger to Meals Regularly**:
  - » Both garlic and ginger have powerful antiviral properties. Adding these ingredients to meals daily can strengthen immunity and help prevent viral infections.
  - » **Tip**: Use garlic and ginger in salad dressings, soups, stir-fries, or herbal teas.
- **Create Nutrient-Dense Alkaline Salads**:
  - » Alkaline salads are a simple way to increase nutrient intake and support immune health. Base salads on leafy greens, add colorful vegetables, and top with avocado and a citrus-based dressing for added vitamin C.
  - » **Example**: A salad with spinach, cucumbers, bell peppers, avocado, and a dressing made from olive oil, lemon, and garlic can provide both immune-boosting and anti-inflammatory benefits.

- **Use Sea Moss as a Daily Supplement**:
  - Sea moss is a versatile ingredient that can be added to smoothies, soups, or even as a thickener in sauces. Its high mineral content supports overall immunity, while its antiviral properties help manage respiratory infections.
  - **Tip**: Prepare sea moss gel at home by soaking and blending the sea moss, then storing it in the fridge. Use 1–2 tablespoons daily for best results.

5. SAMPLE ALKALINE MEAL PLAN FOR VIRAL MANAGEMENT

Following an alkaline meal plan can help ensure you're consistently supporting immune health and managing the body's pH balance. Here's a sample day:

- **Morning**:
  - Start with a glass of warm lemon water to support liver detoxification and maintain an alkaline start to the day.
  - **Breakfast**: Green smoothie with spinach, kale, avocado, blueberries, ginger, and a tablespoon of sea moss gel. Blend with alkaline water or coconut water for hydration and added minerals.
- **Mid-Morning Snack**:
  - Enjoy a handful of raw almonds and an apple, both of which are alkalizing and provide essential nutrients for immunity.
- **Lunch**:
  - Salad with mixed greens, cucumbers, bell peppers, and a dressing of olive oil, lemon, and crushed garlic. Add sliced avocado and a handful of sprouts for extra nutrients.
- **Afternoon Snack**:
  - Herbal tea with ginger and a squeeze of lemon. This tea supports hydration, provides antioxidants, and has immune-boosting properties.
- **Dinner**:
  - Steamed vegetables (broccoli, Brussels sprouts, zucchini) with quinoa and a side of sea moss soup for added minerals. Season with herbs and a sprinkle of turmeric for anti-inflammatory benefits.
- **Evening**:
  - Finish the day with a soothing chamomile tea to support relaxation and immune recovery, helping the body rest and restore itself.

Following an alkaline diet rich in nutrient-dense, immune-supporting foods creates an internal environment that helps the body manage and resist viral infections. Dr. Sebi's approach emphasizes these principles, helping you take control of your health by aligning diet with immune resilience. Consistent daily habits, from eating leafy greens and berries to avoiding processed foods and refined sugars, reinforce the immune system, reduce inflammation, and offer a natural path to enhanced viral resistance.

CHAPTER 2
HERBS FOR IMMUNE BOOSTING

Herbal remedies have been used for centuries to support the immune system, helping the body naturally defend itself against infections. Specific herbs are known for their immune-boosting, antiviral, and anti-inflammatory properties, making them valuable allies for those looking to strengthen their defenses. This chapter introduces some of the best immune-boosting herbs, along with practical ways to incorporate them into your daily routine.

1. ELDERBERRY: NATURE'S IMMUNE PROTECTOR

Elderberry has gained widespread recognition for its immune-boosting properties, particularly its effectiveness against viral infections. Elderberries are rich in antioxidants, especially anthocyanins, which help reduce inflammation and combat oxidative stress.

- **Benefits of Elderberry**:
  - **Antiviral Properties**: Elderberry has been shown to inhibit viral replication, making it effective for preventing and managing colds and the flu.
  - **Rich in Antioxidants**: Elderberries are high in vitamin C and other antioxidants that support immune function.
  - **Reduces Inflammation**: Its anti-inflammatory effects help relieve symptoms associated with viral infections.
- **How to Use Elderberry**:
  - **Elderberry Syrup**: Elderberry syrup is a popular way to take this herb, especially during cold and flu season. Take 1–2 teaspoons daily for prevention, or increase to 1–2 teaspoons every few hours when feeling under the weather.
  - **Elderberry Tea**: Brew dried elderberries in hot water for 10–15 minutes, strain, and enjoy as a warming tea to boost immunity.

2. ECHINACEA: THE IMMUNE STIMULATOR

Echinacea is well-known for its immune-stimulating properties. It activates various immune cells, helping the body respond more effectively to infections. Echinacea is most effective when taken at the first signs of illness or as a preventive measure during peak viral seasons.

- **Benefits of Echinacea**:
  - **Enhances Immune Response**: Echinacea stimulates immune cells, including macrophages and lymphocytes, which fight infections.
  - **Anti-inflammatory Properties**: It helps reduce inflammation, supporting the body's ability to manage symptoms during an infection.
  - **Antiviral Effects**: Echinacea has mild antiviral properties, helping reduce the severity and duration of colds and flu.
- **How to Use Echinacea**:
  - **Echinacea Tea**: Steep 1 teaspoon of dried echinacea in hot water for 10–15 minutes. Drink 1–2 cups daily as a preventive measure or up to three cups when experiencing symptoms.
  - **Echinacea Tincture**: Take 1–2 droppers full of echinacea tincture daily as an immune booster, especially during cold and flu season.

3. ASTRAGALUS: THE DEEP IMMUNE TONIC

Astragalus is an adaptogenic herb known for its immune-strengthening properties. It helps the body resist infections by supporting both the immune and respiratory systems, making it a valuable herb for long-term immune support.

- **Benefits of Astragalus**:
  - **Immune Tonic**: Astragalus supports the immune system at a deep level, making it ideal for those looking to build long-term immunity.
  - **Supports Respiratory Health**: It strengthens the lungs and respiratory tract, which are often affected by viral infections.
  - **Antioxidant-Rich**: Astragalus contains antioxidants that protect cells from damage and support overall vitality.
- **How to Use Astragalus**:
  - **Astragalus Tea**: Simmer 1 tablespoon of dried astragalus root in water for 20–30 minutes. Drink one cup daily as a tonic to strengthen immunity.
  - **Astragalus Powder**: Add astragalus powder to smoothies or soups as a daily immune booster.

4. GARLIC: THE POTENT ANTIVIRAL

Garlic is a powerful herb with antiviral, antibacterial, and immune-stimulating properties. Its active compound, allicin, is known to enhance immune cell function and help fight off infections. Garlic is most effective when consumed raw or lightly cooked to preserve its immune-boosting properties.

- **Benefits of Garlic:**
  - **Antiviral and Antibacterial**: Garlic's allicin content helps the body combat various pathogens, including viruses.
  - **Enhances Immune Function**: Garlic stimulates immune cells, boosting the body's response to infections.
  - **Anti-inflammatory Effects**: It helps reduce inflammation, which is beneficial during viral infections.
- **How to Use Garlic:**
  - **Garlic Honey**: Mix chopped raw garlic with raw honey and take 1 teaspoon daily as a preventive measure. This blend is especially effective for sore throats and respiratory infections.
  - **Garlic Tea**: Crush a clove of garlic and steep it in hot water for 5–10 minutes. Add lemon and honey for taste and immune support.

5. GINGER: THE WARMING IMMUNE ALLY

Ginger is a warming herb with antiviral and anti-inflammatory properties, making it ideal for supporting the immune system and reducing inflammation. It is especially effective for respiratory health, as it helps break up mucus and relieve congestion.

- **Benefits of Ginger:**
  - **Antiviral Properties**: Ginger helps inhibit viral replication, making it a supportive herb for managing viral infections.
  - **Supports Respiratory Health**: Its warming effects help relieve congestion and support respiratory function.
  - **Anti-inflammatory and Antioxidant**: Ginger reduces inflammation and supports immune health, especially during viral infections.
- **How to Use Ginger:**
  - **Ginger Tea**: Grate fresh ginger and steep in hot water for 10 minutes. Drink daily for immune support or increase to 2–3 cups per day during illness.
  - **Ginger Shot**: Blend ginger with lemon and a bit of cayenne pepper for a potent immune boost. Take a small shot in the morning to kickstart your immune system.

6. LICORICE ROOT: THE SOOTHING ANTIVIRAL

Licorice root has strong antiviral and anti-inflammatory properties, particularly effective for managing respiratory infections. It also helps soothe sore throats and reduce inflammation, making it a useful herb during viral outbreaks.

- **Benefits of Licorice Root:**
  - **Antiviral**: Licorice root contains glycyrrhizin, a compound known for its antiviral activity, particularly against respiratory viruses.
  - **Soothes Mucous Membranes**: It helps reduce irritation in the throat and respiratory tract, making it useful for coughs and sore throats.
  - **Supports Immune Health**: Licorice root helps regulate the immune response, reducing excessive inflammation during infection.
- **How to Use Licorice Root:**
  - **Licorice Root Tea**: Steep 1 teaspoon of dried licorice root in hot water for 10 minutes. Drink 1–2 cups daily to support immune health and relieve respiratory symptoms.
  - **Licorice Tincture**: Take 1–2 droppers of licorice tincture daily. Avoid long-term use of licorice if you have high blood pressure.

7. TURMERIC: THE ANTI-INFLAMMATORY SUPER HERB

Turmeric, with its active compound curcumin, is a powerful anti-inflammatory herb that supports immune health and helps reduce symptoms associated with viral infections. It can be particularly useful for managing respiratory inflammation and supporting overall immunity.

- **Benefits of Turmeric:**
  - **Anti-inflammatory**: Turmeric's anti-inflammatory properties help reduce immune overactivity, which is beneficial during viral infections.
  - **Antioxidant**: It protects cells from oxidative damage, supporting the immune system in fighting infections.
  - **Supports Respiratory Health**: Turmeric's anti-inflammatory effects can relieve respiratory inflammation, a common issue during viral infections.
- **How to Use Turmeric:**
  - **Turmeric Tea**: Mix 1/2 teaspoon of turmeric powder

with warm water, a pinch of black pepper, and a touch of honey. Drink daily to support immunity.
- » **Golden Milk**: Combine turmeric with warm almond milk, ginger, and honey for a comforting, immune-boosting drink before bed.

8. PRACTICAL TIPS FOR INCORPORATING IMMUNE-BOOSTING HERBS

Including these immune-boosting herbs in your daily routine can be simple and effective. Here are a few practical tips for making herbal support a consistent part of your lifestyle:

- **Create a Daily Herbal Tea Routine**:
  - » Choose 1–2 herbs each day to make a supportive tea. For example, combine elderberry with ginger for a warming, immune-boosting blend, or pair licorice root with turmeric to soothe and support immunity.
- **Incorporate Herbs into Meals**:
  - » Herbs like garlic, ginger, and turmeric can be easily added to meals, enhancing flavor and providing immune support. Use garlic in sauces, add ginger to stir-fries, and sprinkle turmeric on vegetables or soups.
- **Use Herbal Tinctures for Convenience**:
  - » Tinctures offer a concentrated way to take herbs without preparation. Tinctures can be taken directly under the tongue or added to a glass of water. Keep a few immune-boosting tinctures on hand, like echinacea and astragalus, for convenient support during peak viral seasons.
- **Make a Weekly Immune-Boosting Syrup**:
  - » Prepare a batch of elderberry syrup or garlic-infused honey to have on hand for daily immune support. These syrups are particularly effective when taken preventatively, especially during times when you're at higher risk of viral exposure.

These herbs, when used consistently, create a strong foundation for immune health, helping the body naturally defend itself against viral infections. Dr. Sebi's approach emphasizes the use of plant-based remedies, and these herbs align with his principles by offering natural, effective immune support without the need for pharmaceuticals. By incorporating immune-boosting herbs into your daily routine, you empower your body to maintain health and resilience against viral threats, enhancing overall wellness and reducing the likelihood of illness.

CHAPTER 3
PROTOCOLS FOR VIRAL CLEANSING

Cleansing the body of viruses requires more than just immune support; it involves detoxification practices and specific herbs that help the body expel toxins and fight viral particles. These protocols are designed to gently cleanse the body, reduce viral load, and strengthen the immune system, making it easier to resist infections and recover from them more quickly.

1. UNDERSTANDING VIRAL CLEANSING AND DETOXIFICATION

When viruses invade the body, they leave behind metabolic byproducts and toxins that can weaken the immune system and contribute to inflammation. Viral cleansing focuses on removing these byproducts, reducing inflammation, and promoting cellular health.

- **Supporting the Liver and Kidneys:**
    - » The liver and kidneys play a central role in detoxifying the body and filtering out toxins. A viral cleanse supports these organs by reducing their workload and promoting efficient waste removal.
- **Eliminating Inflammatory Toxins:**
    - » Viral infections can increase inflammation, which impairs healing and can lead to chronic health issues. A proper cleanse helps flush out inflammatory toxins, reducing overall stress on the body and promoting faster recovery.

2. CORE COMPONENTS OF A VIRAL CLEANSE PROTOCOL

The foundation of a viral cleanse includes an alkaline, nutrient-rich diet, detoxifying herbs, and daily practices that support efficient waste elimination. Here's a breakdown of each component and its role in cleansing the body of viruses.

- **Alkaline Diet:**
    - » An alkaline diet supports a balanced pH, which makes it more difficult for viruses to thrive. By avoiding acidic foods and focusing on alkaline, plant-based options, you help create an internal environment that is less conducive to viral activity.
    - » **Key Foods:** Leafy greens, cucumbers, avocados, and citrus fruits are highly alkaline and packed with vitamins and antioxidants that support cellular health.
- **Hydration with Herbal Teas and Alkaline Water:**
    - » Staying hydrated is essential for effective detoxification. Herbal teas that support the liver and kidneys, such as dandelion root, ginger, and nettle, help the body flush out toxins while providing immune support.
    - » **Suggested Teas:** Drink 2–3 cups of herbal tea daily. Dandelion root supports liver detoxification, nettle provides kidney support, and ginger helps reduce inflammation and cleanse respiratory passages.
- **Daily Practices to Support Detox:**
    - » Incorporating daily detox practices, like dry brushing and gentle movement, encourages lymphatic flow and toxin elimination through sweat and circulation.
    - » **Dry Brushing:** This practice stimulates the lymphatic system, which helps remove waste from the body. Before showering, use a dry brush with upward strokes, focusing on areas where lymph nodes are concentrated.

3. KEY HERBS FOR VIRAL CLEANSING

Certain herbs are particularly effective for cleansing the body of viruses, supporting the liver, and promoting immune function. Incorporating these herbs into a cleansing routine helps target and eliminate viral byproducts and strengthens the body's defenses.

- **Burdock Root:**
    - » Burdock root is known for its blood-purifying properties and helps eliminate toxins from the bloodstream, supporting immune function and reducing inflammation.
    - » **How to Use:** Simmer 1–2 teaspoons of dried burdock root in hot water for 10–15 minutes and drink as a tea once or twice daily.
- **Dandelion Root:**
    - » Dandelion root is a powerful liver cleanser that assists with removing toxins and supports overall immune health, helping the body efficiently detoxify after viral infections.
    - » **How to Use:** Brew dandelion root tea or take it in tincture form. Drink one cup daily as part of your cleansing protocol.
- **Ginger:**
    - » Ginger has anti-inflammatory and detoxifying prop-

erties, helping to reduce respiratory inflammation and expel mucus and viral toxins. It also supports digestion, which is essential for detoxification.
  » **How to Use**: Grate fresh ginger and steep in hot water for 10 minutes. Drink ginger tea 2–3 times per day, especially during active infection periods.
- **Elderberry**:
  » Elderberry not only boosts immunity but also helps the body expel viral particles, supporting a faster recovery and reducing the severity of symptoms.
  » **How to Use**: Take elderberry syrup daily as a preventive measure or increase to 1–2 teaspoons every few hours during an active infection.

4. SAMPLE 3-DAY VIRAL CLEANSE PROTOCOL

A viral cleanse can be short and intensive or part of a longer, more gradual approach to detox. Here is a sample 3-day protocol designed to cleanse the body of viral toxins, promote immune function, and support detoxification organs.

- **Day 1: Alkaline Start and Hydration**:
  » **Morning**: Start with warm water and lemon to stimulate digestion and support liver function. Have a smoothie with spinach, cucumber, ginger, and a tablespoon of sea moss gel.
  » **Mid-Morning**: Drink a cup of dandelion root tea for liver support.
  » **Lunch**: A large salad with mixed greens, avocado, and a lemon-olive oil dressing. Add garlic for antiviral support.
  » **Afternoon Snack**: Enjoy a handful of berries and a cup of elderberry tea for antioxidant and immune support.
  » **Dinner**: Steamed vegetables (broccoli, zucchini) with quinoa. Season with turmeric for added anti-inflammatory support.
  » **Evening**: Wind down with ginger tea to soothe the digestive system and aid in viral cleansing.
- **Day 2: Increasing Detoxification**:
  » **Morning**: Start with lemon water. Follow with a smoothie containing kale, avocado, a handful of berries, and a teaspoon of spirulina for added minerals.
  » **Mid-Morning**: Drink nettle tea to support kidney function and aid in waste removal.
  » **Lunch**: Vegetable broth with cruciferous vegetables (broccoli, Brussels sprouts) and garlic for immune support.
  » **Afternoon**: Dry brushing before a warm shower to stimulate lymphatic circulation.
  » **Dinner**: A hearty salad with leafy greens, cucumber, and grated carrots, topped with avocado. Add apple cider vinegar to promote alkalinity.
  » **Evening**: Chamomile or ginger tea to promote relaxation and support digestion.
- **Day 3: Deep Cleansing and Immune Support**:
  » **Morning**: Start with warm water and lemon. Enjoy a green smoothie with dandelion greens, cucumber, ginger, and elderberry syrup for immune support.
  » **Mid-Morning**: Drink burdock root tea to purify the blood and reduce inflammation.
  » **Lunch**: Quinoa salad with mixed greens, bell peppers, avocado, and lemon dressing. Add garlic for antiviral benefits.
  » **Afternoon Snack**: Drink nettle tea and enjoy a handful of nuts or seeds for energy and protein.
  » **Dinner**: Steamed cruciferous vegetables with a side of wild rice or quinoa and a sprinkle of sea salt for mineral balance.
  » **Evening**: Finish the day with a warm cup of ginger tea to support digestion and prepare for restful sleep.

5. TIPS FOR MAINTAINING LONG-TERM VIRAL HEALTH

After completing a cleanse, it's important to continue supporting the body to prevent future viral infections. Here are some tips for maintaining long-term viral health:

- **Stay Consistent with Alkaline Foods**: Include leafy greens, cucumbers, and citrus fruits in daily meals to keep the body's pH balanced and reduce viral susceptibility.
- **Practice Routine Herbal Support**: Keep using immune-boosting and antiviral herbs, like elderberry and ginger, throughout the year to support immunity.
- **Prioritize Rest and Relaxation**: Adequate sleep and stress management play a vital role in maintaining immune health. Ensure you're giving your body time to rest, recover, and resist infections.
- **Stay Hydrated**: Hydration helps the kidneys and liver flush out toxins more effectively. Include herbal teas, such as nettle or ginger, and aim for 8–10 cups of fluids daily.
- **Incorporate Movement**: Gentle exercises like walking, yoga, and tai chi help improve circulation, support lymphatic function, and promote overall immune health.

By following these protocols, you're supporting the body's natural cleansing processes, helping to remove viral toxins, and reducing the body's susceptibility to infections. Dr. Sebi's approach emphasizes the importance of creating an alkaline environment and using plant-based support to keep the body resilient. With regular detoxification and supportive herbs, you're giving your body the tools it needs to stay strong, reduce viral load, and maintain optimal health.

BOOK 16
Herbs for Stress and Mental Clarity

Modern life is filled with stressors that impact mental clarity, emotional balance, and overall well-being. Dr. Sebi's holistic approach to mental health emphasizes the use of plant-based remedies to reduce anxiety, enhance mental clarity, and promote a calm, centered state of mind. This book provides an in-depth guide to using herbs to manage stress, support the nervous system, and improve focus naturally.

CHAPTER 1
DR. SEBI'S HERBS FOR ANXIETY

Anxiety affects millions of people worldwide and can disrupt sleep, productivity, and emotional well-being. Dr. Sebi's approach to managing anxiety centers on natural, plant-based remedies that calm the nervous system, reduce stress hormones, and restore balance without the side effects often associated with pharmaceuticals. This chapter introduces the best herbs for managing anxiety, detailing their benefits and offering practical tips for daily use to help calm the mind and reduce stress naturally.

1. UNDERSTANDING ANXIETY AND NATURAL REMEDIES

Anxiety is a complex response involving both the body and mind. It's often triggered by stress, lifestyle factors, or unresolved emotional issues. Chronic anxiety can impact physical health, weakening the immune system and increasing the risk of developing other health issues. Dr. Sebi's approach to managing anxiety focuses on using herbs that address the root causes of stress and anxiety by calming the nervous system, balancing hormones, and supporting mental clarity.

- **The Body's Stress Response**:
  » When stress becomes chronic, the body's fight-or-flight response remains active, releasing stress hormones like cortisol and adrenaline. Over time, this can lead to tension, exhaustion, and an overactive mind, contributing to anxiety.
  » Herbs that support the nervous system and reduce cortisol levels help break this cycle, promoting a state of calm and balance.

- **The Role of Alkaline Balance**:
  » Anxiety can be exacerbated by an acidic diet and lifestyle. Dr. Sebi's emphasis on an alkaline diet helps reduce the body's overall stress load, as alkaline foods are anti-inflammatory and provide essential nutrients that support mental health.
  » Combined with herbs, an alkaline lifestyle promotes an internal environment that supports relaxation and reduces the likelihood of chronic anxiety.

2. KEY HERBS FOR MANAGING ANXIETY

Several herbs align with Dr. Sebi's approach to anxiety management, offering natural support to calm the nervous system, reduce tension, and enhance mental clarity. Each herb has specific properties that make it uniquely beneficial for reducing stress and managing anxiety.

- **Passionflower**:
  » Passionflower is a powerful herb known for its calming effects on the mind and body. It works by increasing levels of gamma-aminobutyric acid (GABA), a neurotransmitter that promotes relaxation and reduces anxiety.
  » **Benefits**:
  - Helps calm an overactive mind and reduces racing thoughts, which can help improve sleep and reduce anxiety symptoms.
  - Gently soothes the nervous system, making it useful for those experiencing tension and nervousness.
  » **How to Use**: Steep 1–2 teaspoons of dried passionflower in hot water for 10–15 minutes to make a calming tea. Drink once or twice daily, especially in the evening to promote relaxation.

- **Ashwagandha**:
  » Ashwagandha is an adaptogen, meaning it helps the body adapt to stress and regulates stress hormones like cortisol. It's particularly useful for those with chronic stress and anxiety, as it supports both mental clarity and emotional resilience.
  » **Benefits**:
  - Reduces cortisol levels, easing the body's stress response and promoting a calmer state of mind.
  - Supports adrenal health, helping those who feel fatigued or "burned out" from chronic anxiety.
  » **How to Use**: Take ashwagandha in capsule or powder form. Mix 1/2 teaspoon of ashwagandha powder into smoothies or warm almond milk. Daily use over several weeks is recommended to see cumulative effects.

- **Valerian Root**:
  » Valerian root is known for its calming and mildly sedative effects, making it ideal for reducing anxiety and promoting restful sleep. Its effects on GABA levels make it effective for calming the mind.
  » **Benefits**:
  - Eases tension and relaxes the nervous system, making it helpful for those who experience anxiety at night.

- Supports sleep quality, which is essential for reducing anxiety over the long term.
  » **How to Use**: Brew valerian root tea by steeping 1 teaspoon of the dried root in hot water for 10–15 minutes. Drink in the evening as it may induce drowsiness. Avoid taking valerian root during the day if it makes you feel too relaxed.
- **Holy Basil (Tulsi)**:
  » Holy basil, also known as tulsi, is a powerful adaptogen that supports emotional resilience and reduces stress. It is used in Ayurvedic medicine for its calming effects and ability to improve mental clarity and reduce anxiety.
  » **Benefits**:
    - Reduces the effects of stress on the body, helping to lower cortisol levels and improve emotional balance.
    - Boosts cognitive function and mental clarity, making it helpful for reducing anxiety and improving focus.
  » **How to Use**: Holy basil can be enjoyed as a tea or taken as a supplement. Brew 1–2 teaspoons of dried tulsi in hot water for 5–10 minutes. Drink up to two cups daily to experience its calming benefits.
- **Lemon Balm**:
  » Lemon balm is a gentle, calming herb that is particularly helpful for those who experience mild to moderate anxiety. Its soothing properties make it useful for relieving stress and promoting mental clarity.
  » **Benefits**:
    - Reduces anxiety without sedating, making it a good option for daytime use.
    - Helps improve mood and mental focus, which can be beneficial for those who experience anxiety-related brain fog.
  » **How to Use**: Brew lemon balm tea by steeping 1–2 teaspoons of dried lemon balm in hot water for 10 minutes. Drink up to three cups daily for consistent, gentle anxiety relief.

3. INCORPORATING DR. SEBI'S HERBS INTO A DAILY ANXIETY-RELIEF ROUTINE

A structured routine incorporating these herbs can provide consistent support for managing anxiety, reducing stress, and improving mental clarity. Here's a suggested daily routine:

- **Morning**:
  » Begin with a warm cup of holy basil tea to start the day with calmness and focus. If you prefer capsules, take one dose of ashwagandha to support stress resilience throughout the day.
  » **Alkaline Breakfast**: Include leafy greens, avocado, and lemon water to reduce inflammation and support mental clarity.
- **Mid-Morning**:
  » Prepare a lemon balm tea or tincture to reduce any mid-morning anxiety and promote focus. Lemon balm is ideal for maintaining calm without causing drowsiness.
- **Afternoon**:
  » For mid-day anxiety, drink a cup of passionflower tea to support relaxation. If work or personal tasks cause stress, passionflower can help calm the mind and prevent afternoon burnout.
- **Evening**:
  » Prepare a cup of valerian root tea or a blend of valerian and passionflower about an hour before bedtime. This combination will help ease any lingering anxiety from the day and promote restful sleep.

4. LIFESTYLE TIPS FOR ENHANCED ANXIETY MANAGEMENT

In addition to herbal support, lifestyle practices aligned with Dr. Sebi's philosophy can further reduce anxiety and improve mental clarity. Here are a few tips:

- **Practice Mindful Breathing**:
  » Simple breathing exercises can calm the nervous system and reduce anxiety quickly. Try taking five deep breaths, inhaling for a count of four and exhaling for a count of six.
  » Regular mindful breathing helps regulate stress hormones and supports a relaxed state.
- **Eat Alkaline Foods**:
  » Foods high in magnesium, potassium, and B vitamins support nerve health and mental clarity. Foods like leafy greens, avocados, nuts, and seeds are particularly calming and nutrient-dense.
  » Alkaline foods also reduce the body's overall stress load, promoting a balanced mood and energy levels.
- **Limit Caffeine and Sugar**:
  » Both caffeine and sugar can increase anxiety by stimulating the nervous system. They create spikes and crashes in energy levels, which can worsen anxiety symptoms.
  » Opt for herbal teas like lemon balm or holy basil instead of coffee, and replace sugary snacks with fresh fruits or a handful of nuts.

- **Incorporate Gentle Exercise**:
  - » Physical activity helps release endorphins, which improve mood and reduce anxiety. Gentle exercises like yoga, walking, or stretching are particularly beneficial for stress relief without causing overstimulation.

5. SAMPLE WEEKLY ROUTINE FOR ANXIETY MANAGEMENT WITH HERBS

To maximize the benefits of Dr. Sebi's herbs for anxiety, consider a weekly schedule that balances various herbs and practices:

- **Monday**:
  - » **Morning**: Holy basil tea for a calm start to the week.
  - » **Evening**: Passionflower tea to unwind and relax after the day.
- **Tuesday**:
  - » **Morning**: Ashwagandha powder in a smoothie to support stress resilience.
  - » **Evening**: Valerian root tea for deep relaxation and restful sleep.
- **Wednesday**:
  - » **Morning**: Lemon balm tea for daytime calmness and focus.
  - » **Evening**: Holy basil tea for continued relaxation and reduced stress.
- **Thursday**:
  - » **Morning**: Ashwagandha capsule to build resilience.
  - » **Afternoon**: Lemon balm tea for midday stress relief.
- **Friday**:
  - » **Morning**: Passionflower tea for calm focus.
  - » **Evening**: Valerian root tea to relax and release any week-related stress.
- **Saturday and Sunday**:
  - » Use a combination of lemon balm, holy basil, and passionflower as desired, alternating teas for a relaxed and balanced weekend.

By following this routine, incorporating Dr. Sebi's herbs, and practicing mindful habits, you can manage anxiety naturally, reduce stress, and promote mental clarity. These herbal remedies not only support the nervous system but also align with Dr. Sebi's holistic approach to wellness, providing a foundation for long-term emotional and mental health.

CHAPTER 2
ALKALINE FOODS FOR EMOTIONAL BALANCE

Our diet directly impacts our emotional and mental well-being. Emotions are influenced not only by external stressors but also by the internal environment of the body, including its biochemical balance. Dr. Sebi's emphasis on an alkaline diet stems from the belief that maintaining a balanced pH helps reduce internal stress, supports stable mood levels, and promotes mental clarity. By incorporating alkaline foods, we can create an environment that supports emotional balance, enhances focus, and fosters a calm state of mind.

1. THE BIOCHEMICAL CONNECTION BETWEEN DIET AND EMOTION

Understanding the connection between diet and mood involves recognizing how certain foods impact blood sugar levels, neurotransmitter production, and hormonal balance. Consuming an alkaline diet composed of nutrient-dense, plant-based foods can help stabilize blood sugar, prevent spikes in cortisol (the body's main stress hormone), and support the production of neurotransmitters like serotonin and dopamine, which are essential for emotional well-being.

- **Blood Sugar Stability**:
    » Blood sugar fluctuations contribute to mood swings, irritability, and anxiety. By choosing foods that release energy steadily, we prevent sudden blood sugar dips that can lead to stress and emotional instability.
    » Alkaline foods like leafy greens, nuts, and seeds help maintain stable blood sugar levels, providing sustained energy and balanced emotions throughout the day.
- **Hormone Regulation**:
    » Cortisol and adrenaline are hormones released during times of stress. If consistently high, they can lead to heightened anxiety, fatigue, and mood imbalance. Alkaline foods help lower inflammation, supporting a healthy hormonal balance that reduces stress response.
- **Neurotransmitter Support**:
    » Neurotransmitters like serotonin and dopamine are critical for feelings of happiness, relaxation, and motivation. Nutrients found in alkaline foods, such as magnesium, B vitamins, and antioxidants, support the production and function of these mood-regulating chemicals.

2. KEY NUTRIENTS IN ALKALINE FOODS FOR EMOTIONAL BALANCE

Certain nutrients are especially important for mental health, as they play a direct role in regulating stress and maintaining emotional equilibrium. Here are some of the most important nutrients and how they help support a calm, balanced mood:

- **Magnesium**: Known as the "relaxation mineral," magnesium is essential for calming the nervous system and managing stress. Deficiency in magnesium is linked to anxiety and poor sleep quality.
- **Omega-3 Fatty Acids**: Found in certain seeds and nuts, omega-3s are anti-inflammatory and support brain health. They have been shown to reduce symptoms of depression and anxiety.
- **Vitamin B6 and Folate**: These B vitamins are essential for producing serotonin, the "feel-good" neurotransmitter. Low levels of these vitamins are linked to increased stress and mood instability.
- **Antioxidants**: Foods rich in antioxidants, like berries and leafy greens, protect brain cells from oxidative stress, which is often associated with mood disorders.

3. BEST ALKALINE FOODS FOR EMOTIONAL BALANCE

Incorporating the following alkaline foods into your diet can have a positive effect on mood, helping to create a sense of calm and reduce stress. Each of these foods is nutrient-rich, anti-inflammatory, and supports overall mental wellness.

- **Leafy Greens (Spinach, Kale, Swiss Chard)**:
    » Leafy greens are abundant in magnesium, B vitamins, and antioxidants. They support brain health and help reduce stress. Their high fiber content also stabilizes blood sugar, which is crucial for emotional stability.
    » **How to Use**: Add leafy greens to salads, smoothies, or lightly sauté them with olive oil and garlic. A handful of greens daily can make a noticeable difference in stress levels and energy.
- **Avocado**:
    » Avocados are rich in healthy fats that nourish the brain and improve cognitive function. They're also

high in B vitamins and potassium, which help reduce anxiety and keep cortisol levels stable.
  - **How to Use**: Slice avocado onto toast, add it to salads, or blend it into smoothies for a creamy texture. Its versatility makes it easy to include in various meals.
- **Berries (Blueberries, Blackberries, Strawberries)**:
  - Berries are high in antioxidants, particularly vitamin C, which reduces oxidative stress in the brain. Their natural sweetness and fiber help satisfy sugar cravings without causing blood sugar spikes.
  - **How to Use**: Enjoy a handful of berries with breakfast, add them to smoothies, or use them as a topping for oatmeal or chia pudding.
- **Bananas**:
  - Bananas contain tryptophan, an amino acid that helps produce serotonin. They are also a good source of potassium and magnesium, which support relaxation and heart health.
  - **How to Use**: Enjoy a banana as a snack, add slices to smoothies, or pair with almond butter for a mood-boosting treat.
- **Seeds and Nuts (Chia Seeds, Flaxseeds, Almonds, Walnuts)**:
  - Seeds and nuts provide essential omega-3 fatty acids, protein, and magnesium. They are also rich in fiber, helping to keep blood sugar steady.
  - **How to Use**: Add seeds to smoothies, oatmeal, or salads. A small handful of nuts or a tablespoon of chia seeds daily can support emotional well-being.
- **Citrus Fruits (Lemon, Lime, Oranges)**:
  - Citrus fruits are rich in vitamin C, which helps reduce stress and strengthens the immune system. Their alkalizing properties help balance the body's pH, reducing acidity-related stress.
  - **How to Use**: Start the day with warm lemon water, add lime to salads, or enjoy an orange as a refreshing snack.

4. HOW TO INCORPORATE ALKALINE FOODS FOR DAILY EMOTIONAL SUPPORT

Implementing alkaline foods into your daily routine doesn't have to be complicated. Here are practical ways to incorporate these foods consistently, helping you maintain a balanced, nutrient-rich diet that supports emotional wellness:

- **Begin with an Alkaline Breakfast**:
  - Starting the day with a green smoothie made from spinach, avocado, banana, and a handful of berries provides a nutrient-dense foundation for mood stability.
  - **Recipe Example**: Blend spinach, half an avocado, a banana, and a handful of berries with a splash of almond milk for a creamy, satisfying breakfast smoothie.
- **Midday Snack to Balance Blood Sugar**:
  - Snack on a handful of nuts or seeds to maintain energy and prevent blood sugar crashes. Pair with a citrus fruit like an orange or a slice of apple with almond butter.
  - **Snack Example**: Mix almonds with dried blueberries or have a banana with a small spoonful of chia seeds for a fiber-rich, mood-supporting snack.
- **Nutrient-Dense Lunch with Leafy Greens and Healthy Fats**:
  - A salad rich in leafy greens, avocado, cucumber, and citrus dressing provides essential vitamins and minerals for emotional support. Top with seeds for an added nutrient boost.
  - **Salad Idea**: Mixed greens with sliced avocado, cucumber, a sprinkle of chia seeds, and a lemon-tahini dressing for a balanced, mood-boosting meal.
- **Evening Meals to Promote Relaxation**:
  - A warm meal of steamed vegetables, quinoa, and a handful of walnuts or almonds helps to reduce cortisol levels and promote relaxation before bed.
  - **Dinner Example**: Steam a mix of vegetables (broccoli, carrots, zucchini) and serve over quinoa. Add a drizzle of olive oil and a few slices of avocado for a calming, nutrient-rich dinner.

5. SAMPLE ALKALINE MEAL PLAN FOR EMOTIONAL BALANCE

Here is a sample day-by-day alkaline meal plan that focuses on incorporating foods for emotional support and mood balance.

- **Day 1**:
  - **Breakfast**: Smoothie with spinach, avocado, banana, and blueberries.
  - **Lunch**: Salad with mixed greens, cucumber, bell pepper, seeds, and a lemon dressing.
  - **Dinner**: Quinoa bowl with steamed vegetables and a handful of nuts.
- **Day 2**:
  - **Breakfast**: Chia pudding with almond milk and a topping of berries and sliced banana.
  - **Lunch**: Mixed greens with avocado, citrus dressing, and a side of hummus with sliced veggies.

- **Dinner**: Stir-fried leafy greens with garlic, served with roasted sweet potatoes.
- **Day 3**:
  - **Breakfast**: Warm oatmeal topped with almond slices, berries, and a drizzle of honey.
  - **Lunch**: Vegetable soup with leafy greens, carrots, and a sprinkle of flaxseeds.
  - **Dinner**: Baked squash with a salad of mixed greens, walnuts, and avocado.

6. ADDITIONAL TIPS FOR EMOTIONAL BALANCE WITH ALKALINE FOODS

To maintain emotional balance consistently, incorporate the following tips into your routine:

- **Mindful Eating**:
  - Eating slowly and savoring each bite can help reduce stress and improve digestion. Take time to enjoy meals without distractions to maximize nutrient absorption and promote a calm state.
- **Stay Hydrated**:
  - Drinking plenty of water and herbal teas supports detoxification and prevents dehydration, which can cause irritability and fatigue. Begin the day with warm lemon water to promote an alkaline state.
- **Avoid Processed Foods and Sugars**:
  - Processed foods and sugars can lead to mood crashes, stress, and anxiety. Replace sugary snacks with fresh fruits or a handful of nuts to maintain steady energy.
- **Consistent Routine**:
  - Try to maintain regular mealtimes to stabilize blood sugar and avoid mood swings. Consistency is key to balancing energy levels and emotional well-being.

By incorporating these alkaline foods into your daily life, you're supporting the body's ability to maintain emotional stability, reduce stress, and enhance mental clarity. Dr. Sebi's emphasis on an alkaline diet aligns with the goal of emotional balance by nourishing the body and mind through whole, nutrient-dense foods. This approach creates a foundation for ongoing mental and emotional health, helping you manage stress naturally and feel more centered and calm in your daily life.

CHAPTER 3
DETOX FOR MENTAL CLARITY

Mental clarity and cognitive health are foundational to a balanced, fulfilling life. In our daily routines, the brain is constantly working, processing thoughts, emotions, and decisions. However, the accumulation of toxins—from processed foods, environmental pollutants, stress, and even mental fatigue—can hinder cognitive function, leading to brain fog, lack of focus, and mental fatigue. Dr. Sebi's detox approach emphasizes creating a clean internal environment that supports optimal brain function and enhances mental clarity.

1. HOW TOXINS AFFECT MENTAL CLARITY AND BRAIN HEALTH

Toxins can accumulate in the body through various sources: the food we eat, air we breathe, and products we use. Over time, these toxins affect brain function by causing oxidative stress, inflammation, and disruption in neurotransmitter balance. Key sources of toxins affecting brain health include:

- **Processed Foods and Additives**:
  - Chemicals, preservatives, and artificial ingredients in processed foods introduce toxins that the body struggles to break down. These chemicals can cross the blood-brain barrier, leading to inflammation and impairing cognitive function.
- **Environmental Pollutants**:
  - Heavy metals like mercury and lead, found in water and certain foods, as well as air pollutants, can accumulate in the body and impact brain health. Heavy metal toxicity is linked to memory problems, anxiety, and impaired mental clarity.
- **Hormonal Disruptors**:
  - Certain chemicals, like BPA found in plastics, mimic hormones in the body and interfere with natural hormone function. This hormonal imbalance can impact mental clarity and mood regulation.
- **Mental Fatigue from Chronic Stress**:
  - Chronic stress increases cortisol, a hormone that, when elevated over time, negatively impacts cognitive function and reduces the brain's ability to process information efficiently.

2. THE IMPORTANCE OF DETOX FOR MENTAL CLARITY

Detoxification for mental clarity involves removing harmful substances from the body and supporting the body's natural elimination processes. A detox regimen targets the liver, kidneys, lymphatic system, and digestive system, helping to cleanse the bloodstream and reducing the toxic burden on the brain. Benefits of a detox for mental clarity include:

- **Reduced Brain Fog**:
  - Detoxing removes substances that cloud cognition, allowing the brain to process information more efficiently.
- **Improved Memory and Focus**:
  - By eliminating toxins that disrupt neurotransmitters, detox can enhance focus, mental sharpness, and memory retention.
- **Enhanced Mood Stability**:
  - Clearing out toxins helps balance hormones and neurotransmitters, reducing mood swings, anxiety, and depression.

3. CORE DETOX PRACTICES FOR MENTAL CLARITY

A structured detox routine that supports the body's natural cleansing pathways can make a noticeable difference in mental clarity. Here are some effective detox practices recommended by Dr. Sebi:

- **Alkaline Diet for Mental Clarity**:
  - An alkaline diet is central to detox, as alkaline foods are rich in antioxidants, vitamins, and minerals that support cellular repair and cleanse the bloodstream. Dr. Sebi's recommended foods, such as leafy greens, fruits, and sea vegetables, help neutralize acidity and reduce inflammation.
  - **Key Foods**:
    - **Leafy Greens**: Rich in chlorophyll, which purifies the blood and removes toxins.
    - **Sea Moss**: Contains essential trace minerals that bind to toxins and heavy metals, helping to remove them from the body.

- **Berries**: High in antioxidants, which combat oxidative stress and support brain health.
- **Hydration with Alkaline Water**:
  » Proper hydration is essential for detox as it helps flush out toxins through the kidneys. Alkaline water, with its higher pH, aids in maintaining a balanced pH in the body and supports cognitive health.
  » **How to Use**: Aim for 8–10 cups of water daily, with an emphasis on alkaline water. Start the day with a glass of warm water and lemon to stimulate digestion and support liver detoxification.
- **Incorporating Detoxifying Herbal Teas**:
  » Certain herbal teas support detoxification by stimulating the liver, kidneys, and lymphatic system, helping remove toxins from the body. Dandelion root, burdock root, and nettle are particularly beneficial for detoxifying the body and supporting mental clarity.
  » **Suggested Teas**:
    - **Dandelion Root Tea**: Supports liver detoxification, clearing toxins that can impair brain function.
    - **Burdock Root Tea**: Aids in blood purification, supporting the removal of heavy metals and other toxins.
    - **Nettle Tea**: Rich in minerals and antioxidants, nettle tea supports kidney health and mental clarity.
- **Intermittent Fasting for Brain Reset**:
  » Fasting allows the digestive system to rest, giving the body more energy to focus on cleansing and repairing cells. Intermittent fasting also promotes autophagy, a process where cells break down and remove damaged components, supporting brain health.
  » **How to Implement**: A 16:8 fasting approach (fasting for 16 hours and eating within an 8-hour window) is effective. During fasting hours, stay hydrated with alkaline water and herbal teas.

4. KEY HERBS AND FOODS FOR DETOX AND MENTAL CLARITY

Incorporating specific detoxifying herbs and nutrient-rich foods into a daily routine can amplify detox results, helping to clear toxins more efficiently and support mental clarity. Here are some of the most beneficial herbs and foods:

- **Dandelion Root**:
  » Known for its liver-supporting properties, dandelion root helps flush toxins from the liver and improves digestion. This herb's cleansing effect on the blood can enhance mental clarity and energy levels.
  » **How to Use**: Brew dandelion root tea or take it as a tincture. Drink one cup daily as part of a regular detox routine.
- **Burdock Root**:
  » Burdock root is a potent blood purifier, helping to remove heavy metals and environmental toxins. Its anti-inflammatory properties also support cognitive function and brain health.
  » **How to Use**: Brew a tea using dried burdock root, or add burdock root powder to smoothies. Drink 1–2 cups of tea daily.
- **Sea Moss**:
  » Sea moss is packed with essential trace minerals, including iodine, which supports cognitive health and mental clarity. It also binds to heavy metals and toxins, helping to eliminate them from the body.
  » **How to Use**: Add sea moss gel to smoothies or teas. A tablespoon daily can provide the minerals needed for optimal brain function.
- **Cilantro**:
  » Cilantro has powerful chelation properties, meaning it can bind to heavy metals like mercury and lead and aid in their removal from the body. Reducing heavy metal accumulation is beneficial for mental clarity.
  » **How to Use**: Add fresh cilantro to salads, smoothies, or juice it with other vegetables for a potent detox drink.
- **Ginger**:
  » Ginger is both a digestive aid and an anti-inflammatory, helping reduce inflammation in the body and the brain. It also supports circulation, which is essential for transporting oxygen and nutrients to brain cells.
  » **How to Use**: Add ginger to teas, smoothies, or juices. Consuming ginger daily helps support detoxification and mental clarity.

5. SAMPLE 3-DAY DETOX FOR MENTAL CLARITY

Here's a sample 3-day detox plan designed to promote mental clarity, reduce brain fog, and support cognitive health. This plan includes nutrient-dense, alkaline foods and detoxifying herbs to help eliminate toxins and enhance brain function.

- **Day 1: Alkaline Start and Hydration**:
  » **Morning**: Start with a glass of warm lemon water. Follow with a green smoothie made with spinach, cucumber, ginger, and sea moss gel.
  » **Mid-Morning**: Drink a cup of dandelion root tea to support liver function.

- **Lunch**: A salad with mixed greens, cucumber, cilantro, avocado, and lemon-tahini dressing.
- **Afternoon**: A handful of berries and a cup of nettle tea for hydration and detox support.
- **Dinner**: Steamed vegetables (broccoli, zucchini) with a side of quinoa and a sprinkle of burdock root powder.
- **Evening**: A calming ginger tea to promote relaxation and support detox before bed.

- **Day 2: Supporting Detox Pathways**:
  - **Morning**: Begin with warm water and lemon. Smoothie with kale, avocado, sea moss, and a handful of berries.
  - **Mid-Morning**: Nettle tea to support kidney function and hydration.
  - **Lunch**: Quinoa salad with mixed greens, bell peppers, and a lemon-cilantro dressing.
  - **Afternoon**: Drink burdock root tea and snack on a handful of nuts or seeds.
  - **Dinner**: Vegetable soup with leafy greens, carrots, garlic, and a pinch of sea salt for mineral balance.
  - **Evening**: Ginger and turmeric tea for anti-inflammatory and detox support.

- **Day 3: Deep Cleansing and Mental Clarity Support**:
  - **Morning**: Warm lemon water, followed by a smoothie with dandelion greens, cucumber, and sea moss gel.
  - **Mid-Morning**: Burdock root tea to purify the blood and reduce inflammation.
  - **Lunch**: Large salad with mixed greens, avocado, cucumber, and a citrus-based dressing.
  - **Afternoon Snack**: A small bowl of fresh berries and a cup of ginger tea for brain-boosting antioxidants.
  - **Dinner**: Steamed vegetables (cauliflower, carrots) with a side of wild rice, topped with fresh herbs.
  - **Evening**: Chamomile tea to relax the mind and body before sleep.

6. POST-DETOX TIPS FOR SUSTAINED MENTAL CLARITY

After completing a detox, it's essential to continue supporting brain health and mental clarity by incorporating routine practices and maintaining a nutrient-rich, alkaline diet.

- **Maintain Alkaline Eating Habits**:
  - Continue consuming leafy greens, berries, and nutrient-dense foods that support detoxification and cognitive health.
- **Use Detoxifying Herbs Regularly**:
  - Keep including detox-supportive herbs like dandelion root and cilantro to prevent toxin accumulation and support ongoing brain health.
- **Practice Mindful Hydration**:
  - Staying hydrated is essential for mental clarity and energy. Drink plenty of alkaline water daily, and consider adding lemon to boost detoxifying benefits.
- **Limit Processed Foods and Sugars**:
  - Processed foods and sugars can quickly disrupt brain function and reduce mental clarity. Aim to reduce or eliminate them from your diet, replacing them with whole, unprocessed foods.

Through a detox for mental clarity, you are creating an environment where the brain can function optimally, free from the burden of toxins and inflammation. By following Dr. Sebi's approach, which emphasizes alkaline foods, detoxifying herbs, and regular hydration, you can naturally improve focus, reduce brain fog, and achieve a clearer state of mind. This approach helps you feel energized, mentally sharp, and emotionally balanced, supporting overall well-being and resilience against daily stressors.

BOOK 17
Digestive Health and Dr. Sebi's Methods

Digestive health is at the core of Dr. Sebi's philosophy for overall well-being. When the gut is healthy, nutrients are absorbed more effectively, the immune system is strengthened, and the body's internal environment is balanced. An alkaline diet supports the gut by creating a favorable environment for beneficial bacteria, reducing inflammation, and aiding the elimination of toxins. This book outlines the importance of digestive health and how Dr. Sebi's methods offer a natural approach to nurturing the gut.

CHAPTER 1
ALKALINE FOODS FOR GUT HEALTH

The digestive system is crucial for overall health, as it processes food, absorbs nutrients, and eliminates waste. However, when the gut becomes imbalanced due to poor diet, stress, or environmental factors, it can lead to digestive issues such as bloating, constipation, acid reflux, and even contribute to conditions like leaky gut. An alkaline diet emphasizes whole, plant-based foods that support gut health by reducing acidity, promoting the growth of beneficial gut bacteria, and minimizing inflammation. This chapter explores how alkaline foods can optimize gut function and provides practical tips for incorporating these foods into your daily diet.

1. THE ROLE OF GUT HEALTH IN OVERALL WELLNESS

Gut health is foundational to every aspect of physical and mental well-being. Often referred to as the "second brain," the gut contains millions of nerve cells and a complex ecosystem of bacteria, known as the gut microbiome, that influence mood, immunity, and even cognitive function.

- **The Gut Microbiome**:
  - » The gut microbiome is a diverse community of bacteria and other microorganisms that play an essential role in digestion, immune function, and mental health. A diet high in processed foods, sugar, and acidity can disrupt this microbiome, leading to imbalances that impact digestion and overall health.
- **Digestive Health and Immune Function**:
  - » Around 70% of the immune system is located in the gut, where beneficial bacteria help protect against harmful pathogens. An alkaline diet strengthens these beneficial bacteria, which in turn supports immune defenses.
- **Gut Health and Mental Clarity**:
  - » The gut-brain connection, often called the gut-brain axis, highlights the link between gut health and mental well-being. By supporting gut health with alkaline foods, we can reduce inflammation, improve nutrient absorption, and experience better mental clarity and emotional stability.

2. BENEFITS OF AN ALKALINE DIET FOR GUT HEALTH

An alkaline diet helps reduce inflammation and acidity, two factors that contribute to digestive discomfort and imbalances in the gut microbiome. By consuming alkaline foods, the digestive system functions more smoothly, inflammation is reduced, and beneficial bacteria can thrive.

- **Reduced Inflammation**:
  - » Inflammation in the gut can cause discomfort, bloating, and even more severe issues over time. Alkaline foods help reduce inflammation, creating a calming environment within the digestive tract.
- **Improved pH Balance**:
  - » A more alkaline environment in the gut discourages the growth of harmful bacteria and yeast, such as Candida, which thrive in acidic conditions. Alkaline foods help maintain an optimal pH level in the gut.
- **Enhanced Nutrient Absorption**:
  - » When the digestive system functions efficiently, nutrients from food are more readily absorbed. Alkaline foods, rich in vitamins, minerals, and antioxidants, support gut health and ensure that the body receives the nutrients it needs.

3. KEY ALKALINE FOODS FOR SUPPORTING GUT HEALTH

Here are some of the most beneficial alkaline foods for gut health, each offering specific nutrients and properties that support digestion, reduce inflammation, and nourish the gut microbiome.

- **Leafy Greens (Spinach, Kale, Swiss Chard)**:
  - » Leafy greens are highly alkaline and rich in fiber, magnesium, and antioxidants. Fiber supports regular bowel movements, while magnesium helps relax the digestive tract, reducing symptoms of bloating and constipation.
  - » **How to Use**: Incorporate leafy greens into salads, smoothies, or lightly sauté them as a side dish. Aim to consume at least one serving of leafy greens daily to support gut health.
- **Cucumber**:

- Cucumber is hydrating and has a high water content, which supports digestion and prevents constipation. Its alkaline nature helps balance the pH in the digestive system.
- **How to Use**: Add cucumber slices to salads, infuse in water, or eat as a refreshing snack. Its mild taste makes it versatile and easy to include in meals.

- **Avocado**:
  - Avocado is rich in healthy fats and fiber, both of which support digestion. The fiber promotes healthy bowel movements, while the fats nourish the gut lining and reduce inflammation.
  - **How to Use**: Add avocado to salads, toast, or blend into smoothies for a creamy texture. Its nutrient density makes it a powerful addition to an alkaline diet.

- **Ginger**:
  - Ginger is known for its anti-inflammatory and digestive benefits. It helps reduce bloating, stimulates digestion, and soothes the digestive tract, making it ideal for managing symptoms of indigestion and acid reflux.
  - **How to Use**: Fresh ginger can be added to teas, smoothies, or grated into dressings. Drinking ginger tea before meals can also stimulate digestion and promote gut health.

- **Bananas**:
  - Bananas are slightly alkaline and are rich in potassium and fiber. They help reduce acidity in the stomach, relieve symptoms of acid reflux, and support healthy bowel movements.
  - **How to Use**: Add bananas to smoothies, oatmeal, or enjoy as a snack. They are particularly helpful for reducing stomach acidity and soothing the gut.

- **Aloe Vera**:
  - Aloe vera is highly alkaline and contains enzymes that aid digestion. It soothes the lining of the digestive tract, reduces inflammation, and is helpful for conditions like acid reflux and irritable bowel syndrome (IBS).
  - **How to Use**: Aloe vera juice can be taken on an empty stomach in the morning. Look for organic, pure aloe vera juice for best results.

- **Sea Moss**:
  - Sea moss provides essential minerals and has mucilaginous properties, meaning it forms a gel-like substance that soothes the digestive tract. It promotes healthy gut bacteria and reduces inflammation.
  - **How to Use**: Add sea moss gel to smoothies or teas. A tablespoon daily supports gut health and provides trace minerals essential for digestion.

4. PRACTICAL TIPS FOR INCORPORATING ALKALINE FOODS INTO DAILY MEALS

Including alkaline foods in every meal can make a substantial difference in gut health and overall wellness. Here are some tips for integrating these foods consistently:

- **Start the Day with Alkaline Hydration**:
  - Begin the day with warm lemon water to stimulate digestion and create an alkaline environment. Adding lemon helps promote liver detoxification, which supports gut health.
  - **Tip**: Drink a glass of warm lemon water on an empty stomach every morning for optimal results.

- **Include Leafy Greens in Every Meal**:
  - Leafy greens are highly versatile and can be added to smoothies, salads, or stir-fries. Their fiber content and alkaline nature make them ideal for supporting digestion.
  - **Tip**: Rotate between spinach, kale, and Swiss chard to get a variety of nutrients and flavors.

- **Add Fermented Foods for Probiotic Support**:
  - Although not strictly alkaline, fermented foods like sauerkraut and kimchi provide beneficial bacteria that support gut health. Adding a small amount to meals can boost beneficial gut flora.
  - **Tip**: Include a tablespoon of sauerkraut or kimchi with your meals to support a balanced microbiome.

- **Snack on Hydrating Foods**:
  - Cucumber, watermelon, and celery are hydrating and gentle on the digestive system. These snacks not only support hydration but also help alkalize the body.
  - **Tip**: Keep sliced cucumber or celery sticks on hand for an easy, alkaline snack.

5. SAMPLE ALKALINE MEAL PLAN FOR GUT HEALTH

Here's a sample day of alkaline meals that support gut health, emphasizing nutrient-dense, plant-based foods to promote digestion and reduce inflammation.

- **Breakfast**:
  - **Green Smoothie**: Blend spinach, cucumber, avocado, banana, and sea moss gel with a splash of almond milk. This smoothie provides fiber, healthy fats, and antioxidants to support gut health.
  - **Ginger Tea**: Enjoy a warm cup of ginger tea to stimulate digestion and soothe the stomach.

- **Lunch**:
  - **Alkaline Salad**: Mixed greens, cucumber, shredded carrots, and sliced avocado with a lemon-tahini dressing. This salad provides fiber, healthy fats, and hydration.
  - **Add Fermented Foods**: Top with a tablespoon of sauerkraut for added probiotics.
- **Afternoon Snack**:
  - **Fresh Fruit**: A banana or apple with a handful of nuts. This combination provides fiber, potassium, and healthy fats to maintain steady energy and support digestion.
- **Dinner**:
  - **Steamed Vegetables and Quinoa**: Steamed zucchini, broccoli, and bell peppers over a bed of quinoa, seasoned with herbs like basil and parsley.
  - **Optional**: Include a cup of aloe vera juice before dinner to soothe the digestive tract and support regularity.
- **Evening**:
  - **Chamomile or Peppermint Tea**: These calming teas help relax the digestive system and promote restful sleep.

6. ADDITIONAL LIFESTYLE PRACTICES FOR ENHANCED GUT HEALTH

In addition to an alkaline diet, certain lifestyle practices can further support gut health, helping to optimize digestion and prevent common digestive issues.

- **Mindful Eating**:
  - Eating slowly and chewing thoroughly helps ease the digestive process, allowing nutrients to be absorbed more effectively. Avoid distractions while eating to fully engage in the experience and support optimal digestion.
- **Regular Movement**:
  - Physical activity promotes circulation and aids in moving food through the digestive tract, reducing bloating and supporting regular bowel movements. Gentle exercise like walking or yoga can be especially beneficial for digestion.
- **Stress Management**:
  - Chronic stress can disrupt digestion, increasing the risk of conditions like IBS and acid reflux. Practice relaxation techniques such as deep breathing, meditation, or journaling to reduce stress levels and support gut health.
- **Stay Hydrated**:
  - Proper hydration is essential for digestion. Drinking water throughout the day supports the body's ability to break down food and absorb nutrients, reducing the risk of constipation and promoting gut health.

By incorporating these alkaline foods and lifestyle practices, you can support gut health naturally, helping to maintain a balanced microbiome, reduce inflammation, and promote regular digestion. Dr. Sebi's approach to an alkaline diet emphasizes whole, plant-based foods that work harmoniously with the body to create an internal environment that supports digestive health. Following these principles consistently can help improve not only gut health but also overall wellness, setting a strong foundation for vitality and mental clarity.

CHAPTER 2
REMEDIES FOR DIGESTIVE ISSUES

Digestive issues can significantly affect daily life, causing discomfort, fatigue, and even impacting mood and productivity. From occasional bloating to more persistent problems like acid reflux or constipation, each digestive issue has unique causes and, fortunately, natural solutions. Dr. Sebi's approach focuses on plant-based, alkaline remedies that help soothe the digestive system, reduce inflammation, and improve overall gut health. This chapter explores effective remedies for common digestive problems using simple, natural ingredients and easy-to-follow practices.

1. UNDERSTANDING COMMON DIGESTIVE ISSUES AND THEIR CAUSES

Digestive issues can arise from poor diet, stress, lack of hydration, or an imbalanced gut microbiome. Addressing these problems naturally involves not only treating the symptoms but also understanding their root causes and using holistic remedies to support the body's digestive processes.

- **Bloating and Gas**: Often caused by gas buildup from undigested food, bloating can result from eating too quickly, consuming carbonated beverages, or eating foods that the digestive system struggles to break down.
- **Constipation**: This occurs when the digestive tract moves too slowly, often due to insufficient fiber, lack of hydration, or a sedentary lifestyle.
- **Acid Reflux and Heartburn**: When stomach acid flows back into the esophagus, it causes discomfort and a burning sensation. Acid reflux is commonly triggered by certain foods, eating late at night, or stress.
- **Indigestion**: Symptoms like fullness, nausea, or discomfort after eating can be signs of indigestion. It may be caused by overeating, poor food combinations, or low stomach acid.

2. HERBAL REMEDIES FOR DIGESTIVE SUPPORT

Several herbs can naturally soothe and support digestion, addressing issues like bloating, acid reflux, and indigestion. Here are some of the most effective herbs in Dr. Sebi's approach:

- **Ginger**:
  » Ginger is known for its anti-inflammatory and digestive properties. It helps stimulate the digestive enzymes, reduces bloating, and relieves nausea and indigestion.
  » **How to Use**: Fresh ginger tea is one of the best ways to soothe digestive discomfort. Steep a few slices of fresh ginger in hot water for 10 minutes and sip slowly after meals. Ginger can also be added to smoothies or meals.
- **Peppermint**:
  » Peppermint relaxes the muscles of the digestive tract, making it useful for relieving gas, bloating, and cramps. It's also effective in soothing acid reflux and reducing nausea.
  » **How to Use**: Drink peppermint tea after meals to help with digestion and relieve any bloating. Avoid peppermint if you experience acid reflux frequently, as it can sometimes relax the esophageal sphincter, which could worsen symptoms.
- **Dandelion Root**:
  » Dandelion root stimulates the liver, aiding in the production of bile, which is essential for fat digestion. It also helps relieve constipation and supports detoxification.
  » **How to Use**: Brew dandelion root tea by steeping a teaspoon of dried root in hot water for 10–15 minutes. Drink before meals to improve digestion and ease constipation.
- **Fennel**:
  » Fennel has carminative properties, meaning it helps reduce gas and bloating. It also supports digestion by relaxing the muscles in the gut and easing cramps.
  » **How to Use**: Chew a few fennel seeds after meals to prevent gas and freshen your breath. Alternatively, make fennel tea by steeping crushed fennel seeds in hot water.
- **Licorice Root**:
  » Licorice root is soothing to the digestive tract and helps reduce inflammation in the stomach lining. It's beneficial for acid reflux, as it forms a protective layer over the stomach lining.
  » **How to Use**: Deglycyrrhizinated licorice (DGL) tablets can be chewed before meals for acid reflux relief. Alternatively, licorice tea can be enjoyed to soothe the stomach, though avoid if you have high blood pressure.

3. ALKALINE FOODS FOR RELIEVING DIGESTIVE ISSUES

An alkaline diet not only supports gut health but also provides relief from common digestive problems. Certain alkaline foods are especially effective at reducing acidity, easing bloating, and supporting regular bowel movements.

- **Aloe Vera**:
  » Aloe vera is highly alkaline and has soothing, anti-inflammatory properties that can help with acid reflux, indigestion, and constipation.
  » **How to Use**: Drink 1–2 ounces of aloe vera juice (without added sugars) before meals to soothe the digestive tract. Aloe vera is also useful for relieving constipation due to its mild laxative effect.
- **Cucumber**:
  » Cucumber is hydrating and rich in fiber, making it beneficial for preventing constipation and reducing bloating. Its cooling properties are helpful for calming acid reflux as well.
  » **How to Use**: Add cucumber to salads or snack on slices throughout the day to keep the digestive tract hydrated and supported.
- **Papaya**:
  » Papaya contains an enzyme called papain, which aids digestion by breaking down proteins. This can help reduce bloating and ease digestion after a heavy meal.
  » **How to Use**: Eat fresh papaya as a snack or add it to smoothies. Consuming papaya before a meal can help prepare the digestive system for protein-rich foods.
- **Bananas**:
  » Bananas are slightly alkaline and contain fiber, potassium, and natural antacid properties that help soothe acid reflux and support regular bowel movements.
  » **How to Use**: Eat a banana when experiencing heartburn or bloating, or add it to your breakfast to support digestion throughout the day.
- **Chia Seeds**:
  » Chia seeds are rich in fiber, which promotes regular bowel movements and reduces constipation. When soaked, they create a gel-like substance that soothes the digestive tract.
  » **How to Use**: Soak a tablespoon of chia seeds in water or almond milk and add them to smoothies, oatmeal, or yogurt for added digestive support.

4. SIMPLE HOME REMEDIES FOR COMMON DIGESTIVE ISSUES

In addition to herbs and alkaline foods, there are practical home remedies you can incorporate to ease common digestive problems:

- **Warm Lemon Water for Digestion**:
  » Drinking warm lemon water on an empty stomach helps stimulate the liver and prepares the digestive system for the day. Lemon's acidity turns alkaline in the body, promoting an ideal environment for gut health.
  » **How to Use**: Squeeze the juice of half a lemon into a glass of warm water and drink it first thing in the morning.
- **Apple Cider Vinegar for Acid Reflux**:
  » Despite its acidity, apple cider vinegar helps balance stomach acid and can alleviate symptoms of acid reflux.
  » **How to Use**: Mix one tablespoon of apple cider vinegar with a cup of water and drink before meals to aid digestion and reduce acid reflux symptoms.
- **Chamomile Tea for Indigestion**:
  » Chamomile tea has calming properties that soothe the digestive tract and relieve symptoms of indigestion and bloating.
  » **How to Use**: Steep a chamomile tea bag in hot water for 5–10 minutes and drink after meals to calm the stomach.
- **Activated Charcoal for Gas Relief**:
  » Activated charcoal absorbs gas and toxins, making it an effective remedy for bloating and gas discomfort.
  » **How to Use**: Take activated charcoal in capsule form according to the product's instructions, typically when experiencing gas or after eating gas-producing foods.

5. LIFESTYLE TIPS FOR SUPPORTING DIGESTIVE HEALTH

Good digestive health is supported not only by what we eat but also by our daily habits and routines. Here are a few tips to help maintain a balanced digestive system:

- **Eat Mindfully**: Chew food thoroughly and eat slowly to give the digestive system time to process food efficiently, which can help prevent bloating and indigestion.
- **Stay Hydrated**: Drinking enough water throughout the day keeps the digestive system hydrated, aiding in the breakdown of food and preventing constipation.
- **Incorporate Movement**: Regular physical activity, such

as walking or yoga, helps stimulate digestion and reduce bloating. Gentle movement after meals can be especially beneficial.
- **Limit Processed Foods**: Processed foods can disrupt the gut microbiome and increase acidity in the digestive system. Instead, focus on whole, unprocessed foods that support a balanced pH.
- **Avoid Eating Close to Bedtime**: Eating late at night can lead to acid reflux and indigestion. Aim to finish meals at least 2–3 hours before lying down to allow for proper digestion.

By using these plant-based remedies, you can support a healthy digestive system and alleviate common issues like bloating, acid reflux, and constipation. Dr. Sebi's approach to digestive health emphasizes the power of natural remedies, herbs, and alkaline foods to create a balanced, resilient gut. By incorporating these practices into your routine, you're not only addressing symptoms but also fostering long-term digestive wellness and comfort.

CHAPTER 3

DETOX PROTOCOLS FOR DIGESTIVE SUPPORT

A healthy digestive system is foundational for optimal health. Toxins, processed foods, and environmental stressors can build up in the digestive tract, leading to issues like bloating, constipation, and sluggish digestion. Dr. Sebi's approach emphasizes detox protocols that use natural, alkaline ingredients to cleanse and rejuvenate the digestive system. These protocols not only aid in the elimination of toxins but also help restore gut balance, promoting better digestion and overall vitality.

1. UNDERSTANDING THE NEED FOR DIGESTIVE DETOXIFICATION

Our bodies encounter toxins daily through food, water, air, and even stress. Over time, these toxins accumulate in the digestive system, affecting its ability to function optimally. A detox protocol can help:

- **Eliminate Toxins**: Flushes out harmful substances that disrupt gut health.
- **Improve Digestion**: Clears waste buildup, which can otherwise lead to bloating and constipation.
- **Support Gut Flora**: Creates a balanced environment for beneficial bacteria to thrive.
- **Enhance Nutrient Absorption**: Detoxification removes barriers to nutrient absorption, ensuring the body receives essential vitamins and minerals.

2. CORE ELEMENTS OF A DIGESTIVE DETOX PROTOCOL

A successful detox protocol for digestive support includes the following key components:

- **Alkaline, Fiber-Rich Foods**: Foods high in fiber help sweep waste and toxins from the digestive tract. Alkaline foods further reduce acidity and inflammation, promoting an environment where gut bacteria can thrive.
- **Hydration**: Proper hydration helps move toxins through the body, supporting kidney and liver function, which are integral to detoxification.
- **Herbal Teas**: Teas made from herbs like dandelion root, burdock root, and ginger aid detoxification by stimulating liver and kidney function, promoting bowel movements, and reducing inflammation in the digestive tract.
- **Gentle Movement and Rest**: Physical activity and relaxation support circulation and digestion, aiding the body's natural detox processes.

3. STEP-BY-STEP DIGESTIVE DETOX PROTOCOL

This three-day detox protocol provides a structured approach to cleanse the digestive system, relieve discomfort, and promote a balanced gut. The program includes alkaline meals, detoxifying beverages, and helpful lifestyle practices to ensure a thorough yet gentle cleanse.

Day 1: Preparing the Body

The first day focuses on preparing the digestive system for detoxification by incorporating hydrating and fiber-rich foods.

- **Morning**:
  - **Warm Lemon Water**: Start the day with a glass of warm lemon water to stimulate digestion and alkalize the body. Lemon also supports liver detoxification.
  - **Green Smoothie**: Blend a handful of spinach, cucumber, ginger, and a tablespoon of sea moss gel with water or almond milk. This smoothie is rich in fiber, minerals, and antioxidants that prepare the digestive system for cleansing.
- **Mid-Morning**:
  - **Herbal Tea**: Sip on a cup of dandelion root tea to stimulate liver function and support the elimination of toxins.
- **Lunch**:
  - **Alkaline Salad**: Prepare a salad with mixed greens, cucumber, shredded carrots, and avocado. Top with a lemon-tahini dressing. This meal provides fiber and hydration, helping to keep the digestive tract moving.
- **Afternoon Snack**:
  - **Fresh Fruit**: Choose a hydrating fruit like watermelon or berries, which are alkaline and easy on the digestive system.
- **Dinner**:
  - **Steamed Vegetables and Quinoa**: Lightly steam zucchini, broccoli, and bell peppers, and serve over a bed of quinoa. This meal is nutrient-dense, low in fat, and easy to digest.
- **Evening**:
  - **Ginger Tea**: End the day with ginger tea to soothe the stomach, reduce inflammation, and promote restful digestion.

Day 2: Active Detoxification

The second day emphasizes flushing out toxins with fiber, hydration, and detox-supportive foods.

- **Morning**:
  » **Warm Water with Aloe Vera**: Start with a glass of warm water mixed with 1–2 ounces of aloe vera juice to soothe the digestive tract and promote regularity.
  » **Green Juice**: Make a juice using cucumber, celery, lemon, and a small piece of ginger. This juice is hydrating and provides nutrients that cleanse the digestive system.
- **Mid-Morning**:
  » **Nettle Tea**: Nettle tea is rich in minerals and supports kidney function, which plays a role in flushing out toxins.
- **Lunch**:
  » **Vegetable Broth**: Prepare a light, homemade vegetable broth with carrots, celery, parsley, and garlic. This provides essential minerals and supports the body's detox pathways.
- **Afternoon Snack**:
  » **Chia Pudding**: Soak chia seeds in almond milk and let them form a gel. Chia seeds are high in fiber, promoting bowel regularity and gently cleansing the digestive tract.
- **Dinner**:
  » **Steamed Vegetables and Millet**: Choose light, alkaline vegetables like carrots, broccoli, and kale, and serve them with a small portion of millet. This meal is easily digestible and rich in fiber.
- **Evening**:
  » **Peppermint Tea**: Peppermint tea helps relax the digestive muscles, reducing any discomfort from gas or bloating.

Day 3: Restorative Cleansing

The final day focuses on gentle cleansing and restoring gut balance by including probiotic foods and hydrating, soothing meals.

- **Morning**:
  » **Warm Lemon Water with a Pinch of Sea Salt**: This helps rehydrate and supports electrolyte balance.
  » **Green Smoothie with Probiotics**: Blend spinach, cucumber, a small green apple, and a tablespoon of sea moss. Add a spoonful of coconut yogurt or a probiotic supplement to support gut flora.
- **Mid-Morning**:
  » **Burdock Root Tea**: This tea helps cleanse the blood and support liver function, promoting full-body detox.
- **Lunch**:
  » **Alkaline Soup**: Prepare a soup with alkaline vegetables like zucchini, cauliflower, and herbs like parsley. Add a tablespoon of chia seeds for fiber, which helps sweep toxins out of the intestines.
- **Afternoon Snack**:
  » **Sliced Cucumber and Fresh Mint Leaves**: This hydrating snack is easy to digest and refreshing.
- **Dinner**:
  » **Steamed Sweet Potatoes with a Side of Leafy Greens**: Sweet potatoes are gentle on the stomach and provide fiber to support bowel movements. Pair with lightly steamed kale or spinach.
- **Evening**:
  » **Chamomile Tea**: Chamomile is calming and supports relaxation, helping the digestive system wind down and process the detox.

4. POST-DETOX PRACTICES FOR CONTINUED DIGESTIVE SUPPORT

After completing the detox, it's essential to reintroduce regular foods gradually and maintain some of the detox practices to keep the digestive system healthy.

- **Incorporate Fiber-Rich Foods**:
  » Keep including fiber-rich, alkaline foods like leafy greens, chia seeds, and cucumbers to support daily detox and regularity.
- **Stay Hydrated**:
  » Proper hydration is key for moving waste through the digestive tract. Aim for 8–10 cups of water daily, and continue drinking herbal teas that support digestion.
- **Use Detoxifying Herbs Regularly**:
  » Incorporate dandelion root, ginger, and peppermint teas regularly to support liver function and digestive health.
- **Limit Processed Foods and Sugars**:
  » Processed foods and added sugars can disrupt gut bacteria and increase acidity in the digestive tract. Focus on whole, unprocessed foods for sustained digestive health.
- **Practice Mindful Eating**:
  » Take time to chew food thoroughly and eat without distractions to improve digestion and reduce bloating.

Following Dr. Sebi's detox protocols can effectively support and rejuvenate the digestive system, helping to remove built-up toxins, reduce bloating, and promote gut balance. Through these simple but powerful steps, you can experience improved digestion, enhanced nutrient absorption, and a refreshed sense of vitality. With regular detoxification and mindful dietary choices, you are setting a foundation for long-term digestive health and overall wellness.

BOOK 18
Kidney Health Support

The kidneys are essential for filtering waste and maintaining electrolyte balance, playing a critical role in overall health. By removing toxins from the bloodstream and balancing fluids, the kidneys support a clean, efficient internal environment. However, modern lifestyles, processed foods, and environmental toxins can strain the kidneys, leading to compromised function and even chronic kidney issues. Dr. Sebi's approach to kidney health emphasizes natural, plant-based remedies that support the kidneys' cleansing functions and promote long-term vitality. This book provides a comprehensive guide to natural kidney care, focusing on herbal protocols and alkaline practices.

CHAPTER 1

HERBAL PROTOCOLS FOR KIDNEY HEALTH

The kidneys serve as the body's natural filtration system, removing waste, balancing electrolytes, and regulating fluid levels. Given their importance, keeping the kidneys healthy is critical for overall wellness. Herbs play a unique role in supporting kidney health by helping to cleanse the kidneys, reduce inflammation, and prevent buildup that can lead to kidney stones or infection. Dr. Sebi's philosophy focuses on using specific, alkaline herbs that support kidney function, relieve strain, and optimize filtration.

1. UNDERSTANDING THE IMPORTANCE OF KIDNEY HEALTH

The kidneys process about 150 quarts of blood daily, filtering out toxins, waste, and excess fluid. When the kidneys are overworked or compromised, it can lead to various health issues, including high blood pressure, fluid retention, and imbalances in electrolytes. Herbal support is particularly valuable for the kidneys, as it helps relieve their workload and offers protective benefits against long-term damage.

- **Detoxification**: By filtering out toxins and waste, the kidneys help prevent toxic buildup in the bloodstream. Herbs that support this function aid in reducing the toxic load on the body.
- **Fluid and Electrolyte Balance**: The kidneys regulate sodium, potassium, and fluid levels in the body. Herbal diuretics assist in maintaining this balance, reducing bloating, and relieving water retention.
- **Prevention of Kidney Stones and Infections**: Certain herbs help prevent calcium and other mineral deposits from forming kidney stones, while others have mild antimicrobial properties that protect against infections in the urinary tract.

2. KEY HERBS FOR KIDNEY HEALTH AND THEIR BENEFITS

Dr. Sebi's approach to kidney health includes specific herbs known for their ability to support, cleanse, and protect the kidneys. Here are some of the most effective herbs for promoting kidney function, along with practical tips for incorporating them into your routine.

- **Dandelion Root**:
  - » Dandelion root is a powerful diuretic that helps flush out toxins, reduce fluid retention, and cleanse the kidneys. It also stimulates bile production, which aids in digestion and further supports the body's detox processes.
  - » **How to Use**: Brew a tea with dandelion root by steeping 1–2 teaspoons of dried root in hot water for 10–15 minutes. Drink this tea once or twice daily to support kidney health and relieve bloating.
- **Nettle Leaf**:
  - » Nettle is rich in antioxidants, minerals, and anti-inflammatory compounds. It supports kidney function by acting as a gentle diuretic and reducing inflammation, which helps alleviate the strain on the kidneys.
  - » **How to Use**: Nettle tea can be made by steeping 1–2 teaspoons of dried nettle leaves in hot water. Drink a cup daily for ongoing kidney support, or up to three cups during a detox period.
- **Parsley**:
  - » Parsley is a natural diuretic and helps flush out excess fluid and toxins. It is also high in vitamins A, C, and K, which provide antioxidant protection to the kidneys.
  - » **How to Use**: Fresh parsley can be blended into smoothies, juiced, or steeped as a tea. Drinking parsley tea or juice a few times a week helps maintain kidney health and supports detoxification.
- **Marshmallow Root**:
  - » Known for its soothing, mucilaginous properties, marshmallow root helps calm the urinary tract and prevent infections. It also supports kidney health by providing a protective coating to the bladder and kidneys.
  - » **How to Use**: Steep 1 tablespoon of dried marshmallow root in cold water for several hours (ideally overnight). Strain and drink as a cooling, soothing kidney tonic once daily.
- **Hydrangea Root**:
  - » Hydrangea root has been traditionally used to dissolve kidney stones and prevent their formation. It helps maintain a healthy mineral balance in the kidneys, reducing the risk of deposits.
  - » **How to Use**: Hydrangea root tea can be prepared by simmering 1 teaspoon of dried root in water for 15 minutes. Drink this tea 1–2 times per week as a preventive measure for kidney stones.
- **Celery Seed**:

- » Celery seeds act as a diuretic and support kidney function by flushing out toxins and excess fluid. They are also known for their anti-inflammatory properties.
- » **How to Use**: Crush a teaspoon of celery seeds and steep in hot water for 10 minutes. Drinking this tea once a day can help prevent fluid retention and support kidney cleansing.

3. SAMPLE KIDNEY HEALTH PROTOCOL USING DR. SEBI'S HERBS

This protocol provides a structured approach to support kidney health over a one-week period. By incorporating these herbal remedies and lifestyle practices, you can naturally support kidney function, promote detoxification, and maintain long-term kidney health.

Day 1–3: Preparatory Phase

- **Morning**:
  - » **Dandelion Root Tea**: Start each morning with a warm cup of dandelion root tea to stimulate detoxification and kickstart kidney support.
  - » **Warm Lemon Water**: Follow with a glass of warm water and lemon to further support liver and kidney detox.
- **Mid-Morning**:
  - » **Nettle Tea**: Nettle provides gentle kidney support, reducing inflammation and promoting fluid balance. Enjoy a cup of nettle tea mid-morning.
- **Afternoon**:
  - » **Parsley Smoothie**: Blend fresh parsley with cucumber, celery, and a squeeze of lemon for a refreshing, kidney-supporting smoothie.

Day 4–6: Active Cleansing Phase

- **Morning**:
  - » **Dandelion and Nettle Tea Combo**: Prepare a mix of dandelion root and nettle tea for enhanced diuretic and anti-inflammatory effects.
  - » **Aloe Vera Juice**: Drink 1-2 ounces of aloe vera juice to soothe the digestive tract and support kidney function.
- **Mid-Morning**:
  - » **Marshmallow Root Infusion**: Sip on a cool marshmallow root infusion to protect the urinary tract and aid in kidney function.
- **Lunch**:
  - » **Alkaline Salad**: Make a salad rich in kidney-supporting ingredients like cucumber, parsley, celery, and leafy greens.
- **Dinner**:
  - » **Hydrangea Root Tea**: End the day with a mild hydrangea root tea to help prevent mineral deposits and support mineral balance in the kidneys.

Day 7: Restorative Phase

- **Morning**:
  - » **Celery Seed Tea**: Drink a cup of celery seed tea for mild diuretic effects and detoxification support.
  - » **Smoothie**: Prepare a smoothie with spinach, avocado, a bit of sea moss gel, and a handful of parsley for balanced kidney and electrolyte support.
- **Evening**:
  - » **Peppermint or Chamomile Tea**: These calming teas relax the body and provide gentle support to the digestive and urinary systems.

4. LIFESTYLE PRACTICES TO SUPPORT KIDNEY HEALTH

In addition to herbal protocols, certain lifestyle practices help maintain kidney health and support the kidneys' natural detoxification processes.

- **Stay Hydrated**:
  - » Drinking plenty of water is essential for kidney health, as it helps flush out toxins and prevents the formation of kidney stones. Aim for at least 8–10 cups of water daily, with a focus on alkaline or filtered water.
- **Limit Processed Foods and Sodium**:
  - » Processed foods and high sodium intake put additional strain on the kidneys, potentially leading to high blood pressure and kidney dysfunction. Focus on whole, plant-based foods and limit processed options to reduce kidney strain.
- **Exercise Regularly**:
  - » Physical activity supports blood circulation, which is essential for kidney function. Gentle exercises like walking, yoga, and stretching also help reduce stress on the kidneys.
- **Manage Stress**:
  - » Chronic stress releases hormones that can impact kidney function and overall health. Practice stress-management techniques such as meditation, deep breathing, or journaling to support kidney health.
- **Limit Caffeine and Alcohol**:

- » Both caffeine and alcohol can dehydrate the body and strain the kidneys. Reducing or eliminating these substances can relieve stress on the kidneys and improve detoxification.

By following these herbal protocols and incorporating kidney-supportive lifestyle practices, you can maintain healthy kidney function and support the body's natural filtration processes. Dr. Sebi's approach to kidney health highlights the importance of natural, plant-based remedies that work harmoniously with the body, allowing the kidneys to perform their crucial role in cleansing and balancing the internal environment. Through consistent kidney care, you're setting a foundation for long-term wellness, improved energy, and resilience against daily stressors.

CHAPTER 2
PREVENTING KIDNEY STONES

Kidney stones are small, hard mineral deposits that form in the kidneys and can cause severe pain, discomfort, and even complications if left untreated. They develop when the concentration of certain minerals in the urine—such as calcium, oxalate, and uric acid—becomes too high, leading to crystallization. While there are various types of kidney stones, all are associated with dehydration, dietary habits, and imbalances in body chemistry. Following Dr. Sebi's principles of an alkaline, plant-based lifestyle can significantly reduce the risk of developing kidney stones. This chapter explores preventive strategies that focus on maintaining proper hydration, balancing dietary intake, and incorporating herbs to support kidney health and prevent stones.

1. UNDERSTANDING KIDNEY STONES: TYPES AND CAUSES

Kidney stones form when minerals in the urine crystallize and combine to form hard deposits. There are different types of stones, each associated with unique causes and dietary factors:

- **Calcium Oxalate Stones**: The most common type of kidney stone, these stones form when calcium combines with oxalate, a compound found in foods like spinach, nuts, and chocolate. High calcium or oxalate intake and dehydration can contribute to their formation.
- **Uric Acid Stones**: These stones form when the urine becomes too acidic, typically due to a high intake of purine-rich foods like red meat, shellfish, and alcohol. High uric acid levels can lead to crystal formation in the kidneys.
- **Struvite Stones**: Less common, struvite stones usually form in response to urinary tract infections. These stones are composed of magnesium, ammonium, and phosphate.
- **Cystine Stones**: These rare stones form due to a genetic condition that causes cystine to leak into the urine, leading to crystallization.

Understanding these types and their causes helps in adopting effective preventive strategies that align with Dr. Sebi's approach to maintaining kidney health.

2. CORE PRINCIPLES FOR PREVENTING KIDNEY STONES

Preventing kidney stones naturally involves adopting lifestyle and dietary habits that support kidney health and balance mineral levels in the body. Dr. Sebi's approach emphasizes creating an alkaline environment, which reduces the likelihood of mineral crystallization and supports the kidneys' natural detoxification function.

- **Stay Hydrated**:
  » Dehydration is one of the primary causes of kidney stone formation. Proper hydration helps dilute the concentration of minerals in the urine, making it less likely for them to crystallize. Drinking enough water each day flushes the kidneys and prevents the buildup of minerals.
- **Limit High-Oxalate Foods**:
  » Foods high in oxalates, like spinach, beets, nuts, and chocolate, can contribute to calcium oxalate stone formation. While it's not necessary to avoid them entirely, balancing their intake and combining them with calcium-rich foods can reduce the risk of crystallization.
- **Alkalize the Diet**:
  » An alkaline diet helps balance the body's pH and reduces the acidity in the urine, particularly helpful in preventing uric acid stones. Focus on alkaline foods like leafy greens, cucumbers, and citrus fruits to maintain a balanced internal environment.
- **Reduce Salt Intake**:
  » Excessive sodium can lead to higher calcium levels in the urine, increasing the risk of kidney stones. Reducing salt intake helps prevent calcium from accumulating in the urine.
- **Limit Animal Protein**:
  » Animal protein, particularly red meat and shellfish, increases uric acid levels in the body, promoting stone formation. Opting for plant-based protein sources like lentils, chickpeas, and hemp seeds reduces this risk.

3. ALKALINE FOODS AND BEVERAGES TO PREVENT KIDNEY STONES

Adopting an alkaline diet is a cornerstone of Dr. Sebi's approach to kidney health. By including alkaline, mineral-rich foods, we can prevent the crystallization that leads to kidney stones while supporting overall kidney function.

- **Cucumber**:

- » Cucumber is hydrating, alkaline, and high in water content, making it an ideal food for preventing kidney stones. It supports kidney health by promoting hydration and helping to flush out toxins.
- » **How to Use**: Add cucumber to salads, smoothies, or infuse it in water for a refreshing and hydrating beverage.
- **Lemon and Lime**:
  - » Lemon and lime contain citric acid, which binds with calcium and helps prevent stone formation. Their alkalizing effect reduces urine acidity, particularly beneficial for those prone to uric acid stones.
  - » **How to Use**: Start each day with warm lemon water, and add fresh lemon or lime juice to water throughout the day to support hydration and prevent stones.
- **Celery**:
  - » Celery is naturally hydrating, diuretic, and rich in minerals that promote kidney health. It helps reduce the concentration of stone-forming minerals in the urine.
  - » **How to Use**: Juice celery, add it to salads, or snack on raw celery to support kidney function and prevent dehydration.
- **Watermelon**:
  - » Watermelon is hydrating, alkaline, and supports kidney health by providing natural electrolytes and reducing urine concentration. Its high water content helps flush the kidneys.
  - » **How to Use**: Eat fresh watermelon or blend it into a juice for hydration and kidney support.
- **Basil**:
  - » Basil has mild diuretic properties that aid in flushing out the kidneys. It also helps reduce uric acid levels, which can prevent the formation of uric acid stones.
  - » **How to Use**: Add fresh basil to salads, make basil tea, or add basil leaves to smoothies for gentle kidney support.

4. HERBAL REMEDIES TO PREVENT KIDNEY STONES

Several herbs can naturally prevent kidney stones by helping the kidneys flush out excess minerals, reducing inflammation, and maintaining a balanced mineral environment. Incorporating these herbs into your routine can support ongoing kidney health and stone prevention.

- **Hydrangea Root**:
  - » Hydrangea root has traditionally been used to dissolve and prevent kidney stones. It helps maintain mineral balance and prevents the formation of crystal deposits in the kidneys.
  - » **How to Use**: Brew hydrangea root tea by simmering 1 teaspoon of dried root in water for 10–15 minutes. Drink this tea a few times a week for preventive kidney health.
- **Dandelion Root**:
  - » Dandelion root is a natural diuretic that helps flush out the kidneys and prevents the accumulation of minerals that form stones. It also supports liver health, which indirectly benefits kidney function.
  - » **How to Use**: Make a tea with dried dandelion root, drinking one cup daily to support detoxification and prevent kidney stones.
- **Horsetail**:
  - » Horsetail is high in silica, a mineral that helps strengthen kidney tissue and prevent stone formation. It has diuretic properties, helping the kidneys remove waste efficiently.
  - » **How to Use**: Steep horsetail as a tea by using 1–2 teaspoons of dried horsetail in hot water. Drink once daily for kidney support.
- **Marshmallow Root**:
  - » Marshmallow root has a soothing effect on the urinary tract and helps prevent irritation from passing small stones. It promotes urine flow, helping the kidneys flush out excess minerals.
  - » **How to Use**: Soak marshmallow root in cold water for several hours, strain, and drink as a refreshing, hydrating tonic. This can be consumed daily during detox periods.
- **Uva Ursi (Bearberry)**:
  - » Uva ursi has mild antiseptic properties and helps maintain an alkaline environment in the urinary tract. It prevents the formation of stones by reducing acidity and flushing the kidneys.
  - » **How to Use**: Uva ursi tea can be consumed for a few days at a time as a preventive measure against kidney stones.

5. SAMPLE DAILY ROUTINE FOR KIDNEY STONE PREVENTION

By incorporating specific foods, herbs, and hydration practices, you can create a daily routine that supports kidney health and helps prevent stones. Here's a sample routine that incorporates the principles and remedies discussed:

- **Morning**:
  - » **Warm Lemon Water**: Start the day with a glass of

- warm lemon water to support kidney function and reduce urine acidity.
  » **Hydrangea Root Tea**: Brew a cup of hydrangea root tea to promote mineral balance and prevent stone formation.
- **Mid-Morning**:
  » **Celery and Cucumber Juice**: Blend celery and cucumber with a splash of lemon juice for a hydrating, kidney-supporting beverage.
- **Lunch**:
  » **Alkaline Salad**: Include hydrating, alkaline ingredients like cucumber, celery, basil, and leafy greens. Add a light olive oil and lemon dressing for extra kidney support.
- **Afternoon Snack**:
  » **Watermelon**: A bowl of fresh watermelon hydrates and supports kidney health, helping to flush out toxins and excess minerals.
- **Dinner**:
  » **Steamed Vegetables with Fresh Basil**: Steam vegetables like zucchini and asparagus, and add fresh basil for flavor and kidney support.
- **Evening**:
  » **Dandelion Root or Horsetail Tea**: Drink a cup of tea made from dandelion root or horsetail to support gentle kidney detoxification overnight.

6. ADDITIONAL TIPS FOR LONG-TERM KIDNEY STONE PREVENTION

In addition to dietary and herbal approaches, certain lifestyle practices can support kidney health and reduce the risk of stone formation:

- **Stay Consistently Hydrated**:
  » Dehydration increases the concentration of minerals in the urine, which can lead to stone formation. Aim to drink 8–10 cups of water daily, with an emphasis on alkaline or lemon-infused water.
- **Limit Processed Foods and Sugars**:
  » Processed foods and sugary drinks can increase uric acid and calcium levels in the urine, raising the risk of kidney stones. Choose whole, unprocessed foods as often as possible.
- **Maintain a Balanced Diet**:
  » A balanced intake of calcium and oxalate is essential to prevent calcium oxalate stones. Pairing high-oxalate foods with calcium-rich options (such as sesame seeds) helps prevent oxalate absorption.
- **Exercise Regularly**:
  » Physical activity supports kidney health and improves circulation, aiding in the prevention of kidney stones. Aim for moderate exercise like walking or stretching to support kidney function.

By incorporating these natural practices and herbs into your daily routine, you can effectively prevent kidney stones and support long-term kidney health. Dr. Sebi's approach, which emphasizes an alkaline diet and herbal remedies, provides a powerful, plant-based foundation for maintaining balanced kidney function, reducing the risk of stone formation, and promoting overall well-being. With consistent hydration, mindful dietary choices, and targeted herbal support, you can keep your kidneys healthy and free from painful kidney stones.

CHAPTER 3
NATURAL DETOX FOR KIDNEY SUPPORT

The kidneys work continuously to maintain a clean, balanced internal environment by filtering waste, balancing electrolytes, and removing excess fluids. Over time, exposure to environmental toxins, processed foods, and stress can place a heavy load on the kidneys, impacting their ability to function efficiently. Regular detoxification practices support kidney health by reducing the buildup of harmful substances, aiding in the removal of waste, and preventing the formation of kidney stones and other complications. This chapter provides a comprehensive guide to natural kidney detoxification, using plant-based foods, herbs, and lifestyle practices to rejuvenate and sustain kidney health.

1. WHY KIDNEY DETOXIFICATION IS ESSENTIAL

Kidneys play a central role in the body's detoxification system. They filter approximately 50 gallons of blood daily, removing waste and regulating levels of electrolytes like sodium, potassium, and calcium. When toxins accumulate or the kidneys become overworked, the risk of kidney stones, infections, and other health complications increases. Detoxification for kidney support aims to:

- **Eliminate Toxins**: Aid the kidneys in removing accumulated toxins, promoting a cleaner internal environment.
- **Reduce Strain**: Relieve the kidneys by supporting their natural filtration process, reducing the burden of processing toxins and waste.
- **Prevent Kidney Stones**: Alkaline foods and specific herbs can prevent mineral buildup that contributes to kidney stones.
- **Enhance Fluid Balance**: Proper hydration and detoxification practices support the kidneys' role in regulating body fluids.

2. KEY ALKALINE FOODS FOR KIDNEY DETOX

An alkaline diet is central to Dr. Sebi's approach and provides a natural way to detoxify the kidneys. Alkaline foods help neutralize acidity, reduce inflammation, and prevent the crystallization of minerals, which can lead to kidney stones. The following foods are particularly beneficial for kidney detox:

- **Cucumber**:
  » Cucumber is high in water content, hydrating the body and aiding in the removal of waste. Its natural diuretic properties encourage urination, which helps the kidneys flush out toxins.
  » **How to Use**: Enjoy cucumber slices in salads, infuse in water, or add to smoothies for a refreshing and hydrating boost.
- **Watermelon**:
  » Watermelon is not only hydrating but also rich in antioxidants and natural electrolytes that support kidney function. Its high water content makes it an excellent food for flushing out toxins.
  » **How to Use**: Eat fresh watermelon as a snack, blend into a juice, or freeze for a cooling treat during a detox period.
- **Celery**:
  » Celery acts as a natural diuretic and helps remove excess fluids from the body, reducing the kidneys' workload. It also contains anti-inflammatory compounds that support kidney health.
  » **How to Use**: Juice celery, add it to salads, or snack on it raw. A daily serving of celery helps support kidney detoxification.
- **Cilantro**:
  » Cilantro is known for its chelation properties, meaning it binds to heavy metals and helps remove them from the body. This is beneficial for reducing toxic buildup in the kidneys.
  » **How to Use**: Add fresh cilantro to salads, blend in smoothies, or juice it with other greens to promote kidney cleansing.
- **Dandelion Greens**:
  » Dandelion greens are rich in potassium, which helps regulate kidney function and prevent fluid retention. Their mild diuretic effect encourages toxin removal.
  » **How to Use**: Use dandelion greens in salads, green juices, or smoothies. They pair well with other leafy greens and provide a potent boost for kidney health.
- **Lemon and Lime**:
  » Lemons and limes help alkalize the body and stimulate digestion. Their citric acid content reduces the likelihood of stone formation by preventing mineral crystallization in the kidneys.
  » **How to Use**: Start the day with warm lemon water,

and add fresh lemon or lime juice to water throughout the day to support kidney detoxification.

3. HERBAL REMEDIES FOR KIDNEY DETOX

In addition to alkaline foods, specific herbs play a crucial role in detoxifying the kidneys. These herbs work synergistically with the body, promoting toxin elimination, reducing inflammation, and supporting the kidneys' natural cleansing functions.

- **Dandelion Root**:
  - » Dandelion root is a powerful detox herb that supports liver and kidney function. It acts as a diuretic, promoting urine production and helping the kidneys flush out waste more efficiently.
  - » **How to Use**: Brew dandelion root tea by steeping 1–2 teaspoons of dried root in hot water. Drink this tea once daily as part of a kidney detox protocol.
- **Nettle Leaf**:
  - » Nettle leaf is rich in minerals and has diuretic properties that support kidney function. It helps flush out toxins, reduce inflammation, and maintain a balanced mineral environment in the kidneys.
  - » **How to Use**: Nettle tea can be made by steeping 1–2 teaspoons of dried nettle leaves in hot water. Drink one cup daily for gentle kidney support or up to three cups during an active detox.
- **Parsley**:
  - » Parsley is a natural diuretic, helping the kidneys eliminate waste more efficiently. Its high vitamin and mineral content also provides antioxidant support to protect the kidneys.
  - » **How to Use**: Add fresh parsley to smoothies, salads, or infuse in water for a kidney-supporting tonic. Drinking parsley tea is also effective for kidney detoxification.
- **Marshmallow Root**:
  - » Marshmallow root has soothing properties that protect the urinary tract, reducing irritation and promoting healthy urine flow. It aids in flushing out toxins and prevents urinary tract infections.
  - » **How to Use**: Soak marshmallow root in cold water for several hours, strain, and drink as a hydrating, kidney-soothing tonic. This can be consumed once daily for kidney support.
- **Burdock Root**:
  - » Burdock root helps cleanse the blood and supports kidney health by promoting toxin elimination. Its anti-inflammatory properties also help reduce kidney strain.
  - » **How to Use**: Burdock root tea can be prepared by simmering 1–2 teaspoons of dried root in water for 15 minutes. Drink this tea a few times a week to aid kidney detox.

4. SAMPLE 3-DAY KIDNEY DETOX PLAN

This three-day kidney detox plan includes a variety of alkaline foods and herbs to support kidney health, reduce toxin buildup, and improve overall kidney function. This plan is designed to be gentle yet effective in providing the kidneys with the support they need for efficient detoxification.

Day 1: Hydration and Preparation

- **Morning**:
  - » **Warm Lemon Water**: Start the day with a glass of warm lemon water to alkalize the body and stimulate the kidneys.
  - » **Dandelion Root Tea**: Brew a cup of dandelion root tea to support kidney function and promote gentle detoxification.
- **Mid-Morning**:
  - » **Celery and Cucumber Juice**: Blend celery and cucumber for a hydrating, kidney-supporting juice. Drink slowly to enjoy its benefits.
- **Lunch**:
  - » **Alkaline Salad**: Prepare a salad with dandelion greens, cucumber, celery, and a lemon-tahini dressing for a nutrient-rich meal that supports kidney health.
- **Afternoon Snack**:
  - » **Watermelon**: Enjoy a bowl of fresh watermelon to stay hydrated and support the kidneys in flushing out toxins.
- **Dinner**:
  - » **Steamed Vegetables with Cilantro**: Lightly steam zucchini, broccoli, and bell peppers, and garnish with fresh cilantro for kidney-supportive nutrients.

Day 2: Active Detoxification

- **Morning**:
  - » **Nettle Tea**: Start with a cup of nettle tea to promote diuresis and cleanse the kidneys.
  - » **Green Smoothie**: Blend dandelion greens, cucumber, parsley, and lemon juice for a nutrient-dense smoothie that supports kidney detox.
- **Mid-Morning**:

- » **Parsley Water**: Infuse water with fresh parsley and sip throughout the day to support kidney detoxification.
- **Lunch**:
  - » **Vegetable Broth**: Prepare a light vegetable broth using celery, carrots, and parsley. This provides hydration and supports the kidneys.
- **Dinner**:
  - » **Steamed Sweet Potatoes and Spinach**: Steamed sweet potatoes with a side of sautéed spinach provide kidney-supporting potassium and antioxidants.

Day 3: Restorative Phase

- **Morning**:
  - » **Marshmallow Root Infusion**: Drink a cold infusion of marshmallow root to soothe and protect the kidneys and urinary tract.
  - » **Green Juice**: Make a juice with cucumber, lemon, and cilantro for hydration and mineral support.
- **Lunch**:
  - » **Alkaline Soup**: Prepare a soup with zucchini, dandelion greens, and a pinch of sea salt for mineral support and gentle detox.
- **Dinner**:
  - » **Hydrating Salad with Basil**: Create a salad with mixed greens, cucumber, fresh basil, and lemon dressing for a light, kidney-supportive meal.

5. ADDITIONAL LIFESTYLE PRACTICES FOR LONG-TERM KIDNEY HEALTH

Detoxification is not a one-time event but a consistent practice. Supporting kidney health long-term requires ongoing dietary and lifestyle habits that reduce strain and provide nutrients necessary for kidney function.

- **Regular Hydration**:
  - » Drinking enough water is essential for kidney health. Proper hydration flushes out toxins, reducing the likelihood of stone formation and maintaining fluid balance.
- **Limit Processed Foods and Excess Salt**:
  - » Processed foods and high-sodium diets strain the kidneys. Focus on whole, unprocessed foods and use natural herbs and spices for flavor.
- **Incorporate Physical Activity**:
  - » Gentle exercise like walking, yoga, or swimming promotes circulation and supports kidney function by aiding in detoxification.
- **Manage Stress**:
  - » Chronic stress releases hormones that can impact kidney function. Engage in relaxation practices like meditation, breathing exercises, or journaling to support overall health.

Through the regular practice of natural detox protocols, you can effectively support and maintain kidney health. Dr. Sebi's approach emphasizes the use of alkaline foods, targeted herbs, and lifestyle practices that work together to reduce the toxic burden on the kidneys and promote a clean internal environment. By adopting these detox practices, you help your kidneys perform their crucial role in detoxification, ultimately enhancing energy, vitality, and resilience against daily stressors.

BOOK 19
Cancer Prevention and Management

Cancer is a complex disease influenced by genetic, environmental, and lifestyle factors. While no single approach can guarantee cancer prevention, adopting a lifestyle centered on balanced nutrition, low stress, and regular detoxification can significantly reduce cancer risk. Dr. Sebi's focus on an alkaline, plant-based diet aligns with the belief that a balanced internal environment can inhibit cancer cell growth and create a foundation for long-term health. This book provides readers with an understanding of how natural, holistic practices can aid in cancer prevention and offers tools to manage health through mindful dietary choices.

CHAPTER 1
ROLE OF ALKALINE FOODS IN CANCER PREVENTION

In recent years, the connection between diet and cancer has received increasing attention. Research supports the idea that certain foods can help create an internal environment that discourages cancer cell growth. Dr. Sebi's approach to cancer prevention focuses on consuming alkaline foods that help maintain a balanced pH in the body, reduce inflammation, and strengthen immune function. By following an alkaline diet, we can create conditions that make it challenging for cancer cells to thrive, promoting overall wellness and resilience against disease.

1. UNDERSTANDING PH BALANCE AND CANCER PREVENTION

The pH level of the human body affects numerous bodily functions. A balanced pH helps sustain healthy cells, while an overly acidic environment can contribute to inflammation, weaken immunity, and increase the risk of chronic diseases, including cancer. Here's how pH balance plays a role in cancer prevention:

- **Cancer Cells and Acidic Environments**:
  » Cancer cells tend to thrive in acidic environments, where oxygen is limited, and acidity is high. Acidic conditions can weaken cells, impairing their ability to function and resist disease. Alkaline foods, on the other hand, help neutralize acidity and provide the nutrients needed for healthy cell function.

- **Oxygen and Cell Health**:
  » A more alkaline internal environment improves oxygen levels in tissues, supporting cellular health and vitality. Cancer cells do not fare well in oxygen-rich, alkaline environments, which can inhibit their growth and spread.

- **Alkalinity and Immune Response**:
  » Alkaline foods support a strong immune system by reducing inflammation and providing antioxidants, vitamins, and minerals that enhance immune response. A healthy immune system is essential in identifying and destroying abnormal cells, including those with cancerous potential.

2. KEY NUTRIENTS IN ALKALINE FOODS FOR CANCER PREVENTION

Alkaline foods are rich in nutrients that combat inflammation, support immunity, and protect cells from damage. Here are some of the most important nutrients in an alkaline diet and how they contribute to cancer prevention:

- **Antioxidants**:
  » Antioxidants protect cells from oxidative stress, which damages DNA and can lead to abnormal cell growth. Foods rich in antioxidants, such as berries and leafy greens, neutralize free radicals that contribute to cellular damage and cancer.

- **Phytonutrients**:
  » Phytonutrients are compounds found in plants that have cancer-fighting properties. Cruciferous vegetables, such as broccoli and kale, are particularly high in phytonutrients like sulforaphane, which has been shown to inhibit cancer cell growth.

- **Fiber**:
  » High-fiber foods support healthy digestion and help eliminate toxins from the body. Fiber also helps balance blood sugar levels, which is crucial since high blood sugar can increase inflammation and cancer risk.

- **Minerals (Calcium, Magnesium, Potassium)**:
  » Minerals found in alkaline foods, like calcium, magnesium, and potassium, help maintain pH balance and cellular health. These minerals reduce acidity and inflammation, contributing to a less hospitable environment for cancer cells.

- **Chlorophyll**:
  » Chlorophyll, abundant in green leafy vegetables, detoxifies the body and supports oxygenation. It helps cleanse the blood and provides an alkaline boost, protecting cells from potential damage that can lead to cancer.

3. BEST ALKALINE FOODS FOR CANCER PREVENTION

Certain alkaline foods are particularly effective at creating an anti-cancer environment. These foods are nutrient-dense, low in acidity, and high in protective compounds. Here are some of the top alkaline foods for cancer prevention:

- **Leafy Greens (Kale, Spinach, Swiss Chard):**
  - Leafy greens are high in chlorophyll, antioxidants, and fiber, all of which support detoxification and immune health. They neutralize acidity in the body and help maintain an alkaline pH.
  - **How to Use:** Add leafy greens to salads, smoothies, or sauté with garlic for a nutrient-packed side dish.
- **Cruciferous Vegetables (Broccoli, Cauliflower, Cabbage):**
  - Cruciferous vegetables contain compounds like sulforaphane and indole-3-carbinol, which have been shown to inhibit cancer cell growth. These vegetables are alkaline-forming and support liver detoxification.
  - **How to Use:** Steam or roast broccoli and cauliflower, add shredded cabbage to salads, or blend these vegetables into soups for maximum benefits.
- **Berries (Blueberries, Blackberries, Strawberries):**
  - Berries are rich in antioxidants, vitamins, and fiber, which help protect cells from damage and promote detoxification. They also have anti-inflammatory properties, making them a valuable addition to an anti-cancer diet.
  - **How to Use:** Enjoy berries fresh as a snack, add to smoothies, or use as a topping for oatmeal or chia pudding.
- **Citrus Fruits (Lemon, Lime, Grapefruit):**
  - Although acidic outside the body, citrus fruits have an alkalizing effect once metabolized. They are high in vitamin C and other antioxidants that support the immune system and reduce inflammation.
  - **How to Use:** Start the day with warm lemon water, add citrus juice to dressings, or enjoy fresh grapefruit as a snack.
- **Sea Vegetables (Sea Moss, Nori, Kelp):**
  - Sea vegetables are high in minerals that promote alkalinity and detoxification. They support thyroid function and provide essential trace minerals that protect cells from oxidative damage.
  - **How to Use:** Add nori to salads or wraps, mix sea moss gel into smoothies, or use kelp flakes as a seasoning.
- **Garlic and Onions:**
  - Both garlic and onions contain sulfur compounds that help detoxify the body, reduce inflammation, and enhance immune function. Garlic, in particular, has been shown to have anti-cancer properties, especially in relation to stomach and colorectal cancers.
  - **How to Use:** Add garlic and onions to stir-fries, soups, or roasted vegetable dishes to boost flavor and health benefits.

4. CREATING A DAILY ALKALINE ROUTINE FOR CANCER PREVENTION

Incorporating alkaline foods into your daily routine is a powerful step toward cancer prevention. Here's a sample routine that includes a variety of anti-inflammatory, nutrient-rich foods to maintain an alkaline environment:

- **Morning:**
  - **Warm Lemon Water:** Begin the day with warm water and lemon to alkalize the body, support liver detoxification, and promote hydration.
  - **Green Smoothie:** Blend spinach, kale, cucumber, a handful of berries, and a scoop of sea moss gel with water or almond milk for a nutrient-dense, alkaline breakfast.
- **Mid-Morning Snack:**
  - **Berries and Chia Seeds:** Enjoy a bowl of fresh berries with a sprinkle of chia seeds, which provide fiber and antioxidants.
- **Lunch:**
  - **Alkaline Salad:** Create a salad with mixed greens, cruciferous vegetables like broccoli and cabbage, sliced avocado, and a lemon-tahini dressing. Top with pumpkin seeds or nuts for added minerals and healthy fats.
- **Afternoon Snack:**
  - **Fresh Veggies with Hummus:** Snack on cucumber, bell peppers, and carrots with a side of hummus for a filling, alkalizing snack that provides fiber and protein.
- **Dinner:**
  - **Steamed Vegetables with Garlic and Herbs:** Lightly steam vegetables like cauliflower, zucchini, and asparagus, and season with fresh garlic, parsley, and a squeeze of lemon. Pair with a side of quinoa for a complete, balanced meal.
- **Evening:**
  - **Herbal Tea:** End the day with an herbal tea like cham-

omile or ginger, which supports digestion and reduces inflammation.

5. ADDITIONAL LIFESTYLE PRACTICES FOR CANCER PREVENTION

While an alkaline diet is central to Dr. Sebi's approach to cancer prevention, other lifestyle practices can further support immune function, reduce stress, and maintain an internal environment that discourages cancer cell growth.

- **Stay Hydrated**:
  - » Proper hydration is essential for flushing out toxins and maintaining cellular health. Aim for at least eight cups of water daily, with an emphasis on filtered or alkaline water.
- **Reduce Processed Foods and Sugars**:
  - » Processed foods and added sugars increase inflammation and acidity in the body. Choose whole, unprocessed foods whenever possible to support a balanced pH.
- **Exercise Regularly**:
  - » Physical activity enhances circulation, supports detoxification, and reduces inflammation. Aim for moderate exercise like walking, yoga, or cycling for at least 30 minutes most days.
- **Practice Mindful Stress Management**:
  - » Chronic stress impacts the immune system and can increase acidity in the body. Incorporate stress-reducing practices like deep breathing, meditation, and journaling to promote relaxation and mental clarity.
- **Limit Toxins and Environmental Exposures**:
  - » Avoiding environmental toxins whenever possible can reduce the toxic load on the kidneys and liver. Opt for natural cleaning products, avoid plastic containers, and prioritize organic produce to limit pesticide exposure.

6. LONG-TERM BENEFITS OF AN ALKALINE DIET FOR CANCER PREVENTION

Adopting an alkaline diet not only helps prevent cancer but also promotes overall health by reducing inflammation, enhancing immune response, and supporting detoxification. Over time, these benefits extend to multiple areas of health, including energy levels, digestion, mental clarity, and resilience against chronic illnesses.

By consistently incorporating alkaline foods and mindful lifestyle practices, individuals can create a strong foundation for wellness, supporting their body's natural defenses and reducing the risk of cancer and other diseases. Dr. Sebi's approach provides a roadmap for achieving this balance, empowering individuals to take control of their health through natural, plant-based strategies.

Through an alkaline diet focused on nutrient-dense foods, antioxidants, and consistent hydration, you can significantly support your body in its fight against cancer. Dr. Sebi's method encourages creating an internal environment that is inhospitable to cancer cells while simultaneously nurturing overall wellness. Adopting these principles consistently fosters long-term health, enhances resilience, and supports the body's natural ability to prevent and combat disease.

•

CHAPTER 2
HERBS FOR CANCER RECOVERY

Cancer recovery is a holistic journey that involves not only physical healing but also the restoration of balance within the body. For individuals recovering from cancer, supporting the body's detoxification pathways, bolstering immunity, and reducing inflammation are essential. Dr. Sebi's approach to herbal remedies emphasizes using nutrient-rich, alkaline herbs that work with the body's natural healing processes. This chapter provides a guide to some of the most effective herbs for cancer recovery, highlighting their unique properties and benefits, along with practical methods for incorporating them into a supportive daily regimen.

1. THE ROLE OF HERBS IN CANCER RECOVERY

Herbs are powerful allies in cancer recovery due to their ability to strengthen the immune system, cleanse the blood, reduce inflammation, and support cellular health. Many herbs contain antioxidants, vitamins, and minerals that aid the body in healing from the effects of cancer treatments like chemotherapy and radiation, which often leave the body depleted and stressed. In addition, herbs can help alleviate side effects such as nausea, fatigue, and pain, providing a natural way to enhance quality of life during the recovery process.

- **Immune Support**: Herbs like echinacea and astragalus stimulate the immune system, helping the body defend itself against infections and promote healing.
- **Detoxification**: Herbs like dandelion root and burdock root help remove toxins, reducing the strain on the liver and kidneys, which are vital for processing waste and chemicals.
- **Anti-Inflammatory Properties**: Inflammation can hinder recovery, and herbs like turmeric and ginger help reduce inflammation, supporting tissue repair and pain relief.

2. ESSENTIAL HERBS FOR CANCER RECOVERY AND THEIR BENEFITS

Dr. Sebi's approach to herbs emphasizes those that align with an alkaline, plant-based philosophy. The following herbs are particularly beneficial for individuals recovering from cancer, each offering unique properties that aid in healing, detoxification, and immune support.

- **Dandelion Root**:
    - » Dandelion root is a potent detoxifying herb that supports liver function, helping the body remove waste and toxins. It's rich in antioxidants, which combat oxidative stress and aid in cellular repair.
    - » **How to Use**: Brew dandelion root tea by steeping 1–2 teaspoons of dried root in hot water. Drink this tea once daily to support detoxification and aid in liver recovery.
- **Turmeric**:
    - » Known for its powerful anti-inflammatory properties, turmeric contains curcumin, a compound that has been shown to reduce inflammation and support immune function. Turmeric also has antioxidant effects, protecting cells from damage.
    - » **How to Use**: Add a teaspoon of turmeric powder to soups, smoothies, or golden milk lattes. Combining turmeric with black pepper enhances curcumin absorption, making it more effective in the body.
- **Astragalus**:
    - » Astragalus is an adaptogenic herb that strengthens the immune system, helps the body cope with stress, and supports energy levels. It is particularly helpful for individuals recovering from chemotherapy, as it boosts white blood cell count.
    - » **How to Use**: Astragalus can be consumed as a tea, tincture, or in capsule form. Drink one cup of astragalus tea daily or follow the dosage instructions for capsules as recommended.
- **Ginger**:
    - » Ginger is commonly used to reduce nausea, improve digestion, and relieve pain, making it ideal for individuals recovering from the side effects of cancer treatments. It also has anti-inflammatory and antioxidant properties that support healing.
    - » **How to Use**: Fresh ginger can be brewed into a tea by simmering a few slices in hot water, or it can be grated into juices and smoothies. Ginger tea is particularly beneficial for soothing nausea and digestion.
- **Burdock Root**:
    - » Burdock root supports liver function, blood purification, and cellular health. It helps cleanse the blood by removing toxins and has mild diuretic properties that assist the kidneys in eliminating waste.
    - » **How to Use**: Burdock root can be consumed as a tea or tincture. To prepare a tea, simmer 1–2 teaspoons

of dried root in water for 15 minutes and drink once or twice a day.

- **Milk Thistle**:
  - » Milk thistle is widely known for its ability to support liver health. Its active compound, silymarin, helps repair liver cells, reduce inflammation, and improve detoxification, especially important for those recovering from chemotherapy.
  - » **How to Use**: Milk thistle is commonly taken in capsule form, but it can also be consumed as a tea. Take milk thistle supplements as directed, or drink milk thistle tea once daily for liver support.
- **Echinacea**:
  - » Echinacea is an immune-boosting herb that stimulates the production of white blood cells, helping the body fight infections. It is beneficial for recovery from treatments that suppress immunity, such as chemotherapy.
  - » **How to Use**: Echinacea can be consumed as a tea or in capsule form. Drink echinacea tea daily or as needed, especially during the recovery period when immunity is weakened.

3. SAMPLE DAILY ROUTINE FOR HERBAL SUPPORT DURING CANCER RECOVERY

Incorporating these herbs into a daily routine can support recovery by improving immune function, aiding detoxification, and reducing inflammation. Here is a sample routine that combines these powerful herbs with balanced, supportive practices.

- **Morning**:
  - » **Warm Lemon Water with Dandelion Root Tea**: Begin the day with a glass of warm lemon water to support hydration and alkalize the body. Follow with dandelion root tea to promote liver detoxification.
  - » **Astragalus Tea**: Drink a cup of astragalus tea in the morning to support immune function and enhance energy levels throughout the day.
- **Mid-Morning Snack**:
  - » **Ginger and Turmeric Smoothie**: Blend a small piece of fresh ginger, a teaspoon of turmeric powder, a handful of spinach, and a slice of pineapple with almond milk. This smoothie provides anti-inflammatory benefits, immune support, and antioxidants.
- **Lunch**:
  - » **Alkaline Vegetable Soup with Garlic**: Prepare a nourishing vegetable soup with garlic, onions, carrots, and leafy greens. Add a pinch of turmeric for additional anti-inflammatory benefits.
- **Afternoon**:
  - » **Burdock Root Tea**: Brew a cup of burdock root tea to support blood purification and aid kidney detoxification. This tea also provides antioxidants that assist in cellular repair.
- **Evening**:
  - » **Golden Milk**: Prepare a warm golden milk with turmeric, a pinch of black pepper, and almond milk. This soothing drink supports immunity and reduces inflammation, aiding relaxation and recovery before bedtime.

4. LIFESTYLE TIPS TO ENHANCE THE BENEFITS OF HERBAL REMEDIES

In addition to herbal support, there are lifestyle practices that can complement and enhance the benefits of these herbs, creating a well-rounded approach to cancer recovery.

- **Stay Hydrated**:
  - » Proper hydration is crucial during cancer recovery as it aids in toxin elimination and supports kidney function. Drink 8–10 cups of water daily and incorporate herbal teas for additional support.
- **Prioritize Rest and Sleep**:
  - » Quality sleep is essential for recovery and healing, as it allows the body to repair and regenerate cells. Aim for 7–9 hours of sleep each night, incorporating relaxation practices such as deep breathing or meditation.
- **Consume Nutrient-Dense, Alkaline Foods**:
  - » Alkaline foods like leafy greens, fruits, and whole grains provide the vitamins, minerals, and fiber necessary for a balanced recovery diet. Avoid processed foods and sugars, which can increase inflammation and acidity.
- **Incorporate Light Physical Activity**:
  - » Gentle movement, such as walking or yoga, supports circulation, reduces stress, and enhances detoxification. Physical activity can also boost energy levels and improve mood during the recovery period.
- **Limit Toxins and Chemicals**:
  - » Reducing exposure to environmental toxins can relieve strain on the liver and kidneys. Use natural, non-toxic cleaning products, avoid plastics when

possible, and choose organic produce to limit pesticide intake.

5. LONG-TERM BENEFITS OF HERBAL SUPPORT IN CANCER RECOVERY

Incorporating herbs into a cancer recovery plan provides ongoing support for the immune system, helps manage inflammation, and aids in the detoxification process. Over time, these herbs contribute to an overall sense of vitality, enhance resilience against disease, and help individuals regain their energy and strength. By using natural, plant-based remedies, individuals can work harmoniously with their bodies, fostering a balanced internal environment that supports healing and minimizes the risk of recurrence.

PRECAUTIONS AND GUIDELINES FOR USING HERBS DURING CANCER RECOVERY

While herbs are beneficial, it's essential to use them safely, especially during recovery. Here are a few guidelines:

- **Consult Healthcare Providers**: Before starting any herbal regimen, discuss it with your healthcare provider, particularly if you are taking medications. Some herbs may interact with treatments or medications.
- **Start with Small Amounts**: Begin with small doses and monitor how your body responds, gradually increasing if needed and under the guidance of a healthcare provider.
- **Avoid Synthetic or Processed Supplements**: Choose high-quality, organic herbs from reputable sources to ensure purity and potency. Avoid synthetic additives or heavily processed herbal products.

Dr. Sebi's philosophy on cancer recovery emphasizes a holistic approach that incorporates nature's healing powers. Through herbs that support detoxification, reduce inflammation, and strengthen immunity, individuals can provide their bodies with the tools necessary to heal and thrive. By following these practices and incorporating herbs like dandelion root, turmeric, and astragalus, recovery becomes a journey of restoring balance, regaining strength, and fostering resilience. With a mindful approach to diet, hydration, and stress management, you're setting a foundation for long-term health, empowered by the restorative properties of natural remedies.

CHAPTER 3
DETOXIFICATION PROTOCOLS FOR CANCER

Cancer treatments like chemotherapy, radiation, and surgery place a heavy burden on the body, often leading to a buildup of toxins and leaving the immune system weakened. During recovery, detoxification plays a critical role in removing waste, reducing oxidative stress, and supporting organ health. Dr. Sebi's philosophy on cancer detoxification emphasizes gentle, plant-based approaches that work in harmony with the body's natural processes, enhancing vitality, aiding cellular repair, and creating an internal environment that supports long-term health.

1. WHY DETOXIFICATION IS ESSENTIAL DURING CANCER RECOVERY

Detoxification is the body's way of processing and eliminating waste, toxins, and damaged cells. For those in cancer recovery, detoxification helps:

- **Remove Residual Toxins**: Cancer treatments introduce chemicals and byproducts that can linger in the body. Detoxification aids in eliminating these substances, allowing the body to heal more effectively.
- **Reduce Inflammation**: Inflammation often accompanies cancer and its treatments, contributing to discomfort, fatigue, and impaired healing. A detox helps lower inflammation, relieving the strain on organs and tissues.
- **Support Immune Function**: Detoxification supports the immune system by reducing the toxic load and encouraging the removal of damaged cells, which allows immune cells to work more efficiently.
- **Restore Energy and Vitality**: Clearing out toxins helps reduce fatigue, boost energy, and improve mental clarity, which are vital for maintaining a positive outlook and resilience during recovery.

2. KEY COMPONENTS OF DR. SEBI'S DETOX PROTOCOL

Dr. Sebi's detoxification protocol for cancer recovery includes three essential components: alkaline, nutrient-rich foods; detox-supportive herbs; and hydration. Together, these elements create a comprehensive approach to detoxification that supports the body gently and effectively.

- **Alkaline, Plant-Based Foods**: Alkaline foods reduce acidity and inflammation, supporting cellular health. An alkaline diet helps create an internal environment where cancer cells are less likely to thrive.
- **Detoxifying Herbs**: Herbs with detoxifying, anti-inflammatory, and immune-supporting properties aid the liver, kidneys, and lymphatic system in processing and removing waste.
- **Proper Hydration**: Hydration is critical for flushing out toxins and supporting kidney function. Drinking plenty of water, especially with a touch of lemon or herbal infusions, ensures effective detoxification.

3. ALKALINE FOODS FOR CANCER DETOXIFICATION

A plant-based, alkaline diet provides nutrients, antioxidants, and fiber that cleanse the body, aid in detoxification, and nourish cells. Incorporating these foods into a daily regimen supports detox and helps alleviate common side effects of cancer treatments.

- **Leafy Greens (Kale, Spinach, Swiss Chard)**:
  - » Leafy greens are high in chlorophyll, which detoxifies the blood and reduces inflammation. Their alkaline properties neutralize acidity in the body, promoting healing and tissue repair.
  - » **How to Use**: Add leafy greens to salads, smoothies, or lightly sauté them with olive oil and garlic for a nutrient-rich side dish.
- **Beets**:
  - » Beets are rich in antioxidants, fiber, and betalains, which support liver detoxification. They help cleanse the blood and aid in eliminating toxins through the digestive tract.
  - » **How to Use**: Roast beets, juice them, or add grated raw beets to salads for a vibrant detox boost.
- **Berries (Blueberries, Strawberries, Raspberries)**:
  - » Berries are rich in antioxidants and anti-inflammatory compounds, which protect cells from oxidative stress and support immune function. Their natural sweetness also makes them a pleasant addition to a detox routine.
  - » **How to Use**: Enjoy berries fresh as a snack, add them to smoothies, or use as a topping for chia pudding.
- **Cucumber**:
  - » Cucumber is hydrating, cooling, and alkaline, helping

to flush toxins and maintain kidney health. Its high water content makes it an ideal detox food.
- » **How to Use**: Slice cucumber into water for a refreshing drink, add to salads, or blend in smoothies.
- **Lemon and Lime**:
  - » Although acidic outside the body, citrus fruits like lemon and lime have an alkalizing effect once metabolized. Their vitamin C content supports immune health and helps the liver with detoxification.
  - » **How to Use**: Start each day with warm lemon water to alkalize the body and promote hydration, or squeeze lemon juice over salads and into smoothies.

4. DETOXIFYING HERBS FOR CANCER RECOVERY

In addition to alkaline foods, certain herbs support the body's detoxification pathways, helping remove residual chemicals, toxins, and waste from cancer treatments. These herbs can be incorporated as teas, tinctures, or supplements.

- **Dandelion Root**:
  - » Dandelion root supports liver function, assisting in the breakdown and removal of toxins from the body. It is also a mild diuretic, which aids in kidney health and fluid balance.
  - » **How to Use**: Brew dandelion root tea by steeping 1–2 teaspoons of dried root in hot water. Drink this tea once daily to support liver detoxification.
- **Milk Thistle**:
  - » Milk thistle contains silymarin, an antioxidant that protects and regenerates liver cells. It helps the liver process waste and reduces inflammation, making it especially beneficial after chemotherapy.
  - » **How to Use**: Milk thistle can be taken as a tea or in capsule form. Drink milk thistle tea once a day, or follow dosage instructions on supplements for liver support.
- **Burdock Root**:
  - » Burdock root purifies the blood and aids in detoxification by supporting liver and kidney function. Its antioxidants help neutralize free radicals, which is beneficial for individuals recovering from cancer treatments.
  - » **How to Use**: Brew burdock root tea by simmering 1–2 teaspoons of dried root in water for 15 minutes. Drink this tea once or twice daily during the detox period.
- **Red Clover**:
  - » Red clover has natural detoxifying properties and helps purify the blood. It supports lymphatic health, which is essential for eliminating waste and toxins.
  - » **How to Use**: Red clover tea can be brewed by steeping 1–2 teaspoons of dried blossoms in hot water. Drink once daily to support lymphatic detox.
- **Ginger**:
  - » Ginger is anti-inflammatory and aids digestion, making it helpful for relieving nausea and reducing inflammation. It also supports circulation, which is essential for effective detoxification.
  - » **How to Use**: Add fresh ginger to smoothies, make ginger tea, or add grated ginger to meals. Drinking ginger tea before meals can help stimulate digestion and support the detox process.

5. SAMPLE 3-DAY DETOX PROTOCOL FOR CANCER RECOVERY

A three-day detox protocol provides a structured approach to cleanse the body and support recovery. This gentle protocol uses nutrient-rich foods, detoxifying herbs, and proper hydration to promote a clean internal environment, alleviate inflammation, and aid healing.

Day 1: Hydration and Alkalization

- **Morning**:
  - » **Warm Lemon Water**: Begin the day with a glass of warm lemon water to stimulate digestion and alkalize the body.
  - » **Dandelion Root Tea**: Drink a cup of dandelion root tea to support liver detoxification.
- **Mid-Morning**:
  - » **Green Smoothie**: Blend spinach, kale, cucumber, a handful of berries, and a slice of ginger for a nutrient-dense, alkaline smoothie.
- **Lunch**:
  - » **Alkaline Salad**: Prepare a salad with leafy greens, cucumber, grated beets, and a lemon-tahini dressing for a fiber-rich, detox-supporting meal.
- **Afternoon Snack**:
  - » **Fresh Berries**: Enjoy a bowl of fresh berries to provide antioxidants and support immune health.
- **Dinner**:
  - » **Steamed Vegetables with Burdock Root Tea**: Steam vegetables like broccoli, zucchini, and carrots. Pair with burdock root tea to support blood purification and detoxification.

Day 2: Detoxification and Immune Support

- **Morning**:
  - **Milk Thistle Tea**: Begin the day with milk thistle tea to promote liver detoxification and cellular repair.
  - **Green Juice**: Make a juice with cucumber, celery, lemon, and a handful of parsley for hydration and mineral support.
- **Lunch**:
  - **Vegetable Broth**: Prepare a light broth using celery, carrots, garlic, and red clover. This provides hydration and supports the lymphatic system.
- **Afternoon Snack**:
  - **Cucumber Slices with Hummus**: Snack on hydrating cucumber slices with hummus for a filling, alkaline snack.
- **Dinner**:
  - **Quinoa and Steamed Greens**: Pair cooked quinoa with steamed greens like Swiss chard and dandelion greens. Add a drizzle of lemon juice for extra alkalinity.

Day 3: Restorative Detox and Inflammation Reduction

- **Morning**:
  - **Warm Lemon Water with Ginger Tea**: Start the day with lemon water and ginger tea to soothe the stomach and support detox.
  - **Chlorophyll Smoothie**: Blend spinach, cucumber, lime, and a spoonful of chlorophyll for a hydrating, detoxifying drink.
- **Lunch**:
  - **Alkaline Soup**: Prepare a soup with zucchini, leafy greens, and a pinch of turmeric. This provides anti-inflammatory support and gentle nourishment.
- **Dinner**:
  - **Steamed Sweet Potatoes with Ginger and Fresh Herbs**: Steamed sweet potatoes provide fiber and minerals to support digestion and detoxification.

6. LONG-TERM DETOX PRACTICES FOR CANCER RECOVERY

Detoxification for cancer recovery doesn't end after a few days; incorporating gentle, ongoing practices supports long-term health and vitality. Here are some daily habits that maintain a clean, balanced internal environment:

- **Continue to Hydrate**: Drink alkaline water or herbal teas throughout the day to stay hydrated and support kidney function.
- **Prioritize Sleep**: Quality sleep is essential for cellular repair and immune function. Aim for 7–9 hours of sleep each night.
- **Incorporate Alkaline Foods Daily**: Maintain a plant-based, alkaline diet that includes leafy greens, fresh fruits, and cruciferous vegetables.
- **Engage in Light Movement**: Gentle exercises like walking and yoga improve circulation and support lymphatic drainage.
- **Limit Processed Foods and Sugar**: Avoid refined sugars and processed foods, which contribute to acidity and inflammation.

Through these detoxification protocols, you can support your body's healing process during cancer recovery. Dr. Sebi's emphasis on natural, plant-based foods and detoxifying herbs creates an environment that reduces inflammation, eliminates residual toxins, and strengthens the immune system. By adopting these practices, you are building a foundation for lasting health, resilience, and renewed energy, empowering your body's ability to heal and thrive.

BOOK 20
Respiratory Health with Alkaline Remedies

The respiratory system is essential for delivering oxygen to the body's tissues and removing carbon dioxide, yet it's frequently exposed to environmental pollutants, allergens, and pathogens. These irritants can compromise lung health, contributing to issues like asthma, bronchitis, or chronic inflammation. Dr. Sebi's holistic approach to respiratory health centers on using plant-based, alkaline remedies to clear the lungs, reduce inflammation, and strengthen respiratory function. This book offers readers a natural, effective path to optimizing lung health, detailing herbal treatments, dietary practices, and lifestyle modifications that support respiratory wellness.

CHAPTER 1
HERBAL TREATMENTS FOR LUNG HEALTH

Herbs have been used for centuries to support respiratory health. Many contain natural compounds that open airways, reduce mucus, fight infections, and promote lung healing. With the right combination of herbs, we can maintain clean, healthy lungs, especially in today's environment, where pollution and respiratory infections are common. Dr. Sebi's approach emphasizes alkaline, nutrient-rich herbs that cleanse the lungs, enhance oxygen flow, and reduce inflammation, creating an internal environment that supports overall respiratory function and resilience.

1. THE IMPORTANCE OF LUNG HEALTH AND HERBAL SUPPORT

The lungs serve as a primary interface with the external environment, absorbing oxygen and expelling carbon dioxide. Over time, exposure to pollutants, allergens, and pathogens can strain lung function and contribute to respiratory issues. Strengthening lung health with natural herbs offers numerous benefits:

- **Clearing Mucus**: Excess mucus can clog the airways and create an environment where pathogens thrive. Certain herbs help thin mucus, making it easier to expel and keep airways clear.
- **Reducing Inflammation**: Inflammation in the respiratory system contributes to breathing difficulties, such as asthma and bronchitis. Anti-inflammatory herbs can soothe inflamed tissues and reduce swelling.
- **Supporting Oxygen Flow**: Herbs that improve circulation and lung capacity help oxygenate tissues, which is vital for overall health and energy levels.
- **Boosting Immunity**: Herbs with antimicrobial properties defend against pathogens, helping to prevent respiratory infections and protect lung health.

2. KEY HERBS FOR LUNG HEALTH AND THEIR BENEFITS

Several herbs align with Dr. Sebi's philosophy for supporting lung health, each offering unique properties that contribute to respiratory wellness. Here are some of the most effective herbs for promoting lung health and their practical uses:

- **Mullein:**
  - » Mullein is known for its soothing effects on the respiratory system. It helps expel mucus from the lungs, reduces inflammation, and opens the airways, making it beneficial for conditions like bronchitis and asthma.
  - » **How to Use**: Brew mullein tea by steeping a teaspoon of dried leaves in hot water for 10–15 minutes. Drink 1–2 cups daily to promote clear, healthy lungs.

- **Eucalyptus:**
  - » Eucalyptus contains compounds that help open the airways and reduce inflammation, making it particularly effective for asthma, cough, and congestion. It also has antimicrobial properties that protect against respiratory infections.
  - » **How to Use**: Eucalyptus can be used as a tea or an essential oil. For inhalation, add a few drops of eucalyptus oil to a bowl of hot water, cover your head with a towel, and breathe deeply for a few minutes to clear the airways.

- **Lobelia:**
  - » Lobelia, often referred to as the "asthma herb," helps relax the respiratory muscles and open the airways, which can ease breathing. It also acts as an expectorant, helping to expel mucus.
  - » **How to Use**: Lobelia is potent, so it's best used in tincture form under guidance from a healthcare professional. A few drops in water can help ease breathing difficulties and open the lungs.

- **Licorice Root:**
  - » Licorice root is an anti-inflammatory herb that soothes the mucous membranes in the lungs and reduces irritation. It also has antiviral and antibacterial properties, making it useful during respiratory infections.
  - » **How to Use**: Brew licorice root tea by steeping 1–2 teaspoons of dried root in hot water for 10 minutes. Drink a cup daily during respiratory issues but avoid long-term use, especially if you have high blood pressure.

- **Thyme:**
  - » Thyme is a powerful antimicrobial herb that helps cleanse the respiratory tract and reduce infection risk. It also acts as an expectorant, clearing mucus from the lungs.
  - » **How to Use**: Make thyme tea by steeping a teaspoon of dried thyme in hot water for 10 minutes. Drink once or twice daily, or use thyme essential oil in steam inhalation for added benefits.

- **Osha Root**:
  » Osha root is native to North America and has been traditionally used for respiratory health. It helps open the bronchial tubes, making breathing easier, and has antiviral properties that protect against infections.
  » **How to Use**: Osha root can be chewed or brewed as tea. It's also available as a tincture; take according to package instructions to support lung function.

3. HERBAL STEAM INHALATION FOR LUNG DETOXIFICATION

Herbal steam inhalation is an effective method to cleanse the lungs, reduce mucus, and open the airways. This technique allows the active compounds in herbs to penetrate directly into the respiratory tract, delivering immediate relief and promoting lung health. Here's a simple herbal steam inhalation method using Dr. Sebi's recommended herbs.

- **Herbal Ingredients**: Eucalyptus leaves, thyme, rosemary, and mullein.
- **Instructions**:
  » Boil water in a large pot and add a handful of herbs (dried or fresh).
  » Remove the pot from heat and place it on a stable surface.
  » Drape a towel over your head, lean over the pot, and inhale deeply for 5–10 minutes, allowing the steam to penetrate your lungs.
  » Repeat this inhalation once daily, especially during cold seasons or when experiencing congestion.

4. SAMPLE DAILY ROUTINE FOR HERBAL LUNG SUPPORT

Incorporating these herbs into a daily routine can support respiratory function, reduce inflammation, and enhance lung health. Here's a sample routine to help you integrate these lung-supportive herbs effectively.

- **Morning**:
  » **Warm Lemon Water with Thyme Tea**: Start the day with warm lemon water to hydrate and alkalize the body, followed by thyme tea to clear the lungs and support immunity.
- **Mid-Morning**:
  » **Mullein and Licorice Root Tea**: Brew a tea combining mullein and licorice root to reduce mucus, soothe lung tissues, and support respiratory health.
- **Lunch**:
  » **Alkaline Vegetable Soup**: Prepare a light vegetable soup with garlic, onions, and greens, adding a pinch of thyme for its respiratory benefits.
- **Afternoon Snack**:
  » **Eucalyptus Steam Inhalation**: Set up a steam inhalation with eucalyptus and thyme to clear the airways and reduce inflammation in the lungs.
- **Evening**:
  » **Golden Milk with Turmeric**: End the day with a warm cup of golden milk (almond milk with turmeric, ginger, and black pepper). This drink provides anti-inflammatory support and helps relax the body for restful sleep.

5. ADDITIONAL LIFESTYLE TIPS FOR SUPPORTING LUNG HEALTH

While herbal treatments are essential, lifestyle practices also play a vital role in supporting respiratory health. Here are some tips that align with Dr. Sebi's holistic philosophy to promote lung health:

- **Stay Hydrated**: Proper hydration helps thin mucus, making it easier to expel from the lungs. Drink 8–10 cups of water daily, focusing on filtered or alkaline water for added benefits.
- **Practice Deep Breathing Exercises**: Breathing exercises improve lung capacity, strengthen the respiratory muscles, and promote oxygenation. Techniques like diaphragmatic breathing, pursed-lip breathing, and deep belly breathing are helpful for lung health.
- **Limit Exposure to Toxins**: Avoid smoking, minimize exposure to air pollution, and use natural cleaning products to reduce lung irritation.
- **Incorporate Physical Activity**: Regular physical activity supports lung function and circulation. Aim for moderate exercises like walking, yoga, or stretching to promote respiratory health.

6. LONG-TERM BENEFITS OF HERBAL LUNG SUPPORT

Using herbs for lung health not only supports respiratory function in the short term but also promotes long-term resilience against respiratory issues. Over time, these herbs strengthen the lungs, reduce the impact of environmental pollutants, and enhance oxygenation, which contributes to overall well-being. Consistent use of herbal remedies, combined with an alkaline diet and healthy lifestyle practices, helps maintain respiratory health and protects against conditions like asthma, bronchitis, and other respiratory illnesses.

PRECAUTIONS AND CONSIDERATIONS FOR HERBAL USE

While herbs offer numerous benefits for lung health, it's essential to use them responsibly. Here are a few precautions to consider:

- **Consult a Healthcare Provider**: Always consult a healthcare professional before beginning any herbal regimen, especially if you have existing respiratory conditions or are taking medications.
- **Avoid Long-Term Use of Certain Herbs**: Herbs like licorice root are highly beneficial but should be used with caution, especially for those with high blood pressure. Use such herbs intermittently or under professional guidance.
- **Choose Organic, High-Quality Herbs**: To ensure potency and safety, select organic herbs from reputable sources, and avoid synthetic or heavily processed herbal supplements.

Incorporating Dr. Sebi's recommended herbs into your daily routine offers a natural and effective way to support lung health. These herbs, including mullein, eucalyptus, and thyme, provide respiratory relief, reduce inflammation, and protect against infections, fostering an internal environment that promotes lung vitality. By integrating these practices into your lifestyle and combining them with an alkaline diet and mindful breathing exercises, you are laying a strong foundation for optimal lung health and resilience. Through consistent herbal support and lifestyle adjustments, you can breathe easier, experience increased energy, and enjoy a healthier, balanced respiratory system.

CHAPTER 2
DETOX PROTOCOLS FOR RESPIRATORY SUPPORT

Our lungs are constantly exposed to environmental pollutants, allergens, pathogens, and airborne irritants, making them particularly vulnerable to buildup over time. This exposure can lead to respiratory issues, compromised immune function, and reduced oxygen flow. Regular detoxification supports lung health by clearing mucus, reducing inflammation, and aiding the body's natural processes to cleanse the respiratory system. Dr. Sebi's detoxification methods focus on gentle, plant-based remedies to improve lung function, enhance immunity, and maintain a balanced, alkaline internal environment that supports respiratory resilience.

1. THE NEED FOR REGULAR RESPIRATORY DETOXIFICATION

Respiratory detoxification helps clear the lungs, remove harmful substances, and enhance overall breathing quality. By supporting the lungs and airways, detoxification can alleviate respiratory issues like congestion, shortness of breath, and chronic cough. For individuals living in areas with high pollution, frequent smokers, or those prone to respiratory issues, detox protocols are particularly beneficial:

- **Reducing Mucus and Congestion**: Mucus buildup can trap dust, pollutants, and pathogens, leading to congestion and reducing oxygen flow. Detoxifying the lungs helps break down and expel excess mucus.
- **Clearing Airway Passages**: Detoxification helps keep airways open and reduces inflammation in bronchial passages, supporting easy and unrestricted breathing.
- **Strengthening Immunity**: By removing toxins, the body can direct more resources to immune function, protecting the respiratory system from infections and irritants.
- **Improving Oxygenation**: Clean lungs enable more efficient oxygen exchange, which is essential for energy, mental clarity, and overall cellular health.

2. ESSENTIAL COMPONENTS OF A RESPIRATORY DETOX PROTOCOL

An effective respiratory detox protocol includes three essential elements: hydrating, mucus-clearing herbs; alkaline foods that support lung health; and deep breathing exercises that enhance lung capacity. Together, these components provide a holistic approach to detoxifying the respiratory system.

- **Mucus-Clearing Herbs**: Herbs that help thin and expel mucus, reduce inflammation, and clear respiratory passages are essential for lung detox.
- **Alkaline Foods**: Alkaline foods provide antioxidants, vitamins, and minerals that support cellular repair, reduce inflammation, and cleanse the respiratory system.
- **Breathing Exercises**: Deep breathing exercises expand lung capacity, improve oxygen flow, and aid in expelling residual carbon dioxide.

3. KEY HERBS FOR LUNG DETOXIFICATION

Dr. Sebi's philosophy includes using herbs that align with an alkaline, plant-based approach to support respiratory health. Here are some of the most effective herbs for lung detoxification:

- **Mullein**:
  » Known for its ability to soothe inflamed respiratory tissues and expel mucus, mullein is one of the best herbs for lung detoxification. It acts as an expectorant, helping clear airways and improve breathing.
  » **How to Use**: Brew mullein tea by steeping 1–2 teaspoons of dried mullein leaves in hot water for 10–15 minutes. Drink once daily during a detox period to help clear mucus.

- **Peppermint**:
  » Peppermint contains menthol, which helps relax the bronchial muscles, reduce congestion, and clear airways. It also has mild antimicrobial properties that protect against respiratory infections.
  » **How to Use**: Brew peppermint tea or add fresh peppermint leaves to hot water for a steam inhalation to open up the airways.

- **Ginger**:
  » Ginger is a potent anti-inflammatory herb that reduces mucus, soothes the airways, and fights respiratory infections. It also improves circulation, which is essential for oxygen delivery to tissues.
  » **How to Use**: Grate fresh ginger into hot water to make a tea or add it to smoothies. Ginger can also be included in meals for a gentle, ongoing detox effect.

- **Licorice Root**:
  - Licorice root soothes respiratory tissues, reduces inflammation, and has mild expectorant properties. It's particularly helpful for individuals with a chronic cough or irritated airways.
  - **How to Use**: Brew a tea by steeping 1–2 teaspoons of dried licorice root in hot water for 10 minutes. Drink once daily during detox but avoid long-term use if you have high blood pressure.
- **Thyme**:
  - Thyme is a powerful antiseptic herb that fights infection, reduces inflammation, and clears mucus. It helps cleanse the lungs and strengthens the respiratory system.
  - **How to Use**: Thyme can be used as tea or added to food for respiratory support. Brew thyme tea by steeping a teaspoon of dried thyme in hot water for 10 minutes, and drink once daily.

4. ALKALINE FOODS FOR RESPIRATORY DETOX

Alkaline foods help maintain a balanced pH, reduce inflammation, and support respiratory detoxification by nourishing lung tissue, enhancing oxygen flow, and reducing mucus. Here are some of the best foods to include in a respiratory detox protocol:

- **Leafy Greens (Kale, Spinach, Swiss Chard)**:
  - Leafy greens are high in chlorophyll, which cleanses the blood and supports lung health. Their high antioxidant content protects lung tissue from oxidative damage and reduces inflammation.
  - **How to Use**: Add leafy greens to salads, smoothies, or lightly sauté for a nutrient-dense side dish.
- **Berries (Blueberries, Blackberries, Raspberries)**:
  - Berries are rich in antioxidants, vitamins, and fiber, all of which support lung health and aid in cellular repair. Their anti-inflammatory properties also reduce irritation in the respiratory system.
  - **How to Use**: Add fresh berries to smoothies, salads, or enjoy them as a snack during detox periods.
- **Citrus Fruits (Lemon, Lime, Grapefruit)**:
  - Citrus fruits contain high levels of vitamin C and antioxidants, which help protect lung tissue from pollutants and boost immunity.
  - **How to Use**: Start the day with warm lemon water or squeeze lemon or lime juice over meals for added flavor and lung support.
- **Pineapple**:
  - Pineapple contains bromelain, an enzyme that reduces mucus and inflammation in the respiratory system. It helps clear airways, making it easier to breathe and enhancing lung function.
  - **How to Use**: Fresh pineapple can be eaten on its own, added to salads, or blended into smoothies for an effective respiratory detox.
- **Cucumber**:
  - Cucumber is highly hydrating, which is essential for thinning mucus and reducing congestion. Its alkaline properties support lung health and overall cellular hydration.
  - **How to Use**: Add cucumber slices to water, include them in salads, or blend into green smoothies.

5. BREATHING EXERCISES FOR RESPIRATORY DETOXIFICATION

Breathing exercises are an integral part of any respiratory detox. They help expand lung capacity, expel residual carbon dioxide, and improve oxygenation throughout the body. Here are some simple yet effective exercises:

- **Diaphragmatic Breathing**:
  - Diaphragmatic breathing (also known as belly breathing) engages the diaphragm, promoting deeper oxygen exchange and reducing stress on the respiratory muscles.
  - **How to Practice**: Lie down or sit comfortably, place one hand on your chest and the other on your belly, and take slow, deep breaths, focusing on expanding the belly rather than the chest. Practice for 5–10 minutes daily.
- **Pursed-Lip Breathing**:
  - This technique helps control the flow of air, improving lung function and oxygenation, especially helpful for individuals with chronic respiratory issues.
  - **How to Practice**: Breathe in slowly through the nose and then exhale slowly through pursed lips, as if blowing out a candle. Repeat for 5–10 minutes.
- **Alternate Nostril Breathing**:
  - Practiced in yoga, alternate nostril breathing (Nadi Shodhana) helps cleanse the respiratory system, balance oxygen levels, and calm the mind.
  - **How to Practice**: Sit comfortably, close one nostril with your thumb, inhale through the open nostril, switch nostrils, and exhale through the opposite side. Continue for 5 minutes, focusing on calm, balanced breaths.

6. SAMPLE 3-DAY RESPIRATORY DETOX ROUTINE

A three-day respiratory detox helps clear out mucus, reduce inflammation, and promote overall lung health. This sample routine incorporates the recommended herbs, foods, and practices for optimal respiratory support.

Day 1: Hydration and Mucus Reduction

- **Morning**:
  - » **Warm Lemon Water with Thyme Tea**: Start the day with warm lemon water to alkalize and hydrate, followed by thyme tea to support mucus reduction.
  - » **Diaphragmatic Breathing**: Spend 5–10 minutes practicing deep, belly breaths to open the lungs.
- **Lunch**:
  - » **Leafy Green Salad with Pineapple**: Create a salad with kale, spinach, cucumber, and fresh pineapple. Add lemon juice and a sprinkle of thyme for flavor and lung support.
- **Afternoon Snack**:
  - » **Peppermint Tea**: Brew a cup of peppermint tea to open airways and support lung detox.

Day 2: Active Detoxification and Lung Clearing

- **Morning**:
  - » **Mullein and Licorice Root Tea**: Brew a combination tea to support mucus clearance and reduce lung inflammation.
  - » **Alternate Nostril Breathing**: Practice for 5 minutes to clear the respiratory system and balance oxygen flow.
- **Lunch**:
  - » **Vegetable Broth**: Prepare a light vegetable broth with garlic, onions, and thyme. This provides hydration and soothing support for lung health.
- **Evening**:
  - » **Steam Inhalation with Eucalyptus**: Boil water and add eucalyptus leaves or essential oil. Inhale the steam deeply to open the airways and reduce congestion.

Day 3: Restorative Detox and Lung Support

- **Morning**:
  - » **Ginger Tea**: Start with ginger tea to support inflammation reduction and improve circulation.
  - » **Pursed-Lip Breathing**: Practice this technique for 5–10 minutes to enhance oxygenation.
- **Dinner**:
  - » **Steamed Vegetables and Citrus Salad**: Pair steamed vegetables with a salad of greens and citrus fruits like grapefruit or orange, which provide vitamin C and antioxidants.

7. LONG-TERM MAINTENANCE FOR RESPIRATORY HEALTH

Detoxifying the respiratory system doesn't end after a few days; maintaining long-term respiratory health involves consistent practices:

- **Stay Hydrated**: Drink alkaline water throughout the day to support lung function and mucus clearance.
- **Incorporate Breathing Exercises**: Regular practice of deep breathing techniques keeps lungs open and oxygen flow efficient.
- **Limit Pollutants and Irritants**: Reduce exposure to smoke, chemicals, and pollution to protect lung health.
- **Continue Alkaline Foods and Herbs**: Include leafy greens, berries, and herbs like mullein and thyme in your regular diet.

Dr. Sebi's approach to respiratory health highlights the importance of natural detox protocols that support lung function, reduce mucus, and enhance oxygenation. By following these practices, you can create a cleaner, healthier respiratory system, fostering a foundation for resilient lung health, increased energy, and improved breathing quality.

CHAPTER 3

PREVENTING RESPIRATORY ILLNESS

Our lungs are exposed to pathogens, pollutants, allergens, and environmental irritants daily, increasing the risk of respiratory illnesses like colds, flu, bronchitis, and pneumonia. By proactively supporting lung health, boosting immunity, and maintaining a clean internal environment, we can effectively prevent respiratory illnesses. Dr. Sebi's approach to respiratory wellness centers on creating an alkaline, nutrient-rich internal environment that enhances the body's natural defenses and keeps the respiratory system clear and healthy.

1. STRENGTHENING IMMUNITY FOR RESPIRATORY PROTECTION

The immune system is the body's first line of defense against respiratory illnesses. Enhancing immune function helps the body identify and eliminate pathogens before they have a chance to cause infections.

- **Herbs for Immunity**:
  - **Elderberry**: Elderberry is rich in antioxidants and has been shown to reduce the severity and duration of cold and flu symptoms by boosting immune response.
  - **Echinacea**: This herb stimulates white blood cell production, aiding in the body's ability to ward off infections. It's particularly beneficial during cold and flu seasons.
  - **Astragalus**: Known for its adaptogenic properties, astragalus strengthens the immune system and helps the body resist stress, which can weaken immune defenses.
- **Nutrient-Rich Foods for Immunity**:
  - **Citrus Fruits**: High in vitamin C, citrus fruits like lemon, lime, and grapefruit support immune function by providing antioxidants that help combat pathogens.
  - **Garlic**: Garlic has antiviral and antibacterial properties, making it an effective natural remedy for preventing respiratory infections.
  - **Ginger**: Anti-inflammatory and antimicrobial, ginger helps soothe respiratory passages and supports the immune system.

2. INCORPORATING ALKALINE FOODS FOR LUNG HEALTH

An alkaline diet plays a significant role in preventing respiratory illnesses. Acidic environments foster inflammation, weaken immunity, and increase the body's susceptibility to infections. By maintaining an alkaline balance, we create an internal environment less hospitable to pathogens.

- **Leafy Greens**:
  - Greens like spinach, kale, and Swiss chard are alkaline, antioxidant-rich, and high in chlorophyll, which aids in cleansing the lungs and reducing inflammation.
  - **How to Use**: Add leafy greens to salads, smoothies, or stir-fries for a simple, lung-supporting addition to daily meals.
- **Berries**:
  - Berries are packed with antioxidants that help the body combat oxidative stress, which can weaken the immune system and respiratory health.
  - **How to Use**: Enjoy berries as a snack, add to smoothies, or sprinkle over oatmeal to boost your respiratory resilience.
- **Cucumber**:
  - Cucumber is highly hydrating, which supports mucus thinning and lung health. Its alkaline properties also help maintain a balanced pH in the body.
  - **How to Use**: Add cucumber to salads, smoothies, or infused water for respiratory support.

3. DAILY PRACTICES TO MAINTAIN CLEAN AIRWAYS

Keeping the airways clear of mucus, irritants, and pathogens is essential for respiratory health. Regular practices can help prevent congestion, ease breathing, and reduce the risk of respiratory infections.

- **Herbal Teas and Steam Inhalations**:
  - **Mullein Tea**: Mullein has expectorant properties that help thin mucus and clear the airways. Drinking mullein tea regularly keeps the respiratory passages clear.
  - **Steam Inhalation with Eucalyptus or Peppermint**: Inhaling steam infused with eucalyptus or peppermint essential oil helps open the airways, reduce congestion, and fight respiratory pathogens.

- **Hydration**:
  - Staying well-hydrated supports mucus thinning, making it easier to clear the respiratory tract. Proper hydration keeps mucus membranes moist, which helps trap pathogens and expel them more effectively.
  - **How to Practice**: Drink 8–10 cups of water daily, with a focus on filtered or alkaline water. Add a slice of lemon for added alkalinity and immune support.
- **Breathing Exercises**:
  - Regular deep breathing exercises help strengthen the lungs, improve oxygen flow, and enhance respiratory capacity. Practices like diaphragmatic breathing and pursed-lip breathing keep airways open and increase lung resilience.
  - **How to Practice**: Spend 5–10 minutes daily practicing deep breathing exercises, focusing on expanding the diaphragm with each breath.

4. AVOIDING RESPIRATORY IRRITANTS AND TOXINS

Environmental toxins, pollutants, and irritants can impair lung function and weaken respiratory health. Taking proactive steps to avoid these substances helps protect the lungs from damage and reduces the risk of respiratory illness.

- **Limit Exposure to Air Pollution**:
  - Try to limit time outdoors on days with high pollution or poor air quality. If you live in a high-pollution area, consider using an air purifier indoors to reduce exposure.
  - **Indoor Air Quality**: Keep indoor spaces well-ventilated and free from chemical cleaners, air fresheners, and smoke, as these can irritate the respiratory tract.
- **Avoid Smoking and Secondhand Smoke**:
  - Smoking introduces toxins into the lungs, weakening respiratory defenses. Avoid smoking, and try to stay away from areas where you may be exposed to secondhand smoke.
- **Use Natural Cleaning Products**:
  - Conventional cleaning products often contain harsh chemicals that irritate the lungs. Opt for natural alternatives like vinegar, baking soda, and essential oils to maintain clean air in your living environment.

5. SEASONAL AND LIFESTYLE PRACTICES TO SUPPORT LUNG HEALTH

Seasonal changes and lifestyle habits impact respiratory health. Adjusting your routine to stay proactive during times of increased risk, like cold and flu season or high pollen months, can make a significant difference in preventing respiratory illness.

- **Practice Good Hygiene**:
  - Wash your hands frequently to avoid spreading pathogens, especially during cold and flu season. Avoid touching your face, as viruses and bacteria often enter the body through the nose, mouth, and eyes.
- **Boost Immune Support Seasonally**:
  - During times of increased illness, incorporate additional immune-supporting herbs like elderberry, echinacea, and astragalus. Drinking a daily immune-boosting tea with ginger, lemon, and honey can also help protect against illness.
- **Exercise Regularly**:
  - Regular physical activity improves lung capacity, strengthens the immune system, and supports circulation. Aim for moderate exercise, such as walking, swimming, or yoga, to support respiratory health without straining the lungs.

6. SAMPLE ROUTINE FOR DAILY RESPIRATORY SUPPORT

A consistent daily routine that incorporates these practices can help prevent respiratory illness and maintain lung health over time. Here's a sample routine for respiratory support:

- **Morning**:
  - **Warm Lemon Water**: Begin the day with warm lemon water to alkalize the body and support hydration.
  - **Breathing Exercise**: Spend 5–10 minutes on diaphragmatic breathing exercises to open the lungs and improve oxygen flow.
- **Mid-Morning**:
  - **Immune-Boosting Tea**: Brew a tea with elderberry, echinacea, and ginger to support immunity. Enjoy with a light snack like berries or an apple.
- **Lunch**:
  - **Alkaline Salad**: Make a salad with leafy greens, cucumber, and bell peppers, topped with lemon juice

and olive oil for a nutrient-packed, respiratory-supporting meal.

- **Afternoon**:
  - » **Herbal Steam Inhalation**: Set up a steam inhalation with eucalyptus essential oil to clear the airways, especially during allergy season or when feeling congested.
- **Evening**:
  - » **Mullein Tea**: Enjoy a cup of mullein tea to keep airways clear and promote restful sleep.

7. LONG-TERM BENEFITS OF A RESPIRATORY HEALTH ROUTINE

Adopting these practices as part of a long-term respiratory health routine helps strengthen the immune system, reduce inflammation, and improve lung function. Over time, these habits contribute to a cleaner, more resilient respiratory system, capable of withstanding seasonal threats, environmental stressors, and common respiratory illnesses.

By consistently integrating herbs, alkaline foods, deep breathing, and toxin avoidance into your daily life, you're creating a supportive foundation for respiratory health. This proactive approach minimizes the risk of respiratory illness and fosters a well-rounded sense of wellness, allowing you to breathe easier and maintain higher energy levels year-round.

EXCLUSIVE INSIGHTS AND BONUS CONTENT

Dear Reader,

Thank you for embarking on this journey through the wisdom of the Dr. Sebi Herbal Bible. Your commitment to health, vitality, and self-discovery is truly inspiring. As a token of gratitude, we are thrilled to offer you a special bonus: a downloadable PDF packed with exclusive content and additional insights to deepen your understanding and application of Dr. Sebi's principles.

In this exclusive bonus, you'll find:

- **Advanced Detox Protocols:** Enhance your cleansing routine with detailed, step-by-step guides.
- **Rare Herbal Combinations:** Discover lesser-known herbal blends for targeted wellness.
- **Expanded Alkaline Recipes:** Delight in new, nourishing meals to keep your alkaline lifestyle exciting.
- **Personalized Health Tips:** Practical advice tailored to specific conditions and goals.

Your health journey deserves continued support and inspiration. Accessing this bonus is simple: just follow the link or scan the QR code provided at the end of this page to download your free content.

Here's to your continued growth and radiant health!

Warm regards,

Luna Maria Soledad

YOUR EXCLUSIVE BONUS

Scan the QR-CODE below to show your video extra contents!

Made in the USA
Monee, IL
26 July 2025